Publishe

Oxfo
Jane
V

ndbooks
Beverley

Oxfo
Sue Bec

Oxford Ha eople's
Edited by Mike nd Jim Ri

Oxford Handbook
Edited by Kate Johnson

Oxford Handbook of Pri
Edited by Vari Drennan and Clso

Oxford Handbook of Gastroin
Edited by Christine Norton, Julia
and Kathy Whayman

Oxford Handbook of Respirato
Terry Robinson and Jane Scullion

Oxford Handbook of Nursing
everley Tabernacle, Marie Barnes,

xford Handbook of Clinical S
queline Randle, Frank Coffey, and

ford Handbook of Emergen
rt Crouch, Alan Charters, Mar

rd Handbook of Dental N
eymour, Dayananda Samarav

Handbook of Diabetes
Avery, Sue Beckwith and J

Handbook of Musculos
usan Oliver

ndbook of Women's
ota, Debra Holloway, ar

dbook of Perioper
es and Andy Mardell

book of Critical C
d Sue Osborne

ook of Neuroscie
nd Cath Waterho

ok of Adult Nu
rge Castledine

LANCHESTER LIBRARY, Coventry University
Gosford Street, Coventry CV1 5DD Telephone 024 7688 7555

KT-472-202

Library

1352

WITHDRAWN

of

This book is due to be returned not later than the date and time stamped above. Fines are charged on overdue books

Oxford Handbook of Emergency Nursing

Edited by

Robert Crouch

Consultant Nurse
Senior Lecturer
Emergency Department
Southampton University Hospitals NHS Trust
and School of Health Sciences
University of Southampton
Southampton, UK

Alan Charters

Consultant Nurse
Emergency Department
Portsmouth Hospitals NHS Trust
Hampshire, UK

Mary Dawood

Consultant Nurse
Emergency Department
Imperial College NHS Trust
St Mary's Hospital
London, UK

Paula Bennett

Nurse Consultant
Emergency Department
Stockport NHS Foundation Trust
Honorary Lecturer
University of Manchester
School of Nursing
Midwifery and Social Work

OXFORD
UNIVERSITY PRESS

100

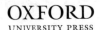

OXFORD
UNIVERSITY PRESS

Great Clarendon Street, Oxford OX2 6DP

Oxford University Press is a department of the University of Oxford.
It furthers the University's objective of excellence in research, scholarship,
and education by publishing worldwide in

Oxford New York

Auckland Cape Town Dar es Salaam Hong Kong Karachi
Kuala Lumpur Madrid Melbourne Mexico City Nairobi
New Delhi Shanghai Taipei Toronto

With offices in

Argentina Austria Brazil Chile Czech Republic France Greece
Guatemala Hungary Italy Japan Poland Portugal Singapore
South Korea Switzerland Thailand Turkey Ukraine Vietnam

Oxford is a registered trade mark of Oxford University Press
in the UK and in certain other countries

Published in the United States
by Oxford University Press Inc., New York

© Oxford University Press, 2009

The moral rights of the author have been asserted
Database right Oxford University Press (maker)

First published 2009

All rights reserved. No part of this publication may be reproduced,
stored in a retrieval system, or transmitted, in any form or by any means,
without the prior permission in writing of Oxford University Press,
or as expressly permitted by law, or under terms agreed with the appropriate
reprographics rights organization. Enquiries concerning reproduction
outside the scope of the above should be sent to the Rights Department,
Oxford University Press, at the address above

You must not circulate this book in any other binding or cover
and you must impose this same condition on any acquirer

British Library Cataloguing in Publication Data
Data available

Library of Congress Cataloging-in-Publication Data
Data available

Typeset by Cepha Imaging Private Ltd., Bangalore, India
Printed in Italy
on acid-free paper by
L.E.G.O. S.p.A. — Lavis TN

ISBN 978–0–19–920349–9

10 9 8 7 6 5 4 3 2 1

Oxford University Press makes no representation, express or implied, that the drug
dosages in this book are correct. Readers must therefore always check the product
information and clinical procedures with the most up-to-date published product information and data sheets provided by the manufacturers and the most recent codes
of conduct and safety regulations. The authors and publishers do not accept responsibility or legal liability for any errors in the text or for the misuse or misapplication
of material in this work. Except where otherwise stated, drug dosages and recommendations are for the non-pregnant adult who is not breast-feeding.

Coventry University Library

Dedication

This handbook is dedicated to the late John Henry, Professor of Emergency Medicine Imperial College London, for his inspirational support and confidence in the skills and abilities of emergency nurses.

Dedication

Contents

Contents

Detailed contents

4 Emergency care of the infant and child   57

9 Musculoskeletal injuries   **255**

10 Gastrointestinal emergencies 315

Contributors

Nicola Adams
(Chapter 20)
Imperial College NHS Trust,
St Mary's Hospital,
London, UK

Nicola Adshead
(Chapter 20)
Emergency Department,
Stockport NHS Foundation Trust,
Stockport, UK

Dawn Atkinson
(Chapter 20)
Emergency Department,
Stockport NHS Foundation Trust,
Stockport, UK

Anne Baileff
(Chapter 14)
Southampton City PCT,
Bitterne NHS Walk-in Centre,
Southampton, UK

Louise Bratt
(Chapter 20)
Emergency Department,
Stockport NHS Foundation Trust,
Stockport, UK

Nick Castle
(Chapter 8, Chapter 20)
Frimley Park Hospital NHS
Foundation Trust, Frimley, UK,
Honorary Research Fellow Durban
University of Technology RSA,
South Africa

Sarah Charters
(Chapter 3)
Emergency Department,
Southampton General Hospital,
Southampton, UK

Andrea Clarke
(Chapter 20)
Emergency Department,
Stockport NHS Foundation Trust,
Stockport, UK

Denise Conyard
(Chapter 20)
Emergency Department,
Stockport NHS Foundation Trust,
Stockport, UK

Nicola Davies
(Chapter 20)
Emergency Department,
Stockport NHS Foundation Trust,
Stockport, UK

Aidan Foley
(Chapter 20)
Imperial College NHS Trust,
St Mary's Hospital,
London, UK

Gerry Gallagher
(Chapter 20)
Imperial College NHS Trust,
St Mary's Hospital,
London, UK

Rebecca Guest
(Chapter 20)
Emergency Department,
Stockport NHS Foundation Trust,
Stockport, UK

Debbie Hancock
(Chapter 20)
Emergency Department,
Stockport NHS Foundation Trust,
Stockport, UK

John Henry[†]
(Chapter 18)
Professor of Accident and
Emergency Medicine,
Imperial College NHS Trust,
St Mary's Hospital,
London, UK

Caroline Hodnett
(Chapter 20)
Imperial College NHS Trust,
St Mary's Hospital,
London, UK

[†]Deceased

Joanna Jarvis
(Chapter 20)
Emergency Department,
Stockport NHS Foundation Trust,
Stockport, UK

Stephanie Lockwood
(Chapter 4)
Emergency Department,
Queen Alexandra's Hospital,
Portsmouth, UK

Clare Long
(Chapter 20)
Emergency Department,
Stockport NHS Foundation Trust,
Stockport, UK

Janet Marsden
(Chapter 13, Chapter 20)
Senior Lecturer, Postgraduate
Programme Leader, Manchester
Metropolitan University,
Manchester, UK

Cathie Marsland
(Chapter 20)
Emergency Department,
Stockport NHS Foundation Trust,
Stockport, UK

Gemma Parr
(Chapter 20)
Emergency Department,
Stockport NHS Foundation Trust,
Stockport, UK

Rachael Pilkington
(Chapter 20)
Emergency Department,
Stockport NHS Foundation Trust,
Stockport, UK

Paula Roderick
(Chapter 20)
Emergency Department,
Stockport NHS Foundation Trust,
Stockport, UK

Audrey Ryan
(Chapter 11)
Imperial College NHS Trust,
St Mary's Hospital,
London, UK

Russell Shaw
(Illustrations Figs. 7.6, 7.8, and 7.9)
Outpatients Department
Stockport NHS Foundation Trust,
Stockport, UK

Clare Taylor
(Chapter 20)
Emergency Department,
Stockport NHS Foundation Trust,
Stockport, UK

Iain Taylor
(Chapter 19)
Imperial College NHS Trust,
St Mary's Hospital,
London, UK

Paul Thirlwell
(Chapter 8)
Coronary Care Unit,
Southampton University Hospitals
NHS Trust,
Southampton, UK

Raynie Thomson
(Chapter 20)
Emergency Department,
Stockport NHS Foundation Trust,
Stockport, UK

Andrew Turvey
(Chapter 20)
Emergency Department,
Stockport NHS Foundation Trust,
Stockport, UK

Chris Walker
(Chapter 16)
Consultant Nurse
Emergency Department
Portsmouth Hospitals Trust,
Hampshire, UK

Jenny Williams
(Chapter 20)
Emergency Department,
Stockport NHS Foundation Trust,
Stockport, UK

Carol Woodward
(Chapter 20)
Imperial College NHS Trust,
St Mary's Hospital,
London, UK

Symbols and abbreviations

↓	decrease
↑	increase
↔	normal
→	leading to
📖	cross reference
▶	important
▶▶	act quickly
⚠	warning
2°	secondary
∴	therefore
~	approx
β	beta
×	multiplication
°	degree
±	plus/minus
☻	paediatric considerations
AAA	abdominal aortic aneurysm
ABC	airway, breathing, circulation
ABCDE	airway, breathing, circulation, disability, exposure
ABG	arterial blood gas
ACF	antecubital fossa
ACJ	acromioclavicular joint
ACL	anterior cruciate ligament
ACS	acute coronary syndrome
ADL	activity of daily living
ADR	adverse drug reaction
AGE	arterial gas embolism
AIDS	autoimmune deficiency syndrome
ALD	alcoholic liver disease
ALP	alkaline phosphatase
ALS	advanced life support
AMD	age-related macular degeneration
AMI	acute myocardial infarction
AMPLE	allergies–medication–past–last meal–events leading up to admission (mnemonic for taking history)

AMS	acute mountain sickness
AOM	acute otitis media
APGAR	American Paediatric Gross Assessment Record
aPTT	activated partial thromboplastin time
ARDS	acute respiratory distress syndrome
ATLS	advanced trauma life support
AV	atrioventricular
AVM	arteriovenous malformation
AXR	abdominal X-ray
bd	twice a day
BiPAP	bilevel positive airway pressure
BLS	basic life support
BMI	body mass index
BNF	British National Formulary
BP	blood pressure
bpm	beats/minute
BTS	British Thoracic Society
BVM	bag–valve–mask
CAP	community-acquired pneumonia
CBG	capillary blood glucose
CCF	congestive cardiac failure
CCU	coronary care unit
CJD	Creatzfeldt-Jakob disease
CK	creatine kinase
CMV	controlled mandatory ventilation
CNS	central nervous system
CO	cardiac output
COPD	chronic obstructive pulmonary disease
CPAP	continuous positive airway pressure
CPR	cardiopulmonary resuscitation
CRF	capillary refill
CRP	C-reactive protein
C & S	culture and sensitivity
CSF	cerebrospinal fluid
C-spine	cervical spine
CSR	central serous retinopathy
CT	computerized tomography
CTPA	computerized tomography pulmonary angiogram
CVA	cerebrovascular accident

CVP	central venous pressure
DCS	decompression sickness
DIC	disseminated intravascular coagulation
DIPJ	distal interphalangeal joint
DKA	diabetic ketoacidosis
DNAR	do not attempt resuscitation
DPL	diagnostic peritoneal lavage
DSH	deliberate self-harm
DVT	deep venous thrombosis
ECG	electrocardiogram
ED	emergency department
ENP	emergency nurse practitioner
ESR	erythrocyte sedimentation rate
EtCO$_2$	end-tidal CO$_2$
ETT	endotracheal tube
FB	foreign body
FBC	full blood count
FEV1	forced expiratory volume in 1 second
FFP	fresh frozen plasma
FOOSH	fall on outstretched hand
GCS	Glasgow Coma Scale
G & S	Group and Save
GFR	glomerular filtration rate
GI	gastrointestinal
GP	general practitioner
GTN	glyceryl trinitrate
GUM	genitourinary medicine
HACO	high altitude cerebral oedema
HAPO	high altitude pulmonary oedema
Hb	haemoglobin
HCG	human chorionic gonadotrophin
HDU	high dependency unit
HEELP	haemolysis, elevated liver enzymes, low platelet count
Hib	*Haemophilus influenzae* type b (vaccine)
HIV	human immunodeficiency virus
HONK	hyperosmolar non-ketotic hyperglycaemia
HR	heart rate
HSV	herpes simplex virus
IBD	inflammatory bowel disease
ICP	intracranial pressure

ICS	intercostal space
ICU	intensive care unit
IDC	indwelling catheter
I:E	inspiration time:expiration time ratio
Ig	immunoglobulin
IM	intramuscular
INR	international normalized ratio
IO	intraosseous
IPJ	interphalangeal joint
IPPV	intermittent positive pressure ventilation
IU	international units
IUCD	intra-uterine contraceptive device
IUD	intrauterine device
IV	intravenous
IVI	intravenous infusion
IVU	intravenous urogram
KUB	kidneys, urine, bladder (X-ray)
LA	left atrium *or* local anaesthetic
LFT	liver function test
LLQ	left lower quadrant (of abdomen)
LMA	laryngeal mask airway
LMP	last menstrual period
LMWH	low molecular weight heparin
LRTI	lower respiratory tract infection
LUQ	left upper quadrant (of abdomen)
LV	left ventricle
LVF	left ventricular failure
MAOI	monoamine oxidase inhibitor
MCPJ	metacarpal phalangeal joint
M, C, & S	microscopy, culture, and sensitivity
MDI	metered dose inhaler
MI	myocardial infarction
MMR	measles, mumps, rubella (vaccine)
MRI	magnetic resonance imaging
MSU	midstream urine
MUA	manipulation under anaesthetic
NAI	non-accidental injury
NBM	nil by mouth
NG	nasogastric
NICE	National Institute for Health and Clinical Excellence

NIV	non-invasive ventilation
NPA	nasopharyngeal airway
NSAIDs	non-steroidal anti-inflammatory drugs
NSTEMI	non ST elevation myocardial infarction
OCD	obsessive compulsive disorder
OCP	oral contraceptive pill
OPA	oropharyngeal airway
OPG	orthopantomogram
ORIF	open reduction and internal fixation
PaO_2	arterial oxygen tension
$PaCO_2$	arterial carbon dioxide tension
PCI	percutaneous coronary intervention
PCL	posterior cruciate ligament
PCO_2	carbon dioxide tension
PCR	polymerase chain reaction
PCT	primary care trust
PE	pulmonary embolism
PEA	pulseless electrical activity
PEEP	peak end expiratory pressure
PEF	peak expiratory flow
PEFR	peak expiratory flow rate
PEP	post-exposure prophylaxis
PERL	pupils equal-sized and reacting to light
PGD	patient group direction
PID	pelvic inflammatory disease
PIPJ	proximal interphalangeal joint
PO_2	oxygen tension
POEC	progesterone-only emergency contraception
POP	plaster of paris
PQRST	provokes–quality–radiates–severity–time (mnemonic for assessing pain)
PR	by rectum
PUD	peptic ulcer disease
PV	by vagina *or* pulmonary vein
qds	four times daily
RA	right atrium
RBC	red blood cell
R.I.C.E.	rest, ice, compression, elevation
RIF	right iliac fossa
RLQ	right lower quadrant (of abdomen)

RR	respiratory rate
RSI	rapid sequence induction
RTC	road traffic collision
rt-PA	recombinant tissue plasminogen activator
RUQ	right upper quadrant (of abdomen)
RV	right ventricle
SA	sinoatrial
SaO_2	arterial oxygen saturation
SARC	sexual assault referral centre
SC	subcutaneous
SIADH	syndrome of inappropriate antidiuretic hormone
SIMV	synchronized intermittent mandatory ventilation
SIPPV	synchronized intermittent positive pressure ventilation
SL	sublingual
SOB	shortness of breath
SpO_2	oxygen saturation measured by pulse oximetry
SSRI	selective serotonin re-uptake inhibitor
STEMI	ST elevation myocardial infarction
STI	sexually transmitted infection
SVT	supraventricular tachycardia
T3	triiodothyronine
T4	thyroxine
TB	tuberculosis
tds	three times a day
TFT	thyroid function test
TIA	transient ischaemic attack
TM	tympanic membrane
TSH	thyroid stimulating hormone
U & E	urea and electrolytes
UPSI	unprotected sexual intercourse
URTI	upper respiratory tract infection
USS	ultrasound scan
UTI	urinary tract infection
VA	visual acuity
VF	ventricular fibrillation
Vt	tidal volume
VT	ventricular tachycardia
WBC	white blood cell
WCC	white cell count

General principles of emergency nursing

Introduction

Emergency nursing is one of the most challenging specialties in nursing. It requires nurses to manage ambiguity and rapid changes in pace and intensity of work and to have a knowledge of a significant number of clinical presentations, diseases, and conditions. The emergency nurse must also be able to relate to and have an understanding of all ages from the very young child to the elderly. Emergency nursing is not for the faint-hearted!

Golden rules of emergency nursing

- An emergency is an emergency. It is only not an emergency in retrospect!
- There is no such thing as a 'minor' injury. Behind any so-called 'minor' presentation there may be a 'major' one masquerading.
- Remember that what looks trivial to you may have significant ramifications for the patient.
- Don't forget the fundamentals—communication and observation.
- Monitors are an adjunct—nurse the patient not the monitor.
- 'If you don't like the patient spend twice as long with them'—that way you will minimize mistakes.[1]
- 'There is no such thing as a poor historian'—it is probably your inability to elicit the history.[1]
- A fall is only a fall after a collapse has been ruled out.
- It may be a common injury or illness to you—remember it may be a first for the patient and carers.
- Have a plan for the worst possible scenario—anything less is a bonus!
- Expect the unexpected.
- If the patient says they feel like they are going to die, believe them and do something about it!
- Common things are common but they can still kill you—you can bleed to death from your nose or a large scalp laceration!
- The patient is not drunk until they have experienced the hangover—do not be misled by the smell of alcohol.
- In a woman of child-bearing age with abdominal pain—actively rule out ectopic pregnancy.
- In all unwell patients—**D**on't **E**ver **F**orget **G**lucose (DEFG).
- When caring for children, toys and distraction are essential tools.
- Do not attribute hyperventilation to hysteria until underlying pathology has been ruled out.
- Do not dismiss or trivialize the frequent attender. They may have an underlying illness.
- Ensure patients re-presenting with the same complaint are seen by someone senior.

Acknowledgement

1 Our thanks to Mike Clancy for these contributions.

Investigations

Biochemical investigations: urea and electrolytes—urea

- Breakdown of protein produces urea.
- 90% excreted by kidneys.
- Urea levels in blood give an indication of kidney function.

Low urea

- Low protein diet/malnutrition.
- In pregnancy due to ↑ blood volume.
- Liver disease.
- Very dilute urine.
- Lower levels can also be seen in infants and small children.

Raised urea—uraemia

- Impaired renal function due to disease or poor blood flow to kidneys.
- Urinary tract obstruction.
- Dehydration.
- High protein diet.
- Extensive tissue damage:
  - necrosis/severe infection.
- Stress/shock due to increased release of adrenaline.
- Medication-induced, e.g. corticosteroids.

Biochemical investigations: urea and electrolytes—calcium

- One of the most important minerals and necessary for:
  - skeletal strength;
  - conduction of impulses from nerve endings for stimulation of muscle contraction;
  - blood clotting;
  - regulation of cell metabolism including sodium shift;
  - cell wall structure and function.
- ↑ calcium level can cause muscle weakness and depress the nervous system.
- ↓ calcium level can lead to overstimulation of muscles by nerve impulses. ▶ Important consideration for cardiac muscle.

Potential causes of hypercalcaemia

- Drug effects, e.g. thiazide diuretics and bendrofluazide.
- Renal problems affecting excretion of calcium.
- Hyperthyroidism.
- Neoplasms.
- High levels of vitamin D.
- Paget's disease.
- Sarcoidosis.

Potential causes of hypocalcaemia

- Reduced dietary intake.
- Vitamin D deficiency.
- Renal-related:
  - nephrotic syndrome (↓ levels of albumin → reduced transport);
  - chronic failure;
  - stones.
- Septic shock.
- Drug induced, e.g. cytotoxic therapy.
- Hypomagnesaemia.

Biochemical investigations: urea and electrolytes—chloride

- Ingested in diet.
- Function in electrolyte balance.
- Component in maintaining acid–base balance.
- Provides osmotic pressure → distribution of extracellular fluid.
- Abnormal chloride levels could → compensatory or abnormal movement of other electrolytes.

Possible causes of hyperchloraemia

- Sodium retention.
- Dehydration.
- Metabolic acidosis.
- Respiratory alkalosis.
- Drug effect, e.g. corticosteroids.

Possible causes of hypochloraemia

- Significant loss of sodium.
- Renal tubular damage leading to loss.
- Heat exhaustion.
- Hypokalaemic acidosis.
- Respiratory acidosis.
- Loss of chloride from GI tract through vomiting, intestinal obstruction, or nasogastric aspiration.
- Drug-induced particularly by diuretics (e.g. furosemide, bendroflumethiazide).

Biochemical investigations: urea and electrolytes—magnesium (Mg)

- A mineral, found in every cell of body.
- Used for energy production, nerve function, and muscle contraction.
- Mg in the body combines with calcium and phosphorus to form bone.
- Only small amount of magnesium in body found in blood.
- Intake of Mg mostly through diet.
- Regulation in body by balance between absorption and excretion/conservation through kidneys.
- Mg deficiencies cause amongst other things cardiac arrhythmia, increased irritability of nervous system with tetany.

Possible causes of hypermagnesaemia

- Renal failure.
- Ketoacidosis
- Addison's disease.
- Medications containing magnesium.
- Hyperparathyroidism.
- Hypothyroidism.

Possible causes of hypomagnesaemia

- Not equivalent to magnesium deficiency.
- Low dietary intake.
- Poor absorption through GI disorders (Crohn's).
- Alcoholism.
- Long-term diuretic use.
- Chronic or prolonged diarrhoea.
- Severe burns.
- Hypoparathyroidism.

Biochemical investigations: urea and electrolytes—sodium

- Plays an important part in regulation of osmotic pressure and the distribution of water within the extracellular compartments of the body.
- Water and sodium balance affected by dietary intake and renal excretion of both.
- Needed for fluid balance, muscle function, and acid–base balance.

Possible causes of hypernatraemia

- Dehydration secondary to ↓ fluid intake, diarrhoea and/or vomiting, or polyuria.
- Pharmacological due to steroids and antibiotics.

Possible causes of hyponatraemia

- Usually excessive loss rather than dietary intake; can include loss from body surface by ↑ sweating or burns.
- Renal disease such as polycystic kidney disease.
- Metabolic disease such as Addison's disease or hypothyroidism.
- ↑ circulatory water caused by excessive fluid intake or oedema.
- Pharmacological due to the effects of diuretics.

Biochemical investigations: urea and electrolytes—potassium (K+)

- Present in all cells.
- Dietary intake (fruit, vegetables, and meat) absorbed through intestinal mucosa.
- Potassium found in plasma and intracellular and extracellular fluid.
- Distribution across cell membranes (i.e. intracellular versus extracellular) and balance between intake and excretion influence the plasma K+ concentration.
- K+ concentrations affect membrane excitability.
  - Hypokalaemia causes ↑ excitability, which can lead to atrial or ventricular arrythmias. ECG changes: small or inverted T waves; prolonged PR interval; ST segment depression; prominent U wave after T.
  - Hyperkalaemia leads to ↓ excitability with ECG changes and can lead to heart block and asystole. ECG changes: tall tented T waves; wide QRS complex; small P wave; VF (📖 see Fig. 2.1).

Possible causes of hyperkalaemia

- ↑ dietary intake.
- ↓ urinary output (renal failure).
- ↓ aldosterone production.
- Excessive use of dietary supplements.
- Cell damage releasing potassium (burns, trauma, severe infection).
- Chemotherapy.
- Metabolic acidosis.
- Insulin deficiency.

Possible causes of hypokalaemia

- ↓ intake.
- Dietary.
- Prolonged ileus.
- Malabsorption.
- Loss from GI tract.
- Diarrhoea.
- Vomiting.

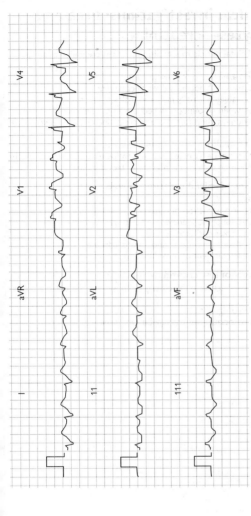

Fig. 2.1 Hyperkalaemia—note the flattening of the P-waves, prominent T-waves, and widening of the QRS complex. (Reproduced with permission from Longmore, M., et al. (2004). *Oxford Handbook of Clinical Medicine*, 6th edn. p. 693. Oxford University Press, Oxford.)

Biochemical investigations: urea and electrolytes—creatinine

- Anaerobic skeletal muscle metabolism produces creatinine as a waste product.
- Normal values are related to muscle mass.
  - ↑ muscle mass → ↑ normal values of creatinine.
  - Creatinine values normally higher in males than females.
- Direct link between amount produced and amount excreted.
- Excreted by kidneys; therefore ↑ blood creatinine levels suggest ↓ renal function.
- Muscle injury may also increase creatinine levels.
- Kidney function can be assessed with a creatinine clearance test, which includes a 24h urine collection and venous blood sample.

Possible causes of raised creatinine levels

- ↑ muscle mass.
- Renal disease or obstruction of renal tract.
- Reduced blood supply to kidneys due to congestive cardiac failure, dehydration, shock, or atherosclerosis.
- Diet high in red meat may cause short-lived increases.
- Drugs causing impairment of renal function.

Possible causes of low creatinine levels

- ↓ muscle mass—such as in the elderly or those with muscular dystrophy.
- Can be seen in pregnancy.
- Occasionally associated with advanced liver disease.

Biochemical investigations: liver function tests—albumin

- One of three main types of plasma protein and the one present in the greatest amount.
- Manufactured by the liver.
- Albumin levels give an indication of liver function.
- Sequential reduced albumin levels may indicate ↓ hepatic funtion.
- Acts as a binding agent for transport of circulating substances such as hormones, bilirubin, and enzymes.
- Half life 20–26 days.
- Physical effects of a low albumin level are delayed.
- Albumin in capillaries provides osmotic pull.
- ↓ albumin will ↑ movement of water into tissues resulting in oedema.
- Albumin may be reduced in:
  - liver disease;
  - nephrotic syndrome;
  - malnutrition;
  - marked inflammatory response;
  - Crohn's disease.
- Albumin may be elevated in:
  - dehydration;
  - inflammatory conditions, e.g. rheumatoid arthritis.

Biochemical investigations: liver function tests (continued)

Alkaline phosphatase (ALP)

- A naturally occurring enzyme.
- Produced by cells in the bile duct (ductoles).
- Normally drains into bile duct.
- In obstructive liver disease (cholestatic) the enzyme will build up in the liver and 'leak' into the circulatory system.
- ALP is also related to bone and placental growth (therefore can be ↑ in pregnancy) and can be produced by tumours.
- Can be ↑ with diseases of the gut such as ulcerative colitis.
- Children can have higher ALP levels due to bone growth.
- Each of the tissues—liver, bone, placenta, and intestine—produce slightly different ALP or isoenzyme.

Bilirubin

This is the major bile pigment; it is a byproduct of haemolysis. Accumulation of bilirubin causes yellow discoloration of sclerae, mucous membranes, and skin (jaundice).

- Destruction of red blood cells by the reticulo-endothelial system releases bilirubin into the blood.
- Bilirubin attaches to plasma proteins—unconjugated or indirect bilirubin. Passes through liver where bilirubin conjugates with glucuronic acid to become conjugated or direct bilirubin.
- Conjugated bilirubin forms part of bile and enters digestive system; partly is excreted in stools and partly in urine.

Possible causes of isolated ↑ in bilirubin

- Haemolysis.
- Ineffective erythropoiesis.
- Immature bilirubin metabolism, e.g. physiological neonatal jaundice; inherited defects in uptake or conjugation, e.g. Gilbert's syndrome.
- Modest elevation of serum bilirubin may be present with disorders such as vitamin B_{12} or folate deficiencies.

Possible causes of ↑ conjugated bilirubin

- Inherited defects in excretion.
- Hepato-cellular disease, post hepatitic disease, or cholestatic disease.
- ↑ faecal and urinary bilirubin can be present in haemolytic anaemias.

Biochemical investigations: blood gases and 'cardiac enzymes'

Bicarbonate

- A measure of the total carbon dioxide in the body.
- Three forms:
  - carbonic acid (H_2CO_3);
  - carbon dioxide (CO_2);
  - bicarbonate (HCO_3^-).
- Main function: acid–base balance or pH.
- Works with potassium, sodium, and chloride to maintain electrical neutrality.
- Test is part of routine U & E testing and also part of ABG testing.

Abnormal findings

↑ Bicarbonate

- Imbalance of body pH through ↑ CO_2 or electrolyte imbalance, particularly potassium (K).
- Particularly with K imbalance, consider diuretics as a cause.
- Can be associated with COPD and conditions/disease causing metabolic alkalosis.

↓ Bicarbonate

- Can be associated with respiratory and or metabolic acidosis, severe dehydration, and renal failure.

Creatine kinase (CK)

- CK is an enzyme found in heart and skeletal muscle.
- Also found in brain.
- Three different forms:
  - CK-MB—mostly found in heart muscle;
  - CK-MM—found in heart and other muscles;
  - CK-BB—mostly found in brain and kidney (not usually found in blood).
- ↑ CK level indicates muscle damage. The type of CK enzyme isolated can indicate which muscles are damaged, e.g. heart or other muscle.
- In chest pain CK-MB rises and falls in 72h, peaking at 24h. A rise can be seen at 4–6h and can be helpful in diagnosis of myocardial infarction.
- CK can also ↑ with heavy/excessive exercise and other forms of muscle damage from falls, etc.
- Excess alcohol intake can lead to a small increase in CK.
- Afro-Caribbeans may have a higher CK than other ethnic groups.
- CK levels may ↓ in early pregnancy.

Biochemical investigations: lipids and other values

Glucose

- Simple sugar used as energy.
- Derived from breakdown of carbohydrate.
- Absorbed in small intestine.
- Required by most cells.
- Brain and CNS rely on glucose. Their functioning is susceptible to fluctuations in glucose levels.
- Insulin required for uptake, metabolism, and storage and mobilization of glucose.
- Glucose measured in the blood; also tested for in urine.
- ↑ blood glucose can lead to excretion in urine through kidneys.
- Ketones present in urine signify metabolism of fat to produce energy, as insulin may not be available to metabolize glucose.
- Ketones in the blood will ↓ pH.
- Respiration rate and depth ↑ in attempt to 'blow off' the CO_2 (📚 see Chapter 16, 'Diabetic ketoacidosis', p.484).
- Both hyper- and hypoglycaemia will affect brain function.

Possible causes of hyperglycaemia

- ↓ insulin production.
- Excessive food intake.
- Diabetes mellitus.
- Pancreatic insufficiency.
- Pancreatitis.
- Cushing's syndrome.
- Pregnancy/eclampsia.
- Hypertension.
- Obesity-induced type 2 diabetes.
- Chronic infection.
- Stress response (raised adrenaline):
  - trauma;
  - sudden illness;
  - seizures.
- Medication-induced, e.g. by corticosteroids.

Possible causes of hypoglycaemia

- ↓ dietary intake:
  - malnutrition;
  - vomiting.
- Exercise.
- Hypothermia.
- Excessive insulin:
  - overadministration;
  - overproduction—pancreatic tumour.
- Endocrine disorders:
  - Addison's disease;
  - hypothyroidism;
  - hypopituitarism.

Amylase

- An enzyme released into the digestive tract used for breaking down starch.
- Found in large quantities in pancreas; lesser quantities in salivary glands.
- Excreted by kidneys; therefore can be found in urine.
- Usually requested as a test with patients presenting with abdominal pain.

Raised amylase (hyperamylasaemia) can be found with:
- acute pancreatitis (serum amylase usually ↑ fourfold);
- diabetic ketoacidosis;
- hepatitis;
- peritonitis;
- renal failure;
- intestinal obstruction/perforation;
- burns;
- infections such as mumps;
- salivary trauma.

C-reactive protein (CRP)

- Protein made by the liver and secreted into blood.
- Elevated in blood after infection or inflammation within a few hours.
- This elevation may precede fever, pain, or other clinical indications.
- There can be a significant ↑ in CRP in response to inflammation; then rapid ↓ as inflammation subsides.
- As CRP responds to both inflammation and infection it is not specific to disease or condition.
- Can be used to monitor reduction in infection or inflammation as it falls quickly in the blood when infection or inflammation subsides.
- CRP ↑ in bacterial infections and ↓ in viral infections.
- Erythrocyte sedimentation rate (ESR) is also used as an adjunct to CRP.

Possible causes of ↑ CRP

- Injury to tissue or necrosis, e.g. pulmonary embolus, myocardial infarction, burns, or necrosis.
- Inflammatory disorders such as Crohn's and arthritis.
- Bacterial infections.
- Neoplastic disease.
- Tissue rejection.

Haematological investigations

Red blood cells (RBC)
- Manufactured by bone marrow.
- Responsible for the transport of oxygen and carbon dioxide.
- RBCs act as an acid–base buffer helping maintain pH balance.
- Lower RBC counts are found in women.
- ↓ RBC with age.
- Hypoxia stimulates the bone marrow to ↑ production of RBC.
- The test counts the number of RBCs per litre of blood.
- Changes in RBC levels have to be interpreted in light of other parameters such as haemoglobin and haematocrit.
- RBC usually requested as part of a full blood count (FBC).
- ↓ RBC > 10% decrease of expected normal value = anaemia.
- ↑ RBC = polycythaemia.
- ↓ RBC may indicate bleeding, anaemia (deficiency, pernicious, aplastic, and haemolytic), renal disease, bone marrow failure, malnutrition.
  - ► Fluid replacement after haemorrhage will reduce RBC volume.
- ↑ RBC may indicate ↓ circulatory volume (possible causes include dehydration, diarrhoea, burns); bone marrow overproduction; prolonged depletion of O_2 in the blood, e.g. in pulmonary disease, heart disease, and at high altitudes.

Haemoglobin
- Important in transportation of oxygen.
- An iron-containing molecule found in RBCs.
- Haemoglobin picks up oxygen as it passes through pulmonary capillary blood vessels.
- Oxygen is transported to cells across arterial capillary walls.
- Haemoglobin levels are adjusted for sex, age, and ethnic origin.
- 📖 See 'red blood cells' above for effects of ↓ haemoglobin and ↑ haemoglobin.

Erythrocyte sedimentation rate (ESR)
- Indirect measure of degree of inflammation caused by disease.
- Not specific to any particular disease.
- Measures rate of settlement (sedimentation) of unclotted blood in a tall thin tube.
- Number of millimetres of clear plasma present at the top of the column at 1h forms the result.
- Normal sample would have a little clear plasma at 1h.
- ↑ sedimentation rate occurs with ↑ red cell weight (increased proteins such as fibrinogen and immunoglobulins as a result of inflammation through disease process increase weight) and causes RBCs to fall more rapidly.
- ESR is affected by age, sex, pregnancy, menstruation, and drugs.

Possible causes of ↑ ESR
- Inflammatory disorder or disease.
- Autoimmune disease.
- Recent trauma.

- Myocardial infarction (early response).
- Anaemia.

Possible causes of ↓ ESR
- Sickle cell.
- Congestive cardiac failure (CCF).
- Hypoproteinaemia.
- Hypofibrinogenaemia.
- Polycythaemia.

Although non-specific, ESR can be helpful in confirming two specific diagnoses: temporal arteritis and polymyalgia rheumatica.

White cell count (WCC)
- Counts and quantifies each type of white blood cell in blood.
- Forms part of the FBC, showing total WCC and 5-part differential count.
- ↑ WCC (leucocytosis) can indicate: inflammation; bacterial infection; leukaemia (raised number of abnormal white cells); or trauma.
- ↓ WCC (leucopenia) can indicate: autoimmune disease (lupus erythematosus); overwhelming bacterial infection; suppression of bone marrow; vitamin B_{12} or folic acid deficiency.
- Stress, exercise, and pregnancy (last trimester) can ↑ WCC.
- Each type of white cell (leucocyte) is expressed as percentage of total count.

Differential white count
- Lymphocytes are formed in lymphoid tissue and bone marrow. Needed for immunity. ↑ lymphocytes indicate stimulation of immune response.
- Eosinophils are related to allergic and parasitic conditions.
- Neutrophils are related to defence against invading organisms. Act by phagocytosis.
- Basophils are primarily related to allergic response. Some defence against parasitic worms. Close relationship to mast cells.
- Monocytes mature into macrophages (in target tissue) in response to infection or inflammation. Macrophages work by phagocytosis, are involved in the generalized systemic reaction to inflammation, and pass information to lymphocytes to produce correct antibodies. Can also destroy tumour cells.

Urinalysis

Used for screening for infection, renal disease, and metabolic disorders. Although commonly conducted, it is often done poorly! Inaccuracies can occur through early reading of screening sticks and the use of out-of-date sticks. Consideration should be given to the sensitivity and specificity of the tests in determining clinical decisions.

Most testing strips will provide data on the following:

pH Measures hydrogen ion concentration in the urine.

Possible causes of ↑ acidity
- Metabolic acidosis: diabetes mellitus; starvation.
- Respiratory acidosis.
- Alkaline loss through diarrhoea.
- Iatrogenic, e.g. ascorbic acid.
- Dietary: high meat content.

Possible causes of ↑ alkalinity
- Metabolic alkalosis.
- Respiratory alkalosis.
- Renal tube defects.
- Loss of acid through vomiting.
- UTI.
- Iatrogenic: sodium bicarbonate.
- Dietary: high vegetable content.

Specific gravity Indicates quantity of dissolved substances in urine. Not accurately recorded via dipstick.

Possible causes of raised specific gravity
- Reduced urine output (more concentrated), dehydration, etc.
- ↑ urea content.
- ↑ glucose content.
- Osmotic diuretics such as mannitol.

Possible causes of lowered specific gravity
- ↓ urea content: low protein diet.
- ↓ sodium concentration.
- ↑ urine output: overhydration; diabetes insipidus.
- Inability of kidney to concentrate urine, particularly in the elderly.

Protein Not normally found in urine. Possible causes of proteinuria (presence of protein in urine) are the following.
- Hypertension
- Heart failure
- Pyrexia
- UTI
- ⚠ Eclampsia.

Very dilute urine may produce false −ve results.

Glucose Not normally found in urine. Possible causes of glycosuria (presence of glucose in urine) include the following.

- Hyperglycaemia (varying causes).
- Reduced renal threshold:
  - pregnancy;
  - ⚠ eclampsia.
- Iatrogenic: corticosteroids; thiazide diuretics.

Ketones Not normally found in urine. Possible causes of presence in urine are:
- Dietary: reduced carbohydrate intake; high fat/protein diet;
- Metabolic: diabetes mellitus; ketoacidosis;
- Pregnancy;
- ⚠ eclampsia;
- Rapid depletion of fat stores: rapid weight loss; ↑ metabolic rate; strenuous exercise.
- ↑ pituitary function.
- ↑ cortisone secretion.

Blood Not normally found in urine.
- Macroscopic blood in the urine will alter its colour to red.
- Microscopic blood may not be visualized.
- Reagent tests normally distinguish haemolysed and non-haemolysed blood.
  - Haemolysed blood identifies free haemoglobin/myoglobin released from breakdown or rupture of red blood cells. May indicate that bleeding occurred in higher urinary tract.
  - Non-haemolysed blood shows intact red blood cells. May indicate that these undamaged RBCs originate from lower down the urinary tract.

Possible causes of haematuria (presence of RBCs)
- Renal disease/trauma.
- Renal calculi.
- Bladder neoplasm; stones.
- Cystitis.
- Prostate gland inflammation or neoplasm.
- Urethritis.
- Menstruation.
- Haemolysed blood external to renal tract excreted through urine.

Nitrites and leucocytes should not be found in the urine.
- Nitrites and leucocytes can be indicative of urine infection.
- Most bacteria, but not all (those that do not have metabolic effect on nitrates) causing UTIs convert nitrates (normal waste product in urine) to nitrites. UTIs cause an inflammatory response ↑ presence of WBCs; ∴ ↑ leucocyte count.
- False +ve and false –ve results are possible.

Urinary chloride
- Chloride excreted by kidneys (also lost through skin in sweat).
- Urinary excretion is a function of balance, affected by pH, sodium, and potassium levels.
- Measured usually through 24h urine collection.

Forms of imaging

X-ray

This is a common investigation in the ED. It is commonly used to detect abnormalities of organs or tissues affected by injury, disease, or degeneration. Also used to confirm or exclude suspicion of a fracture, dislocation, or certain foreign bodies such as glass or metal in wounds, or ingested foreign bodies such as coins.

The densities of the structures inside the body affect the penetration of X-rays and therefore their appearance on the image. For example:

- air-filled spaces such as lungs or gas in bowels allow full passage of X-rays and appear black on the image;
- bones appear white as they are dense and do not permit penetration of X-rays;
- organs and fat, are a darker grey, as they allow some penetration;
- water does not allow much penetration so it looks light;
- specific dyes are used that are impenetrable to X-ray and therefore appear white allowing a contrast to the black image.

X-rays are not without risk as long-term overexposure to radiation can lead to malignancy. Legislation governs the requesting, exposure, and evaluation of the images. Nurses and other allied health professions are, under specific circumstances and local protocol, permitted to refer for a number of X-ray investigations. All referrers must be educated about and conversant with the Ionising Radiation (Medical Exposure) Regulations (IR(ME)R) 2000 regulations.[1]

Computerized tomography (CT)

This form of imaging is commonly used by ED clinicians as a diagnostic tool. In the CT scanner X-rays are used to form three-dimensional images of cross-sections of the body. Early CT scanning is now indicated for a number of conditions including stroke.

Nurses are currently not legally allowed to refer patients for CT scanning. However, nurses have a fundamental role in resuscitation, safe transfer, patient management, and monitoring prior to and during scanning.

CT images are often useful in diagnosis; however the CT scanner is euphemistically referred to as the 'donut of death'! The patient must be adequately resuscitated before transfer to the scanner, in particular, with regards to airway management and fluid resuscitation. An elective rapid sequence induction of anaesthesia to protect the airway of a patient with a reduced Glasgow Coma Score (GCS) in the resuscitation room is preferable to a flustered attempt with a vomiting patient in the CT scanner. Equally, if the patient is haemodynamically unstable, surgery to correct life-threatening haemorrhage may be indicated first before definitive imaging. The ED nurse has a key role in raising questions about safety and appropriateness of transfer of the unstable patient to CT.

Magnetic resonance imaging (MRI)

The use of this form of imaging in the ED setting is increasing. MRI uses magnetic and radiowaves—there is no exposure to X-rays or other damaging rays. As this form of imaging uses magnets the referring clinician must take a history to determine whether the patient has metal implants, clips, or foreign bodies that might be dislodged by the powerful magnets.

The MRI is able to provide images of almost all tissues of the body and is able to make images of tissues that are surrounded by bone. The MRI gives very detailed images, which is particularly useful when imaging the brain and cervical spine. For example, MRI can identify ligamentous involvement in neck injury, which would not be detected on CT. The use of MRI is not limited to areas such as the brain and chest. Small part MRI scanners are proving useful in the early definitive diagnosis of scaphoid fractures. As this imaging modality becomes more common, early imaging of wrists, knees, and ankles may well be a useful adjunct in the management of patients attending the ED with these injuries.

Ultrasound (sonography)

This investigation produces an image by the deflection of ultrasound waves from structures inside the body. It can be used to visualize muscle, tendons, and organs. 'Free fluid' can also be visualized.

Ultrasound can be used for diagnosis as well as guidance of procedures such as the visualization of the venous circulation before insertion of a central venous line.

In trauma, clinicians are being trained in 'focused assessment with sonography for trauma' (FAST). The FAST scan is used to identify fluid in the pericardium, free fluid in the abdominal cavity, and the diameter of the aorta in the abdomen, for example. It is a useful adjunctive scan and can assist in the decision making in both haemodynamically stable and unstable patients. Specific training courses in FAST scanning are available.[2]

Emergency nurse practitioners (ENP) may find ultrasound useful for the assessment of the Achilles tendon when injury is suspected as well as for the identification of foreign bodies that are not radio-opaque such as wood. There is no legislative framework around referral for ultrasound. Referral will be dictated by local agreement.

References

1 For more information on the regulations see 🖰 www.legislation.gov.uk/si/si2000/20001059.htm
2 Further details can be found at 🖰 www.emergencyultrasound.org.uk/index.html

First principles

Surviving an average day

Every day is different, but there are routine things you will do every day. One of the key skills necessary for emergency nursing is anticipation. This applies to the patients you are looking after as well as to the team you are working with. For your patients, given that many will have undifferentiated and undiagnosed problems, anticipating the care, investigations, and treatment they will need is an important component of your role. Emergency care is a team pursuit. Anticipating the needs and actions of the team around you, particularly in an emergency situation, is really important. The skill of anticipation is gained over time, by exposure to many situations, and recognizing the patterns that develop with similar patient presentations and disease/injury processes. Fundamental to this process is knowing the patient outcome; this feedback loop is important in building expertise. This requires discipline in following patients up, seeing how they are progressing, and establishing if your identification of their problems was correct or not.

General assessment of the ED patient

Initial assessment

Do a rapid head to toe visual scan of the patient. Look at:
- respiratory rate and effort
- pallor
- positioning
- perfusion
- haemorrhage—visible signs of blood loss
- signs of distress—physical and psychological.

Teamwork

Emergency care is one area of health care where multidisciplinary team-work is fundamental. For successful teamwork excellent communication and honesty is crucial. Particularly in emergency situations, where antici-pation and proficiency are of utmost importance, training together and rehearsing for incidents can pay dividends in team performance. Clearly defined roles and responsibilities amongst the team can reduce ambiguity and duplication of effort particularly in challenging clinical situations. In the resuscitation room, clear allocation of roles prior to the patient arrival can help with effective resuscitation. Important in developing effective team working is honest appraisal and feedback on performance within the team.

Inappropriate and regular attenders at the ED

Inappropriate attenders

It is easy as health care professionals to make judgements about the reasons for and legitimacy of attendance. Pejorative judgements about patients and their attendance can influence their clinical assessment and ultimately their treatment.

Patients often seek care in an emergency care setting because they have either been unable to contact or are not satisfied with care from other health care providers. They may have sought advice from family or friends as to where they should receive care. Navigating through the health care system, particularly during the 'out of hours' period, can be a challenge. It may well not be the individual who is an inappropriate attender; it may be that the health care system is providing an inappropriate service.

It is important to remember that behind every so-called 'minor' presentation there may be a problem with undetected significant pathology. Be slow to judge the appropriateness of the presentation and take time to explore the real reason for the presentation.

Regular attenders

Every department or emergency service provider has regular attenders, callers, or service users. Many are known by name and are familiar to staff. Their reasons for attendance are often similar, and may appear trivial. It is easy to see these individuals as nuisances or time wasters. They often have complex needs of a physical or psychological nature compounded by challenging social circumstances. The 'regular attenders' are often high users of primary care services as well. They are a vulnerable and at risk group and require extra attention, not dismissal when they attend services.

Amongst the seemingly trivial reasons for attendance may be significant pathology. Remember, just because they are regular attenders does not mean they are not sick or at risk of significant physical and psychological morbidity. One of the 'golden rules' (📖 Golden rules of emergency nursing p.3) applies here: 'If you don't like someone you should spend twice as long with them'. Regular attenders should be seen as part of a vulnerable or at risk group.

Patients with learning disabilities

Patients with learning disabilities require specific attention in the emergency care setting. This setting can cause considerable distress, exacerbating challenges to understanding and communication. Patients with learning disabilities are vulnerable. Staff should be trained to meet their needs and to be able to communicate effectively. Consideration should be given to the environment. The amount of stimulation from noise and human traffic can cause additional stress. Close links should be made with local learning disability specialists to facilitate early expert care.

Close involvement with relatives and carers in the assessment and management of those with learning disabilities is fundamental. Behavioural regression is not uncommon in emergency situations. Working with those who normally care for the individual will be invaluable in managing the situation. A high level of clinical care is required for this vulnerable client group who are particularly at risk in an unfamiliar emergency environment.

Models of unscheduled care delivery

There are a number of new models of service delivery emerging. These include urgent care centres, minor injury units, and NHS walk-in centres. These new models of service delivery are driven by policy changes and clinical developments. The advent of thrombolysis for ischaemic stroke and development of regional centres offering PCI means service reconfigurations are needed. Changes in out of hours service provision by GPs and PCTs have also changed the shape of unscheduled care delivery providing for emergency care providers both challenges as well as opportunities to test new models of service delivery by other professionals such as emergency care practitioners (ECPs). However, many of the models in use have not been thoroughly clinically evaluated.

Fundamental in developing unscheduled services is the provision of consistent access with clear parameters of practice to ensure that the public know where, when, and how to access unscheduled care. Given the current changes in service provision it is likely that formal systems of unscheduled care delivery will emerge such as the development of a trauma network with dedicated trauma centres. The notion of 'super' EDs, providing services for stroke thrombolysis, PCI for cardiac chest pain, and the management of trauma, has been discussed.

Health promotion

This is an important part of emergency care. Patients and relatives are a captive audience. Consultations enable opportunistic health promotion opportunities. However, care must be taken not to be judgemental or to apportion blame for their attendance. Careful judgement of the individual's ability or willingness to accept health promotion information at the time of attendance is necessary.

Having written information that can be taken away is a useful way of providing health promotion. Appropriate information in different areas in the department should be considered for different age groups. It is important to consider access to written information for those whose first language is not English. Written information in the languages spoken by local communities is important.

Thematic displays of relevant health promotion advice and information can be used to good effect in emergency care settings. Patients or relatives may be inclined to seek information about general health and well-being whilst waiting for care.

The role of emergency care settings in surveillance of accident or incident hot spots has been under-recognized. Clear patterns may emerge for road traffic incidents or areas of particular violence or aggression in communities. Monitoring and recording of such incidents can provide useful data in preventing incidents in the future. Careful liaison with local authorities in sharing data can be useful in this respect.

Infection control

Preventing infection is everyone's responsibility. Each health care professional should have an understanding of infection control and be aware of how they can help prevent hospital or community-acquired infection. Key areas for concentration within the emergency setting are reduction of infections related to peripheral IV line insertion, reduction in UTIs (reducing unnecessary uretheral catheterization), and early isolation of patients with diarrhoea and vomiting.

Using personal protective equipment is fundamental to prevent transfer of infection. In an emergency care setting little is known about patients' past medical history. Full protection precautions should be taken with bodily fluids. Given the nature of the working environment and the need to deal with a number of patients at any given time, care must be taken to change gloves and other protective items and clean hands effectively between patients. The importance of hand hygiene can not be over-emphasized.

Notifiable diseases

Health care professionals are required to notify a 'proper officer' of the local authority of suspected cases of certain infectious diseases. This is required under the Public Health (Infectious Diseases) 1988 Act and the Public Health (Control of Diseases) 1988 Act. This information is then passed in turn to the Health Protection Agency. Local information should be available about whom to report to and the information required.

Notifiable infections/poisonings are as follows.[1]

- Acute encephalitis.
- Acute poliomyelitis.
- Anthrax.
- Cholera.
- Diphtheria.
- Dysentery.
- Food poisoning.
- Leptospirosis.
- Malaria.
- Measles.
- Meningitis:
  - meningococcal;
  - pneumococcal;
  - *Haemophilus influenzae*;
  - viral.
- Meningococcal septicaemia (without meningitis).
- Mumps.
- Ophthalmia neonatorum.
- Paratyphoid fever.
- Plague.
- Rabies.
- Relapsing fever.
- Rubella.
- Scarlet fever.
- Smallpox.

- Tetanus.
- Tuberculosis.
- Typhoid fever.
- Typhus fever.
- Viral haemorrhagic fever.
- Viral hepatitis:
  - hepatitis A;
  - hepatitis B;
  - hepatitis C.
- Whooping cough.
- Yellow fever.

Leprosy is also notifiable, but directly to the HPA.

Reference

1 For further information see ⊖ http://www.hpa.org.uk/default.htm

History taking

It is all in the history—spend time getting an accurate history. Vital information is gained from the patient, carers, parents (in the case of children), other family members, and community carers including the general practitioner (GP) and pre-hospital staff.

A general approach to history taking is as follows:

- Presenting complaint (PC). Why the patient has attended the department today, e.g. right wrist injury
- History of presenting complaint (HPC).
  - What happened? e.g. fall on to outstretched hand.
  - How did it happen? e.g. tripped over loose carpet.
  - When did it happen? e.g. this morning at approximately 10.00h.
  - Where did it happen?
  - Any additional information.
- In the case of illness:
  - recent events—any prodromal features; any recent foreign travel?
  - any other members of the family affected?
- Past medical history (PMH): information about previous injuries/illness. It is important to take time to ascertain information about PMH as it may have a direct bearing on the presenting complaint. If, for instance, there is a history of postural hypotension, one might consider asking the patient if they had got up from a chair immediately before they fell.
- Medication (Meds). What medication does the patient take? Ask about:
  - prescribed medication
  - over-the-counter medications
  - complementary medicines
  - recreational drug use.

  Consider:
  - medication as a cause of presentation, particularly polypharmacy in the older person
  - how medications may affect different presentations, e.g. warfarin and head injury
  - in the case of illness, immunization history in particular with children
  - in the case of injury remember to ask about tetanus status.
- Allergies. Both pharmacological and non-pharmacological allergies are important. Medications can have a food base, e.g. eggs in some immunizations.
- Social history (SH).
  - Alcohol consumption and recreational drug use.
  - Smoking status.
  - For children: family structure, e.g siblings; legal guardianships; school/ college.
  - Adults: occupation; accommodation (particularly for the older person when considering mobility issues); hand dominance (important when considering arm/hand injuries).

Findings on examination (O/E)

- Inspection (look).
  - General appearance—do they look unwell? Are they sweaty?

- • Note deformity or discrepancy in contour, bruising, swelling, bleeding. ▶ Compare with unaffected side.
  - • Note scars from previous surgery.
- • Palpation (feel).
  - • Note bony tenderness, crepitus, deformity.
  - • Check circulation distal to injury.
  - • Full systematic systems examination may be required.
- • Auscultation. Evaluation of lung fields, heart sounds, bruits, bowel sounds as appropriate.
- • Percussion. Chest and abdomen as appropriate.
- • Movements. Test range of movement and describe. ▶ Compare with unaffected side.
- • Neurological. Test power, tone, and sensation of affected area ▶ compare with other side.

Impression A note of the impression formed after assessment is important, this can include a differential diagnosis, i.e. a number of diagnostic possibilities that can either be ruled in or excluded when the findings of any investigations are received. Although common things are common it is important to consider rare presentations or conditions.

Plan It is important to have a plan of investigations or plan of care for the patient. Careful documentation is important.

Final impression A clear outline of what you believe to be the problem or diagnosis.

Final instructions

It is helpful to give the patient an outline of what to expect and/or the likely course of their illness or injury recovery. This is helpfully accompanied by instructions about where and when to seek further health care assistance if there is a deviation from this predicted course. This is a safety net for the patient and for you as the clinician.

Careful documentation is a part of good clinical practice.

Documentation

The gold standard for documentation is a contemporaneous record. When this is not possible it is important to make it clear that the notes have been written in retrospect.

Key elements to document

- Time and date seen.
- Person giving the information (i.e. the patient, parent, relative, or carer).
- When using the patient's own words use speech marks.
- Sign, time, and date every entry.
- Avoid using abbreviations.
- Develop a structured approach. This will act as an *aide-mémoire* if you always use the same format.
- Record nursing assessments and interventions, personal care, drinks and meals given, etc.
- Handover of care to other nurses or health care professionals should be recorded.
- Clear discharge instructions and plans for follow-up must be recorded.
- Increasingly, nurses are required to provide statements of events. These may be used in criminal coroner or negligence proceedings—your notes may be scrutinized in court. At the very least you will need to refer to the patient record if you are asked to give evidence. Would your documentation stand up to this scrutiny? Remember you may be asked to account years after the event and will only have your notes.
- Remember the old adage 'If it isn't recorded it didn't happen!'

The handover of care

The handover of information from pre-hospital ambulance personnel to ED staff is crucial, particularly in emergency situations. Each ED should have an agreed process for this. On reception of the patient, the person or persons to take the handover should be identified. Essential care of the patient should continue. Take the history and handover of care given en route. It is good practice to summarize the history and repeat it to the person handing over the patient to ensure salient information is transferred. A written record of pre-hospital care given is essential.

Pre-alerting EDs for patients requiring resuscitation or immediate intervention on arrival is good practice. The commonly used mnemonic 'ASHICE' by ambulance services ensures a concise method of delivering important information from the scene to facilitate correct preparation for trauma patients.

ASHICE

- **A**ge. Patient's age.
- **S**ex. Male or female.
- **H**istory. Synopsis of what has happened, e.g. road traffic collision, head on, combined speed of 80mph.
- **I**njuries sustained, e.g. neck, chest, and pelvis.
- **C**ondition. Vital signs, information about immediate management, etc.
- **E**stimated time of arrival.

Interhospital or intrahospital/care setting handover

Information about the patient can be lost at any stage. Important information about the events preceding admission and events during their treatment in the ED must be handed over to the next team providing care. Ideally, it should be the person who has cared for the patient who hands over care to the next team. If this is not possible a careful briefing should be given. In some settings a written handover of information is considered to be best practice. For critical care transfers particular attention should be paid to preparation for transfer. Checking equipment for battery life, supplementary oxygen, and resuscitation equipment are essential. Preparing for the worst possible scenario in transfer is good practice.

Management of the patient with multiple injuries

Patients with multiple injuries can pose significant challenges in prioritization and management. Adopting a systematic approach is fundamental to ensure that the life- and limb-threatening injuries are managed first. Do not be distracted by obvious non-life-threatening injuries. Following the Advanced Trauma Life Support (ATLS) ABCDE principles will structure your assessment and management. This will consist of a primary and secondary survey. Do not move on to the next principle until you have effectively managed the previous one.

- **A**irway. Is the patient able to talk? Is the airway patent and clear? Remove debris.
- **B**reathing. Are they breathing? Are both sides of the chest rising and falling symmetrically? Any flail segments? Is there good air entry both sides? Is the trachea central in the neck?

- **C**irculation. Is there a pulse? Secure wide bore cannulae access, preferably one line in each arm. Give fluids as indicated by clinical condition and presentation.
- **D**isability. What is the Glasgow coma score? (📖 see Chapter 20, 'Neurological assessment: the Glasgow Coma Score', p.642) Or, in children, AVPU ('alert, verbal, painful, unresponsive'; 📖 see Chapter 4, 'Management of the injured child', p.92).
- **E**xposure. Fully undress the patient to ensure you have not missed any major injury.

▶ Remember not to let them get cold.

Once the primary survey is complete as above and resuscitative measures started, a secondary more detailed survey including a 'log roll' and initial trauma imaging such as lateral C-spine, chest, and pelvis X-rays begins. The secondary survey should not be conducted until the patient has been adequately resuscitated.

In the military or conflict setting the approach has been changed to <C> ABC for patients suffering blast or ballistic injuries. This is in recognition that some deaths are preventable by the control of haemorrhage. The initial C stands for 'catastrophic haemorrhage', and is applied when there is a need to rapidly deal with haemorrhage before ABC. Given the increasing terrorist threats with associated blast and ballistic trauma, this approach should be considered when faced with patients with significant haemorrhage.[1]

Reference

1 Hodgetts, T.J., Mahoney, P.F., Russell, M.Q., and Byers, M. (2006). ABC to <C>ABC: redefining the military trauma paradigm. *Emergency Medicine Journal* **23**, 745–6.

Triage

Triage, determining the urgency of care, is common in UK EDs. The key processes are:
- rapid assessment;
- identifying life- or limb-threatening problems;
- initiation of investigations;
- providing analgesia;
- controlling patient flow.

A national consensus was reached between senior nurses and doctors from professional organizations in the UK in the 1990s about triage categories, times, and nomenclatures (📖 see Table 3.1).

See and treat

Many departments have changed their triage process in recent years to incorporate a 'See and treat' service. See and treat works on the basis of bringing a senior decision maker (an experienced ENP or doctor) close to the triage area to pull out patients who can be seen and treated almost as soon as they arrive. This process allows early management of some of the most straightforward presentations and removes them from the overall queue of patients waiting to be seen. Depending on the case mix of patients presenting, this has helped with managing demand in a number of departments.

Streaming

Many departments have also introduced the concept of streaming patients. This process involves allocating patients to streams of activity within the department or to other service providers from triage. An example of this may be identification of patients at triage who would be suitable for 'See and treat' and directing them to that stream or alternatively to a local walk-in centre from triage. The success of these initiatives relies on effective staffing and management of the streams to which patients are directed to ensure that the patients' journey through the department is as smooth as possible.

Table 3.1 National triage scale

Category	Description	Time frame to be seen
1 Red	Immediate	Immediately
2 Orange	Very urgent	Within 10min of arrival
3 Yellow	Urgent	Within 1h
4 Green	Standard	Within 2h
5 Blue	Non-urgent	Within 4h

Early warning scores (EWS)

EWS and Paediatric EWS (PEWS) are increasingly being recorded in emergency care areas as a means of identifying haemodynamic instability at an early stage. Evidence suggests that hospital staff are slow to recognize signs of early deterioration and intervention is commonly delayed.[1] An EWS/PEWS is calculated by adding together the scores attributed to various haemodynamic parameters. The parameters that are usually measured are: blood pressure, pulse, respiratory rate, GCS, urine output, and temperature. The sum total of each score gives an overall score which subsequent assessment and management is based on. An elevated EWS/PEWS requires intervention from senior staff to identify and treat the cause of the deranged physiology.

Reference

1 Recognition and response to acute illness in adults in hospital (2007). Available at ᐯᐟ http://www. nice.org.uk/Guidance/CGSO

Legal and ethical issues: consent, capacity, and confidentiality

Consent

Traditionally, emergency care practice has relied on the notion of implied consent. If the attendance is voluntary, the consent to examination and, to some extent, to treatment was assumed to be implied by the patient seeking assistance. However, given the increasing litigious nature of society, implied consent is not sufficient. Emergency nurses must have an awareness of the legal framework for practice.

In many cases or procedures, such as the use of wound infiltration with local anaesthetic for exploration and/or closure or local nerve blocks, it is common to gain verbal consent from the patient. However, a full explanation of the procedure including the risks and benefits should be given before proceeding. It is advisable that this process is witnessed. For procedures that require conscious sedation, such as the reduction of a fracture and dislocation, it is advisable to get written consent prior to the procedure. This would also apply to other procedures such as 'Bier's block'.

Capacity

Decision-making capacity is the ability that individuals possess to make decisions or to take actions that influence their life.[1] Under normal circumstances, every adult has the right to decide whether they will accept medical treatment, even if refusal may risk permanent damage to health. Competent adults may refuse treatment for reasons that are rational, irrational, or for no reason.

A person lacks capacity if, at the time a decision needs to be made, they are unable to make or communicate their decision because of an impairment of, or a disturbance in function, of the mind or brain.[2] It may be impaired on a temporary (e.g. mental illness, reduced conscious level, intoxication) or long-term (e.g. dementia, learning disability, brain damage) basis.

Capacity should be assessed in relation to each particular decision that has to be made, rather than making a general assessment. The more serious the consequences of a decision, the greater the level of competence required to make that decision. If capacity is likely to improve, any interventions that are not urgent should be delayed until capacity has been recovered.

The Mental Capacity Act 2005 provides a statutory framework to empower and protect vulnerable people who are not able to make their own decisions.[2] To assess capacity clinicians should ask the following questions.

- Does the patient understand the information relevant to the question?
- Is the patient able to retain that information?
- Is the patient able to use or weigh up that information as part of the decision-making process?
- Is the patient able to communicate their decision?

Confidentiality

This is an absolute right except in exceptional circumstances. Consent from the patient to share information amongst the team should be sought. Relatives or friends may call to enquire if patients are in the department. Consent should be sought from the patient as to what information can be divulged and to whom. In situations where sharing this information outside of the team will have consequence for the patient, their consent must be sought. If they withhold consent, or are not able to give consent, information may only be shared where it can be justified in the public interest or is required by law or an order of court. In situations of child protection local policies and procedures should be followed. For further information see the Nursing and Midwifery Code of Conduct.[3] You may need to defend your actions if you have breached confidentiality.

- In cases of alleged assault considerable care should be taken when handling enquires—the assailant may be interested in where the alleged victim is being treated.
- The press are often interested in incidents or 'celebrity' attendees and will often use a number of ruses or guises to gain information. In sensitive cases it may be appropriate to have a shared password between legitimate contacts to provide some degree of information security. Be aware and brief your staff—reporters or journalists can be very persuasive, inventive, and persistent!
- Inadvertent breaches of confidentiality can occur through corridor conversations. No matter how interesting the case or presentation, the patient has a right to confidentiality.
- Hospital colleagues on occasions injure themselves and become sick. They too have a right to a confidential visit and consultation. It can be easy not to afford them the same rights when enquires are received from concerned colleagues!

References

1 British Medical Association (2007). *The Mental Capacity Act 2005: guidance for health professionals*. Available at ⌂ http://www.bma.org.uk/ap.nsf/Content/mencapact05
2 Department of Health (2005). *Mental Capacity Act*. Department of Health, London.
3 Nursing and Midwifery Council (2007). *The code: standards of conduct, performance and ethics for nurses and midwives*. Available at ⌂ www.nmc-uk.org

Legal and ethical issues: assault and restraint

Assault and battery: supporting the victim

Within criminal law, assault and battery may be components of the same offence.

- Assault is an act that creates fear of imminent battery through intentional and unlawful threat to cause physical injury. No physical contact is involved.
- Battery is the intentional touching of a person against their will by another person, or by an object or substance used by that person, even if no physical injury is caused.

Careful record-keeping during the clinical consultation, including body maps, may support any future legal proceedings. The patient should be asked whether the incident is part of ongoing victimization, such as domestic abuse or hate crime, and offered referral to partner agencies as appropriate. Acute stress reactions may occur as a result of assault and battery. These usually subside over a few days or weeks. If the experiences continue, worsen, or cause marked distress, the patient should be advised to contact their GP or local Victim Support.

Treatment and restraint under the provision of the Mental Capacity Act (2005)

No one can give consent on behalf of an incompetent adult. Treatment may be given under the Mental Capacity Act 2005 if it is necessary to save life or prevent deterioration, if the clinician has a duty of care to the patient and the intervention is in their best interests. However, even if a person lacks capacity, they should still be permitted as far as possible to participate in the decision-making process.[1]

Restraint may only be used if the person using it believes it is necessary to prevent harm to the patient. The restraint used must be proportionate to the likelihood and seriousness of the harm. Restraint is defined as: (1) the use or threat of force when the patient is resisting; or (2) any restriction of liberty of movement whether the patient resists or not.[2] Restraint may be applied via verbal, chemical (rapid tranquillization), or physical means. The minimum level of restraint necessary to protect the patient should be used and physical intervention should only be considered as a last resort.

The NICE guideline: *The short term management of disturbed and violent behaviour in in-patient psychiatric settings and emergency departments* offers helpful guidance on the use of both rapid tranquillization and physical intervention.[3]

A local protocol that covers all aspects of rapid tranquillization and physical intervention should be made available to ED staff. These interventions should only be authorized by a senior clinician. Physical intervention should only be employed by an individual trained to do so, restraint should be applied for no longer than 2–3min, and no direct pressure may be applied to the neck, thorax, abdomen, back, or pelvis. A clinician is to remain responsible for monitoring patient safety and vital signs throughout application of both rapid tranquillization and physical intervention.[3]

Dealing with difficult situations: violence and aggression

Dealing with difficult situations

Challenging or difficult situations are not uncommon in emergency care. Consideration of, and planning for, some of the more predictable situations will be of benefit. Consideration must be given to the patient, carers, and staff dealing with these situations as they may require considerable support.

Violence and aggression towards staff

Each department or setting must have clear guidelines and policies for managing violence and aggression. Patient and staff safety is paramount. Protection of staff is fundamental. This should include adequate provision for calling for assistance in case of danger, as well as provision of training in de-escalation techniques and control and restraint. Key liaison with police and security staff is essential. Planning for and rehearsing responses to violent or aggressive incidents is a useful strategy.

Support frameworks and personnel should be provided for staff who have been involved in violent or aggressive incidents. This should include support from the employing agency to pursue legal redress against the assailant. Inadequate staff support post-incident may lead to long-term problems for those involved.

References

1 British Medical Association (2007). *The Mental Capacity Act 2005: guidance for health professionals.* Available at ⍟ http://www.bma.org.uk/ap.nsf/content/mencapact05
2 Department of Health (2005). *Mental Capacity Act.* Department of Health, London.
3 NICE (2005). *The short term management of disturbed and violent behaviour in in-patient psychiatric settings and emergency departments. NICE Clinical Guideline,* CG25. NICE: London. Available at ⍟ www.nice.org.uk

Dealing with difficult situations: abuse

Domestic abuse

Domestic abuse is 'any incident of threatening behaviour, violence, or abuse (psychological, physical, sexual, financial, or emotional) between adults who are or have been intimate partners or family members, regardless of gender or sexuality'.[1] Health professionals are often the first point of contact for people who have experienced domestic abuse and should be trained to give an appropriate response. The use of routine enquiry about domestic abuse remains controversial. EDs should at least have a policy that supports targeted screening within a safe and supportive environment.

Following disclosure of domestic abuse clinicians should reassure the individual, making it easier for them to talk about their experiences by taking a non-judgemental stance. Assessment of risk to the patient and their children should be undertaken and information about support services provided. Staff should not encourage patients to leave their abusive partner, as only the individual will know when it is safe to do so. However, help should be given with safety planning and clinicians can facilitate access to a refuge if the patient requests it. When domestic abuse is disclosed, clinicians should consider whether adult or child protection factors exist and follow local Protection of Vulnerable Adults and Safeguarding Children guidelines as appropriate. Midwifery services should be advised of women who have been assaulted during pregnancy.

If the patient gives consent, referral to partner agencies, including the police and domestic abuse support services, may help to reduce repeat victimization. It is important that health staff contribute to local multi-agency partnerships to tackle domestic abuse. The government has published helpful guidance for professionals regarding information sharing in the context of domestic abuse.[2] Guidance regarding the care of victims of domestic abuse is also available.[1]

Safeguarding vulnerable adults

Vulnerable adults are at risk of abuse which is often unrecognized and under-reported. The true extent of this abuse is not known. There should be as great a suspicion with vulnerable adults as there is with non-accidental injury in children, particularly if the story or mechanism does not fit with the injury or illness or there are unexplained findings. There are many forms of abuse including:

- Physical: hitting, misuse of medication, restraint.
- Sexual, including sexual assault and rape.
- Psychological, including emotional abuse, humiliation, threats to harm.
- Financial or material, including fraud, theft, misappropriation of benefits.
- Acts of omission or neglect, e.g. ignoring physical or medical needs, delays in seeking care, failure to provide care or seek help.
- Discrimination, including racist, sexual, or disability based comments 📖 see Box 3.1.

Box 3.1 END ABUSE: a guide to intervention[*]

- **E**mpowerment. Enable people to know what their choices are—the choices need to be feasible and practical (information should be made available and known to staff in advance).
- **N**eglect is as much a form of abuse as a violent act. This may be the only sign; when identified it requires action.
- **D**ocumentation. Careful documentation if there is injury and or illness is essential for future reference if legal action is to be taken. Remember to document the patient's own words.
- **A**dvocacy. In the case of a vulnerable elderly person who is either physically or mentally incapacitated and unable to speak for themselves you may have to act as their advocate.
- **B**e aware of the organizations that can assist and have to hand information that can be given to the victim (this may need to be done discreetly).
- **U**nderstanding. Part of the intervention is to help the victim understand that abuse is a crime, that they are a victim (it is not their fault), and that help is available.
- **S**ocial services. Early involvement of social services is essential when abuse is identified.
- **E**ducation of staff in the recognition of elder abuse and the sensitive steps to be taken when identified is fundamental.

[*] Reproduced with kind permission from Crouch, R. (2003) Emergency care of the older person. In *Emergency nursing care: principles and practice* (ed. G. Jones, R. Endacott, and R. Crouch). Greenwich Medical Media, Cambridge University Press, London.

References

1 Department of Health (2005). *Responding to domestic abuse: a handbook for health professionals.* Department of Health, London.
2 Home Office (2004). Safety and justice: sharing personal information in the context of domestic violence—an overview, Development and practice report 30. Available at ⟨ www.homeoffice. gov.uk/rds

Dealing with difficult situations: sexual assault

When caring for a patient who discloses sexual assault, clinicians should ascertain whether vulnerable adult, child, or domestic abuse is a factor and refer to partner agencies accordingly.

Following sexual assault, victims have three main care needs: forensic, medical, and psychosocial.[1] Unless medical problems take precedence, forensic examination should be performed as early as possible.

- If the patient gives consent, they may be referred to the police who will coordinate forensic and legal actions. Whether or not the police are involved, patients can be referred to a Sexual Assault Referral Centre (SARC), which will provide support and services (including forensic medical examination) following rape or sexual assault.[2,3]
- If medical needs predominate, ED staff should optimize preservation of forensic evidence during care provision. Helpful advice regarding preservation of forensic evidence may be gained via ⌀ *wwwcareandevidence. org*.
- Pregnancy testing and postcoital contraception should be offered.
- Sexual health risk factors should be considered; prophylaxis against sexually transmitted illness, including blood borne virus, may be required. Arrangements should be made for follow-up screening by genitourinary medicine staff.
- Referral for counselling via the patient's GP or a voluntary agency may be required. The Rape Crisis service provides face to face and telephone counselling by qualified and trained volunteers.

References

1 Cybulska, B. (2007). Sexual assault: key issues. *Journal of the Royal Society of Medicine* **100** (7), 321–4.
2 Department of Health/Home Office (2005). *National service guideline for developing sexual assault referral centres (SARCs)*. Department of Health, London.
3 Home Office (2006). *Tackling sexual violence: guidance for local partnerships*. Home Office, London.

Dealing with difficult situations: forensic issues

Patients may attend the ED as a result of an incident where criminal proceedings may ensue. Preservation of evidence is of utmost importance. Care should be taken not to dispose of anything that could constitute evidence. Careful documentation of facts is important. Each department should have an agreed process for preservation of evidence and a sufficient supply of materials necessary for the storage of the evidence. A careful record of all personnel interacting with or involved with the case should be kept. They may need to be contacted for witness statements at a later date.

Dealing with difficult situations: resuscitation, death, and communicating bad news

Witnessed resuscitation

In recent years this has become more common practice. Exposure to resuscitation scenes in television dramas appears to have had a role in preparing relatives for what they might witness. Some clinicians are still uncomfortable with the concept of relatives being present whilst resuscitation is being carried out. Experience from practice suggests that relatives are focusing on their loved one and not on all that is going on around them. They often express gratitude and reassurance that it appears all that could be done was done. Preparation and support of the relatives is fundamental. This should include the following.

• Information about their loved one's appearance.
• Brief description and explanation of the equipment, lines, and tubes attached to the patient.
• Brief information about the team.
• Reassurance that they can leave the room at any time.
• An individual member of staff to stay with them and support them at all times.

The team also requires briefing and support before the relatives come in. It can be stressful and emotionally challenging to experience the raw grief sometimes expressed in these circumstances. Senior experienced staff are essential in this situation for both the family and the team.

Bereavement care can be very demanding and time-consuming. Support mechanisms should be in place for staff who have been involved in bereavement support. The hospital chaplaincy team can provide support for relatives, loved ones, and staff involved in these situations.

Sudden death

Dealing with sudden death is common in the ED. It is a sad and traumatic event for the family and loved ones of those involved. Even in circumstances where the death was expected, when the actual death occurs it can still seem sudden and traumatic. Nurses have a key role in breaking bad news and caring for the family and loved ones.

Breaking bad news

This is a key skill that requires preparation and experience. The person to break the bad news should be the person who has established the greatest rapport with the family and loved ones (and who has the greatest experience of breaking bad news). This could be either a nurse or a doctor. It is advisable to have two professional staff present who are able to break the news, provide comfort, and, where possible, answer questions. One person should be the link person and spend time with the family. Breaking bad news is not an exact science—every situation and circumstance is different requiring rapid assessment and decision-making about approach and language to use.

The language used should be clear and unambiguous. Euphemisms, such as 'we lost him' or 'has passed over' or 'gone to a better place', should not be used. Words such as 'has died' or 'is dead' should be used. It is not uncommon to have to repeat these words in the first few sentences.

In situations where you are preparing relatives or loved ones for a poor outlook, again clear language should be used. It is better to be 'up front' with individuals and give the worst possible outcome as well as the most optimistic—but be realistic.

You should be prepared for a wide variety of reactions. These are also culturally dependent. Reactions can include anger, denial, crying, shouting, wailing, laughing, violent outbursts, self-flagellation, and collapse, to name but a few. In the case of sudden death in children, parents have been known to attempt to take their dead child home with them.

A checklist of information and key contacts can be useful in a bereavement situation. No matter how many times you have broken bad news it is still stressful and emotionally challenging. The checklist should ensure that you have relevant contact numbers for follow-up, that correct documentation is given, and that the GP is informed. The necessary arrangements should be made to inform medical records, therefore ensuring that inappropriate letters or appointments are not sent the recently deceased.

▶ Remember to offer the support of spiritual leaders from the patient's faith through either the family's contacts or the hospital chaplaincy team.

Keepsakes
It can be helpful to offer 'keepsakes' to relatives and loved ones. For adults a lock of hair from the deceased nicely presented can be offered. With children, a book of keepsakes can be provided including foot and hand prints, locks of hair, and photographs.

Environment
Providing a quiet area for breaking bad news is important. The area should ideally be close to the resuscitation room, but with sufficient audio/visual separation. Making this area welcoming and comfortable is important.

The provision of a visiting room is highly desirable. The room should accommodate the deceased individual in comfortable surroundings without the equipment found in the clinical area. This area should allow the loved ones to spend time saying goodbye in an unhurried manner. Ideally, this room should be close to the relatives' room and resuscitation room but not in a thoroughfare.

Dealing with difficult situations: tissue and organ donation

There is a UK shortage of organs for donation and, sadly, patients are dying whilst waiting for a transplant. When faced with a sudden or imminent death consideration should be given to raising the issue of organ or tissue donation (check that there are no absolute contraindications first). Although staff are sometimes concerned about raising this issue at a time of significant emotional crisis, experience suggests that many relatives gain some comfort from knowing that others might benefit from the organs or tissues of their loved ones. Recent awareness campaigns about the importance of organ donation have resulted in some families raising the subject of donation when bad news is broken.

There are different types of donation: heart beating donation (where brainstem death has been confirmed); controlled non heart-beating donation; and tissue donation. Local policies and procedures will determine how these processes are enacted.[1]

Organs that may be retrieved from heart-beating donors are: heart and lungs; liver; kidneys; pancreas; and small bowel. Non-heart-beating donation can include liver, kidneys, pancreas, lung, and tissue. Tissues that can be donated include corneas, heart valves, skin, and skeletal tissue (bone, tendon, and ligaments). Tissues can be donated up to 24–48h after death. Absolute contraindications to organ donation are CJD and HIV.

Close liaison with local transplant coordinators is necessary to ensure staff are aware and able to promote organ and tissue donation.

Reference

1 For further information see the following websites: ⋔ http://www.dh.gov.uk/en/Healthcare/
Secondarycare/Transplantation/index.htm
⋔ http://www.uktransplant.org.uk/ukt/

Major incidents and terrorism

A major incident can be described as a situation where the demands imposed by the situation outstrip the resources available. A major incident can be called by an external agency such as the ambulance service or the internal organization. The types and nature of the major incident can be varied. Consideration should be given to your local circumstances. For instance, if your department is near the coast or an airport you could have a major incident related to a coastal event or a aircraft in trouble at landing or take off. In more recent times it has become necessary for heightened consideration to be given to chemical, biological, radiological, or nuclear emergencies (CBRN). Relevant training for dealing with major incidents is mandatory.

Each ED and NHS Trust must have an established major incident plan.

Terrorism

In recent years the threat from terrorist attacks has increased. Heightened awareness is necessary. Any area of mass gathering is a potential target. When considering major incident planning, managing terrorist attacks should form part of the plan. Consideration should be given to different types of injuries/illnesses that could be caused by such attacks, particularly when unfamiliar mechanisms or means are used to cause harm. Special consideration should be given to the preservation of evidence.

Advanced practice

There are a number of advanced roles in emergency care: ENPs; emergency care practitioners (ECPs); clinical nurse specialists; consultant nurses, to name a few. These roles commonly have an element of advance practice using extended patient assessment skills and differential diagnosis. This expansion of practice is currently unregulated. However, registration and regulation of specialist/advanced practice is imminent.[1]

Emergency nurse practitioners (ENPs)

ENPs were introduced in the UK in the 1980s. Most EDs now have ENPs as part of the clinical team. The role involves a more autonomous level of practice including assessment, requesting and interpreting of investigations, differential diagnosis, patient management, and discharge. There is a developing evidence base of effectiveness of the role focused around minor injuries and illnesses. Increasing numbers of departments are now developing a 'major' nurse practitioner role. However, the ENP's role, scope, and effectiveness in this area are largely unevaluated.

There are no UK wide agreements on scope of practice, educational preparation, or standards for testing or examining competence. A national competency framework has been developed, which includes competencies for minor injuries/illness.[2]

Non-medical prescribing

Nurses who have undertaken a specific and recognized programme of education can now be registered as independent and or supplementary prescribers following a change in the law in 2001.[3] From May 2006 the extended formulary was discontinued and qualified nurse independent prescribers were able to prescribe any licensed medication for any medical condition within their competence, this includes limited controlled drugs. Further consultation is underway to expand prescribing powers for controlled drugs. Independent prescribing allows nurses to practise with a greater degree of autonomy and to expand scope of their practice within a competency framework. Advanced and autonomous practice brings with it greater accountability and the potential for litigation.

References

1 See ⁀ www.nmc-uk.org for further information

2 See ⁀ http://www.fen.uk.com

3 Further information about independent and supplementary prescribing can be found in Beckwith, S. and Franklin, P. (2006). *Oxford handbook of nurse prescribing*. Oxford University Press, Oxford and at ⁀ www.dh.gov.uk/en/Policyandguidance/Medicinespharmacyandindustry/ Prescriptions/TheNon-MedicalPrescribingProgramme/index.htm.

Emergency care of the infant and child

Introduction

Many nurses working within the specialty of emergency care feel very anxious about looking after children. This can be for a variety of reasons: they are worried that children 'go off' quickly; they cannot relate to them; or they simply have had no exposure to children within their working career. However, caring for children and their families can be a very rewarding and gratifying experience.

Children are not just little adults. They are different physiologically, psychologically, and anatomically. When assessing children within the emergency setting the nurse must take all of these aspects into account. On assessment the nurse must rely on initial impressions and determine quickly whether the child is distressed or not. Often when screening a child it is the simple subtle clues, such as differing behaviours, non-feeding in infants and no interest in surroundings, that are key. The ability to distinguish the unwell child from the well child is the key to paediatric emergency care and the principal objective of this chapter.

Top 10 principles for assessing a child

- Make friends with parents and child.
- Never take the child away from the parents.
- Get down to the child's level.
- Babies are best examined on a couch; toddlers on parent's lap.
- Be opportunistic.
- Always undress infants fully.
- Always weigh a child and if possible assess a child's growth.
- Do not distress the child with unnecessary investigation.
- Believe the parents.
- Always spend time watching the child whilst taking a history.

The family

When caring for children it is extremely important to remember that you also have to care for the family. Always take siblings into account and be aware of the family dynamics and structure. Careful explanation of the child's condition must be given to the whole family and the subsequent care planned with the family in partnership. Often the siblings get very distressed when their brother or sister is being treated and time should be taken to explain the procedure to them as well as the patient.

Ten tips for play in the ED[1]

- Provide a well-stocked playroom with toys and activities for children of all ages, not forgetting teenagers. Play is a normal and natural part of childhood—children will instinctively play. Encouraging children to play whilst waiting allows them (and their parents) to relax, which in turn will increase the likelihood of their cooperation. Remember, play is *fun!*
- All staff should take time to chat with children. Taking a moment to build a rapport with a child will increase that child's trust in the staff. If a child trusts the staff, they are less likely to resist examination and treatment.
- Children's greatest fear is often the fear of the unknown. The ED is an unfamiliar environment—with strange equipment and strange language. Therefore, take a few minutes to explain procedures to children in child-friendly language and to answer their questions. Remember to reassure parents also—children are receptive to their parents' anxieties and a calmer parent will result in a calmer child. Play specialists can prepare children through play using specially adapted dolls and teddies as well as photo story books. Spending a few minutes preparing a child in this manner increases the child's cooperation with the procedure, which in turn saves valuable time and energy on the part of the staff, as well as making the experience more positive for the child and their parents.
- Distraction therapy offers children a coping mechanism for procedures. Play specialists employ a range of techniques depending on the age and developmental level of the child, as well as the medical procedure being performed. Children do not have a choice over the procedure, so allowing them a choice over distraction technique empowers them to cope as they feel a sense of control. Parents and siblings should also be involved with distraction—again, this encourages parents to stay calm, which helps the child stay calm and cooperative.
- There should be a definite 'finish' to the procedure that is clear to the child. This can be as simple as saying 'all finished', and should involve praise and some form of reward (stickers, certificates, and/or a small prize). 'Finishing' a procedure in such a manner allows everyone to relax.
- Post-procedural play should be offered when a procedure does not go well. Play specialists can talk through the experience with the child and their parents, and allow the child to play through emotions with medical play equipment. Allowing a child a few minutes in the playroom before they leave allows the child to de-stress. Follow-up visits can also be considered. All staff should reflect on such experiences with the aim of avoiding such a situation in the future.

- Read children's body language. Children's primary method of communication is through play. Watching a child at play and taking note of their body language can reveal much about how a child really feels about a procedure. Play specialists can spend time observing children at play, talking and playing with them, and reassuring them about procedures.
- Take time to position children comfortably before beginning a procedure. If the child is comfortable (often on a parent's knee), the child and parent will be more relaxed, increasing the likelihood of the child's cooperation with the procedure. Consider whether the child wants to watch the procedure and take positions accordingly. Remember to make space for the play specialist and distraction therapy.
- Staff must work together as a team. The child is the most important person, and staff should work with the child and their family to ensure the most positive experience in the best interests of the child.
- Play is a natural part of childhood. Children learn much through play, and reach developmental milestones through play. Play specialists can observe children and assess their developmental level through play. Thus, developmental delay can be identified, allowing the child to receive appropriate interventions through referrals to outside agencies.

Reference

1 Stephanie Lockwood, Play Specialist, Portsmouth Hospital's Trust.

The unwell child

One of the most frequent reasons that parents seek health-care advice is that the child or infant has fever or is hot to touch. Mostly the causes are self-limiting, viral infections. However, in young children it can initially be very difficult to distinguish between a serious infection and a self-limiting one. Young infants and children are notoriously difficult to assess when they become unwell. Often the only sign you may get that the infant is unwell is a change in the infant's feeding patterns or the infant sleeping for prolonged periods. The parents know their child better than you, so statements 'that they just aren't themselves' must be believed and taken seriously. Examine the infant fully, paying particular attention to the way they are behaving or handle (📖 see Fig 4.1). All children < 3 years old presenting with a temperature over 38°C should be thoroughly examined and a full infection screen considered. Most febrile illnesses in children will be caused by viruses, usually in the upper respiratory tract. It is important, however, to rule out other causes such as pneumonia, UTI, or septicaemia.

General rules

- Always carry out a full set of observations including respiratory rate, pulse rate, temperature, and capillary refill (📖 see p.682).
- The younger the child, the lower the threshold for seeking senior advice and paediatric referral.
- Always take a urine sample. UTIs are a common cause of infection.
- Always take a blood sugar on children/infants who have a ↓ level of consciousness or a history of a convulsion.
- Regular reassessment must be carried out if the child is not responding to simple measures such as antipyretics and fluids.
- A period of observation within the ED is always useful and should be encouraged.

▶ All children presenting to the ED or primary care centre must undergo a rapid assessment of ABCDE.

Assessment of ABCDE (📖 see p.682)

- Airway and breathing (AB). Assess:
  - work of breathing;
  - respiratory rate (📖 see Table 4.1 for normal values);
  - stridor, wheeze;
  - air entry on auscultation;
  - colour.
- Circulation (C). Assess:
  - heart rate (📖 see Table 4.1 for normal values);
  - pulse volume;
  - capillary refill time;
  - skin temperature;
  - urine output.
- Disability (D). Assess:
  - level of consciousness;
  - posture;
  - pupils;
  - blood sugar.

- Exposure (E). Assess:
  - rash;
  - skin temperature;
  - scars.

Table 4.1 Normal values of respiratory rate (RR) and pulse in children at different ages

Age (years)	RR (breaths/min)	Pulse (beats/min)	Systolic BP (mmHg)
Infant <1 year	30–40	110–160	70–90
Toddler 1–2 years	25–35	100–150	80–95
Preschool 3–4 years	25–30	95–140	80–100
School 5–11 years	20–25	80–120	90–110
Adolescent 12–16 years	15–20	60–100	100–120

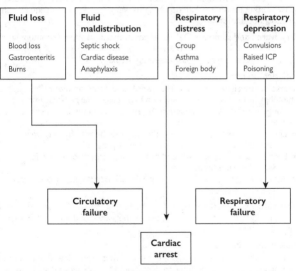

Fig. 4.1 Recognition of acute unwell child. (Adapted from Advanced Life Support Group (2001). *Advanced paediatric life support. The practical approach*, 3rd edn. BMJ Books, London with the kind permission of Wiley–Blackwell Publishing.)

Resuscitation: introduction

Paediatric resuscitation is divided into that for the newborn, infant, and child. International guidelines exist and should be followed.[1] Over the age of 12 years the adult resuscitation guidelines are used.

Resuscitation at birth

Deliveries in the ED or in the community—particularly if it is a concealed pregnancy—should be regarded as high risk, although typically such deliveries are incident free.

Preparation

- Call paediatricians, midwife, and obstetric team.
- Stop obvious draught (e.g. window).
- Prepare resuscitation equipment. Either use a fully stocked resuscitaire (turn on overhead heater) or BVM (500mL), suction, and oxygen.
- Remember to start the timer at the outset of the resuscitation.

Neonatal resuscitation (🕮 see Fig. 4.2) differs significantly from paediatric resuscitation, with the vast majority of neonates recovering following activity stimulus and/or inflation breaths. Very few neonates require compression/intubation/drugs.

Dry, warm, and stimulate Deliver neonate into a warm environment, wrap in a towel, and dry. Remove the wet towel and rewrap; then place on a flat surface. Deliver oxygen whilst assessing the baby.

Inflation breaths

These are designed to open the alveoli and force amniotic fluid out of the lungs as during normal delivery a baby takes a large breath to expand its lungs—if this hasn't happened the resuscitator needs to replicate this process.

- Lie baby flat and open airway—there is little benefit from routine suction of the airway (unless meconium is present).
- Deliver each breath slowly and hold during inspiration phase for 2–3sec. Repeat 5 times.
- Assess response, crying, breathing, HR. Resuscitate as per protocol. (🕮 see Fig. 4.2)

The sustained breaths needed for newborn resuscitation are produced more easily with a 500ml BVM. However, be aware of the risk of increased inflation volume.

Meconium aspiration

The neonate produces meconium (meconium is sterile faecal matter) as a response to distress. Fresh meconium is green in colour and sticky aspiration of meconium leads to pulmonary damage.

- Immediately summon paediatricians.
- Clean face of meconium. There is no proven benefit from applying suction as head is delivered.
- A vigorously breathing/crying baby has not aspirated.
- Floppy baby: suction mouth and nose; attempt to remove all visible meconium.
- If no help has arrived and the baby is apnoeic deliver inflation breaths.

Concerns over ventilating a baby with meconium are understandable, but if all obvious meconium has been removed, the baby remains floppy and apnoeic, and there is no help from an experienced advanced neonatal qualified resuscitator, ventilation becomes an immediate priority.

Compression and ventilation Set at 120/min in a compression:ventilation ratio of 3:1. Preferred method is to use 2 thumbs with hands encircled around the neonate's chest 1 fingerbreadth below the nipple-line. 2 rescuers are required to do this effectively with an adequate respiratory rate. If only 1 rescuer is available compressions using the tips of 2 fingers 1 fingerbreadth below the nipple-line are acceptable.

Reference
1 For more information visit ⊕ www.resus.org.uk

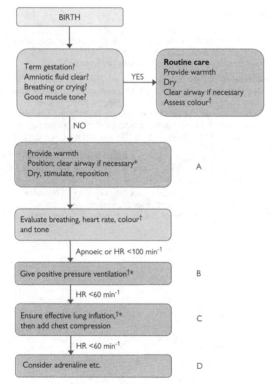

* Tracheal intubation may be considered at several steps
† Consider supplemental oxygen at any stage if cyanosis persists

Fig. 4.2 Newborn life support (Reproduced from *Resuscitation guidelines 2005* with permission of the Resuscitation Council UK ⊕ www.resus.org.uk).

Paediatric basic life support (BLS)

Children are split into infant and child with the only difference in BLS
(📖 see Fig. 4.3) being technique used to provide compression.

- Base your assessment on a high index of suspicion followed by confirmation of unresponsiveness, absence of effective breathing (beware of gasping ventilations), and no pulse (unreliable sign). If in doubt start BLS.
- Get help as soon as you detect a problem *but* note next point.
- Once cardiac arrest is confirmed, early BLS may restore output. If on your own, delay going for help to deliver 1min of CPR (5 cycles).
- Significant numbers of critically ill children arrive by car. The triage nurse must instigate rapid assessment and should deliver the 1st five breaths immediately if cardiac arrest is suspected—before moving to the resuscitation room.

Resuscitation

Open airway (avoid hyperextension). Cover mouth and nose (< 1 year) or cover mouth and occlude the child's nose. Deliver 5 breaths: allow 1sec per breath and allow the child to exhale between breaths. Effective ventilation may reverse respiratory arrest with bradycardia.

Compressions should be instigated if no response to initial 5 breaths. If convinced that there's a pulse > 60bpm, deliver 12–20 breaths/min. If in doubt start compression as the risk of significant injury is low.

- For a child < 1 year use two finger tips one fingerbreadth below the nipple line. The two thumb method used for neonates (📖 see Resuscitation at birth, p.64) is more effective but becomes difficult to perform as the child gets bigger.
- For a child > 1 year use the heel of 1 hand or the adult 2 hand approach in the centre of the child's chest. The aim is to depress the chest wall by 1/3 its diameter, at a rate of 100/min in a compression: ventilation ratio of 15:2 regardless of the child's age. If this proves difficult for a single rescuer to achieve, commence the adult 30:2 ratio, aiming to minimize the delays between breaths and compressions.

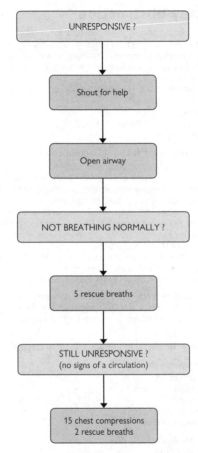

After 1 minute call resuscitation team then continue CPR

Fig. 4.3 Paediatric basic life support (health care professionals with a duty to respond) (Reproduced from *Resuscitation guidelines 2005*, with permission of the Resuscitation Council UK ⁀ *www.resus.org.uk*).

Airway obstruction

Airway obstruction may be due to a foreign body, trauma or infection. Foreign body obstruction tends to occur during play or eating and is therefore rapidly identified. Treatment is based on how the child responds, an effective cough (☐ see Box 4.1) is the most effective technique for clearing the airway.

General signs of foreign body airway obstruction:
- episode is witnessed
- coughing/choking
- sudden onset: no history of illness
- history of playing.

Conscious child with ineffective cough

- Back slaps. Place head down and deliver 5 sharp blows to the back with the heel of the hand in the middle of the shoulder blades. If able, place the child across the rescuer's lap/arm ensuring the child is head-down. In older children help them to lean forward.
- Chest thrusts and abdominal thrusts. In children < 1 year perform chest thrusts once back blows fail. These are performed like cardiac compressions but done slowly with more force. In children > 1 year use the abdominal thrust. Stand behind the child, place a clenched fist between the umbilicus and the xiphoid process, and pull backwards but upwards.
  - ⚠ This technique may cause injury in the young and should only be performed if coughing and back blows have failed.

Continue with back slaps/chest or abdominal thrusts until either the airway is cleared or the child becomes unconscious. Once unconscious instigate BLS regardless of the presence of a pulse.

Box 4.1 Ineffective versus effective cough[1]

Ineffective cough
- Unable to talk
- Quiet/silent cough
- Unable to breathe
- ↓ conscious level
- Central cyanosis

Effective cough
- Crying/talking
- Loud cough
- Able to take breath before coughing
- Fully responsive

Reference

1 Resuscitation Council UK (2005). *Resuscitation guidelines*. Available at ⌁ www.resus.org.uk.

Advanced paediatric life support (APLS)

Cardiac arrest in children is seldom sudden and is typically a deterioration following an overwhelming injury/illness. Therefore outcomes are usually worse than in adult cardiac arrest. Effective compressions and ventilations (avoid hyperventilation) are the principles of paediatric ALS.

- Asystole may be the terminal rhythm following prolonged downtime or a deterioration of bradycardiac pulseless electrical activity (PEA; often 2° to hypoxia), although it maybe a primary arrhythmia following electrocution or drug overdose.
- PEA is a common presenting rhythm. Bradycardia may indicate hypoxia or end-stage hypovolaemia and tachycardic PEA may indicate loss of circulating volume (sepsis, trauma, etc.). To treat loss of circulatory volume, administer a fluid bolus of 20mL/kg.
- VF/VT is relatively rare in paediatric cardiac arrest but may be due to drug overdose, electrolyte imbalance, or congenital abnormality.

Causes of cardiac arrest The four Hs and Ts (📖 see Box 4.2) should be considered in all cardiac arrests regardless of presenting rhythm.

Box 4.2 Causes of cardiac arrest

4 Hs

- Hypoxia: common
- Hypovolaemia: common. Not limited to trauma; can be 2° to dehydration, sepsis. Fluids and possibly blood will be required
- Hyper/hypokalaemia: may cause VF/VT or non-shockable rhythms
- Hypothermia. Prolonged CPR may result in neurologically intact survivor

4Ts

- Tension pneumothorax: not limited to trauma. Consider in asthma. May be bilateral. PEA whilst on a ventilator or following CVP line placement
- Tamponade. Traumatic tamponade = thoracotomy. Tamponade may be medical, e.g. in renal failure
- Toxic/therapeutic cause. Should be considered in all paediatric arrests. It may affect treatment, e.g. role of adrenaline following solvent abuse
- Thromboemboli: rare in young children but possible in young adults

---

Airway and ventilation

- Early supplementary O_2 before cardiac arrest is essential. Once cardiac arrest occurs, effective ventilation with a BVM is the priority—supplement with O_2 as soon as available but don't delay ventilation if O_2 not immediately available.
- The use of oral and nasal airways will assist with effective ventilation. The process of measuring is the same as with an adult. Insert the oral airway with a laryngoscope/tongue depressor to immobilize the tongue. The airway is inserted the 'right way up'. Do not insert and rotate (📖 see Chapter 20 ❶, p.566).

• Suctioning is part of airway management. Use a soft suction catheter to clear nose/mouth of fluid secretions; the ridged Yankauer suction catheter is more effective for vomit and blood. Use with a laryngoscope to minimize airway trauma.

Intubation

There is a significant variation in choice of endotracheal tubes (ETT) for different age groups (⊞ see Box 4.3) but equipment must be checked and available.

Equipment for paediatric intubation should include the following.
• Miller 0 & 1 laryngoscope blade with handle.
• Macintosh 2 & 3 laryngoscope blade with handle.
• Full range of ETTs (2.5–8.0mm including half-sizes).
• Catheter mount: adult and paediatric (make sure it fits ETTs).
• Elastoplast® tape and ETT tie tape.
• EtCO$_2$ monitor.
• Intubating stylet and paediatric bougies.

Box 4.3 Formulae for determining ETT diameter and length*

Internal diameter
• For children aged < 1 year use 2.5–3.5mm ETT
• For children aged 1–10 years: internal diameter (mm) = (age/4) + 4
• For children aged > 10 years use 7.5–8mm ETT

Length of ETT
• For oral tube, length of oral tube (cm) = (age/2) + 12
• For nasal tube, length of nasal tube (cm) = (age/2) + 15

* Numerous charts exist to support the estimation of size. The Broselow tape is popular but be aware of the preferred choice within your ED.

Drug administration in APLS

The two most effective routes for drug administration are IV or intraosseous (IO). Unless an IV was established prior to loss of output, IO should be the preferred drug route due to speed and ease of use.

- There are few contraindications to IO access (particularly during cardiac arrest), but infection, fracture above chosen site, or multiple attempts (always move up the limb) are the main issues with IO access.
- Sites for insertion. The most commonly used site is the proximal tibia 2.5cm below the knee (or one fingerbreadth) on the flat anteromedial surface. Other sites include the calcaneum, distal tibia, distal femur, iliac crest, sternum, and clavicle 📖 see p.624.
- Drugs. The most commonly used resuscitation drugs are adrenaline (epinephrine), saline bolus, sodium bicarbonate, and 10% dextrose. It is vital that the ED nurse is familiar with a drug dosage system (e.g. Broselow tape) for use during emergencies to minimize risk of drug errors.

Adrenaline is administered ever 3–5min at a dose of 10mcg/kg (0.1mL/kg of adrenaline 1:10 000) to improve coronary and cerebral perfusion—there is no evidence of increased survival. The previously recommended high dose adrenaline (100mcg/kg) is no longer routinely recommended. It has a limited role for drugs via the ETT (a discouraged route of drug administration) or during treatment of distributive shock (sepsis or anaphylaxis).

Crystalloid bolus is frequently used during resuscitation. The initial dose is 20mL/kg, which represents 20–25% of a child's circulating volume. The choice of fluid is typically 0.9% saline/Hartmann's. After 2 boluses (40–50% of circulating volume), blood ± intropic support should be considered. A bolus is used to achieve rapid administration. Therefore the bolus should be administered under pressure via a 50 or 20mL syringe.

Sodium bicarbonate is used more often during paediatric resuscitation, as metabolic acidosis is usually an issue before cardiac arrest occurs. There is no evidence of clinical benefit. The dose is 1mmol/kg, which is 1mL/kg of 8.4% sodium bicarbonate. Also consider diluting it in equal parts of 5% dextrose.

Sodium bicarbonate shouldn't be mixed with any other resuscitation drug and the IV/IO line should be flushed prior to the administration of any other drug—use 0.9% saline.

Glucose 10% at a dose of 5mL/kg is the glucose concentration of choice during paediatric emergencies (50% glucose should never be used). During all paediatric emergencies obtain a CBG early to detect hypoglycaemia. Some older Broselow tapes recommend 25% glucose. To avoid confusion use 10% glucose but double the volume.

Amiodarone (5mg/kg) remains an option during VF/VT (but exclude drug overdose if possible first). Consider calcium chloride (10mL/10%) if ↑ potassium/magnesium is expected or following an overdose of a calcium channel blocker. These drugs have very limited roles during paediatric cardiac arrest.

Upper respiratory tract infections (URTIs)

Viruses cause ~90% of URTIs. The upper respiratory tract compromises ears, nose, throat, tonsils, pharynx, and sinuses. While fever is common to all URTIs, remember that it can have many other causes (📖 see Box 4.4).

> **Box 4.4 Causes of fever**
>
> - Upper respiratory tract infections
> - Lower respiratory tract infections
> - Meningitis
> - Gastroenteritis
> - Urinary tract infection
> - Acute abdomen
> - Tropical diseases
> - Leukaemia
> - Autoimmune disorders
> - Allergies

Acute nasopharyngitis Most of the URTIs that occur in children can be classed as acute nasopharyngitis (common cold) of which there are over 200 viral types. However, the majority is caused by the rhinoviruses. Children normally present with a low grade fever, coryza, cough, and general malaise. Symptomatic management is all that is required and reassurance that it will be self-limiting.

Pharyngitis and tonsillitis[1]

- Often children present with a painful throat, low grade pyrexia, and difficulty in taking fluids.
- This is commonly caused by a viral infection, but be aware of group A beta haemolytic streptococcus.
- Children presenting with bacterial infections usually have a higher grade fever, some lymphadenopathy, and severe pain.
- Various diagnostic tools have been developed to assist health professionals make their diagnosis (📖 see 'Mc Isaac score' in Box 4.5).
- Evidence produced by NICE suggests that products such as benzydamine spray can be useful in alleviating some of the pain and thus encouraging the child to take more fluids.

Otitis media

- Children present with a fever and acute pain from the ear involved. They are often very distressed.
- Most inner ear infections are viral in nature but some can be bacterial.
- On examination a red bulging tympanic membrane will be seen, with loss of light reflex.
- Ensure adequate fluid intake and reassurance.
- The tympanic membrane may perforate; this will produce a dramatic relief of the symptoms and will heal spontaneously.

Box 4.5 Mc Isaac score: sore throat or strep throat[2]

This practical tool will help primary care health professionals decide on the management of patients presenting with URTIs and sore throats.

Step 1 Determine the patient's total score by assigning points according to the following criteria

Criterion	Points
Temperature > 38°C	1
No cough	1
Tender anterior cervical nodes	1
Tonsillar swelling or exudates	1
Age 3 > 14 years	1
Age > 45 years	1

Step 2 Suggested management

Total score	Chance of strep infection (%)	Management
0	2–3	No antibiotics required
1	4–6	
2	10–12	Culture all: treat if culture positive
3	27–28	
4	38–36	Antibiotics & culture

Croup (viral laryngotracheobronchitis)

The commonest condition in the child presenting with stridor is viral croup. Most of the episodes are self-limiting and the children get better with limited or no intervention.

- A full history and assessment must be carried out on the child to ensure that the right diagnosis is reached.
- Characteristically the child presents with a barking cough, stridor, and low grade pyrexia.
- Management depends on the symptoms.
  - Admit all children with respiratory distress, cyanosis, and severe stridor and fatigue.
  - There is very good evidence that oral dexamethasone 0.15mg/kg or nebulized budesonide 2mg is beneficial if stridor is present.[3]
  - In severe cases adrenaline via a nebulizer can be beneficial.
- The main priority for the health professionals looking after this child is to try not to upset the child. This means that the child should be nursed in the parent's lap and no attempt should be made to cannulate the child.
- If the stridor does not improve and the child is having some respiratory distress and is becoming exhausted, seek senior support and intensive care.

Acute epiglottitis

Acute bacterial epiglottitis is a rare life-threatening disorder caused almost exclusively by *Haemophilus influenzae* type B. It has become very rare since the introduction of the Hib immunization in the early 1990s. However, with a creeping increase of non-immunization it is sadly on the increase.

- The child presents with a history of a rapid onset high fever and a painful throat. Classically, the children look shocked. They are unable to swallow; they often drool and have a soft inspiratory stridor.
- The treatment is supportive. Do not upset the child in any way, and allow them to find their own airways position.
- Do not attempt to cannulate them.
- You must seek senior anaesthetic, paediatric, and ENT surgical help.
- The child will require intubation and IV antibiotics (third generation cephalosporin as per hospital antibiotic prescribing protocol) for up to 48h.
- Do not allow any one to examine the child's throat, unless they are one of the senior specialists above.

References

1 Scottish Intercollegiate Guidelines Network (2004). *Management of sore throats and indications for tonsillectomy.* Royal College of Physicians, Edinburgh.

2 Mc Isaac, W.J., Goel, V., Tot, T., and Low, D.E. (2000). The validity of the sore throat score in general practice. *Canadian Medical Association Journal* **163**, 811–15.

3 Geelhoed, G.C. and Macdonald, W.B. (1995). Oral dexamethasone in the treatment of croup: 0.15mg/kg versus 0.3mg/kg versus 0.6 mg/kg. *Pediatric Pulmonology* **20** (6), 362–8.

Lower respiratory tract infections (LRTIs)

Pneumonia

Pneumonia is a term used to describe any infection of the lower respiratory tract, either viral or bacterial. Often it can be a very emotive term and, if used, its full meaning must be explained to the child's parent.

- Most LRTIs in children are caused by viruses, the respiratory syncytial virus being the most commonly known (associated with bronchiolitis; see below). Parainfluenza virus, adenovirus, and the Coxsackie virus also cause LRTIs.
- Bacterial causes are *Streptococcus pneumoniae, Haemophilus influenzae, Mycoplasma pneumoniae,* and *group B haemolytic streptococcus* in the newborn.
- Acute presentation usually follows a history of a URTI with the child having a worsening cough, fever, and shortness of breath. Infants are often heard to grunt.
- An X-ray should be performed and blood cultures taken.
- Carry out regular observations and look particularly for signs of increasing respiratory distress and exhaustion. Oxygen may be required to maintain SPO$_2$ >95%.
- Often infants and young children become quite dehydrated and require support with feeding or IV fluids for 24h.
- Administer antibiotics as prescribed and in accordance with local policy.

Bronchiolitis

- Bronchiolitis is commonly caused by the respiratory syncytial virus and occurs in the winter months usually between October and February.
- Annual winter epidemics affect infants < 18 months old.
- Affected infants present to the ED acutely short of breath, coryzal, and with a cough. They are usually exhausted because of the effort required to breathe and feed. They are usually tachypnoeic, wheezy with sub- and intercostal recession.
- Care is supportive. The infants usually require oxygen via either nasal prongs or a head box. Their noses become blocked and require regular clearance. They may require assistance with feeding either via a nasogastric tube or IV therapy. They need to be observed closely and admitted to a paediatric unit 📖 see Table 4.2.

Table 4.2 Bronchiolitis assessment and management*

Severity	Signs	Management
Mild	Alert, pink in air	Manage at home
	Feeding well	Advise parents about course of disease & to return if concerned
	No underlying cardiorespiratory disease	
	SaO_2 > 92%	Reduce quantity of feeds but give often
		Review by GP 24/7
Moderate	Poor feeding	Admit
	Marked respiratory distress, underlying cardiorespiratory disease	Administer O_2 to maintain adequate saturations
	SaO_2 < 92% or aged < 6wks	Reduce quantity of feed but give more frequently
		NG feed or IV fluid maintenance
		Regular observations
Severe	As for moderate with ↑ O_2 requirements	May require CPAP
	Obvious exhaustion	Involve senior paediatric staff
	CO_2 retention	Inform intensive care

* Reproduced with kind permission of the Royal Children's Hospital, Melbourne from South, M. and Young, S. (2002). *Emergency paediatric guidelines.* Royal Children's Hospital, Melbourne.

Asthma

Asthma is the most common respiratory disorder requiring hospital admission in older children. In young children/toddlers it can be very difficult to diagnose. A child with night-time spasmodic cough or a child with difficulty in breathing with no wheeze may indicate the diagnosis of asthma.

Assessment of the child presenting with asthma is extremely important as the severity of the respiratory distress is not always easy to detect (📖 see Table 4.3). On initial assessment, if you are concerned about the child, senior help must be sought and treatment commenced.

Risk factors
- Parental smoking.
- Hospitalized for bronchiolitis.
- Preterm infant.
- Treatment of the acute attack.
- Male.
- Family history.

Immediate management
- High flow oxygen via a non-re-breathe mask.
- Bronchodilator therapy.
- If the child presents with mild to moderate asthma the salbutamol may be administered via a spacer 2–10 puffs depending upon severity.
- If aged <2y, (Ipratropium bromide) 125mcg via nebulizer is sometimes effective. β agonists rarely work in this age group, although it may be worth trying them and assessing their effects.
- >2y–<5y: nebulized salbutamol 2.5mg.
- >5y: nebulized salbutamol 5mg (1mL nebulizer solution with 2mL normal saline) given by mouthpiece or face mask.
- Prednisolone 1–2mg/kg must be given.
  - ⚠ This tastes awful and the child may vomit so try to give it slowly and in the child's own time. Refer to the BTS guidelines for up-to-date drug dosages.

If life-threatening features are present
- Get senior support immediately.
- Prepare an IV infusion of salbutamol 15mcg/kg followed by continuous infusion 1–5mcg/kg/min (dilute to 200mcg/mL).
- Give hydrocortisone 4mg/kg.
- Consider the use of magnesium.
- Consider IV aminophylline 5mg/kg loading dose (omit if on oral theophylline) followed by infusion 1mg/kg per hour.
- Give nebulized β_2 agonist frequently up to every 30min.
- Endeavour to maintain SpO_2 > 92%.
- Watch for exhaustion.

The child should be admitted if
- The attack is very severe when the child arrives at hospital. Initial SpO_2 level is less than 92% in air.
- There is little or no response to 2 doses of nebulized salbutamol after 30min *or* there is response but then rapid deterioration.

- The child is discharged but returns within 4h.
- The child attends late in the evening or the parents are unable to cope.

The child is well enough to go home

- Make sure that the parents understand the instructions you have given about treatment to be taken at home, and record your instructions in the notes.
- Ensure that the child is given a course of oral prednisolone and increase the regular bronchodilator therapy for a couple of days.
- Contact the child's GP or the hospital respiratory team in order to ensure follow-up and further treatment.

Table 4.3 Assessment of asthma*

Moderate	Acute severe	Life-threatening
• $SaO_2 > 92\%$ • No clinical features of severe or life-threatening attack • Peak flow > 50% best or predicted	• Too breathless to feed or complete sentences • Respiratory rate > 30/min (> 5y) *or* > 50/min (2–5y) • Pulse rate > 120/min (> 5y) *or* 130/min (2–5y) • Peak flow < 50%	• Conscious level depressed or agitated • Exhaustion • Poor respiratory effort • $SaO_2 < 92\%$ in air • Silent chest • Peak flow < 33% • Hypotension

* Reproduced with permission from the British Thoracic Society (2003). British guideline on the management of asthma. *Thorax* **58** (Suppl. 1), 1–83.

Meningococcal septicaemia

Meningococcal disease presents in two different ways: meningitis and septicaemia. Early recognition and aggressive management can greatly improve the prognosis. Diagnosis in the early stages of the disease is often problematic. Children present with non-specific febrile illness indistinguishable from a viral URTI or influenza. Health professionals therefore need to be very diligent with their clinical examination and history-taking. If children are sent home following a febrile illness, parents should be advised about what signs and symptoms to look for and told to return immediately if worried.

There are four clinical indicators that health professionals must look out for and manage accordingly.

- Rash. In the early stages the rash may be blanching and maculopapular. It then develops into a non-blanching purpuric rash. Often the rash is a very small subtle rash found in the skin crease. It is very important to undress the patient and to search the skin fully. A rapidly evolving petechial rash is a very worrying sign.
- Shock. Cold hands and feet, fast irregular breathing, tachycardia, and poor capillary refill are all signs of septicaemia (📖 see Box 4.6).
- Decreased level of consciousness. Often subtle signs such as irritability, not feeding, and drowsiness can be indicative of severe sepsis.
- Neck stiffness. This is very difficult to assess in young children, but must be taken seriously when present.

Any child presenting with any of the above symptoms must be very carefully observed. Senior clinical support must be obtained at an early stage and the child cared for in a high dependency area. Early and aggressive intervention is the key to management of any kind of sepsis (📖 see Box 4.7). In symptomatic infants and children lumbar punctures are contraindicated and must not be carried out.

Box 4.6 Signs of early compensated shock

- Tachycardia
- Cool peripheries
- delayed capillary refill
- ↓ level of consciousness
- Tachypnoea
- Poor urine output
- Hypotension

Box 4.7 Management of sepsis

- Senior support early
- ABC and oxygen (100%)
- Blood glucose (treat if below 3 mmol/L)
- Insert two large cannulae
- Send bloods FBC, U+E, glucose, G+S, clotting, PCR, ABE blood, cultures, clotting, calcium+magnesium
- IV cefotaxime or ceftriaxone 80mg/kg
- Volume resuscitation
  - IV fluid 20ml/kg
  - Repeat if necessary
  - Observe closely
- After 40–60mL/kg IV fluid patient will require elective intubation and ventilation
- Continue with fluid boluses 10–20mL/kg
- Consider inotropes
- NG tube and urinary catheter
- Rapid sequence intubation and intubate
- Central venous access
- Correct any electrolyte abnormality

Gastroenteritis

Diarrhoea and vomiting are very common in infants and young children. They are most often caused by viruses such as the rotavirus. However they can be of bacterial origin, e.g. caused by *Campylobacter*, *Shigella*, *Escherichia coli*, and *Salmonella* among others. Key distinguishing factors pointing to a bacterial infection are fever, severe abdominal pain, and blood or mucus in the stool. It is very important to note that there are other causes of diarrhoea and vomiting in infants and children and these must be considered (📖 see Box 4.8). If the vomit is bile-stained, senior clinical advice must be obtained and a surgical opinion sought.

- Most children who have gastroenteritis have a self-limiting condition lasting no longer than 48h.
- They can be simply managed by reducing their milk feed for a small amount of time and encouraging oral dehydration solutions such as Dioralyte®
- It is important to note that early refeeding reduces the duration of the gastroenteritis and therefore should be encouraged.
- Babies who are breast fed should be encouraged to carry on. However, the parents should be encouraged to observe the infant's weight to ensure that they do not become too dehydrated.

Box 4.8 Causes of diarrhoea and vomiting

- Gastroenteritis
- Urinary tract infection
- Febrile illness
- Tonsillitis
- Irritable bowel syndrome
- Gastro-oesophageal reflux
- Small bowel obstruction
- Constipation
- Pyloric stenosis
- Intussusception
- Acute appendicitis
- Sepsis
- Food intolerance
- Metabolic disorders

Dehydration

Dehydration is the major concern in children presenting with gastroenteritis. Assessment should be made as to the degree of dehydration (📖 see Table 4.4).

The most useful assessment of hydration is the comparison of weights. However, this is not always available.

- Mild dehydration (< 5%) can be treated at home using oral rehydration therapy, but the parents must be advised that, if the vomiting persists, they must return. In pre-weaned children milk feeds or breastfeeding should be continued.
- Moderate to severe dehydration requires hospital admission. Infants may require IV fluids to correct any electrolyte imbalance.
  - ⚠ Too rapid rehydration can lead to large shifts in fluids and hyponatraemia.
  - Most infants and young children can be fed via an NG tube, which negates the need for IV fluids, and thus the risks associated with them.
  - Keep careful documentation of the child's fluid balance as well as of the vital signs and weight.

Table 4.4 Assessment of dehydration*

	Mild	Moderate	Severe
Mucous membranes	Dry	Dry	Dry
Urine output	Normal	Reduced	None for 12h
Mental state	Normal	Lethargic	Coma
Pulse rate	Normal	Tachycardia	Tachycardia
Blood pressure	Normal	Normal	Low
Capillary refill	Normal	Delayed	More delayed
Skin & eye turgor	Normal	Reduced	More reduced
Fontanelle	Normal	Sunken	Very much sunken
Dehydration (%)	< 5	5–10	> 10

* Reproduced from Advanced Life Support Group (2001). *Advanced paediatric life support. The practical approach*, 3rd edn. BMJ Books, London, with kind permission of Wiley–Blackwell Publishing.

Urinary tract infections (UTI)

All unwell infants and children presenting to the ED should be tested for a UTI. Although UTIs are relatively common in young infants and toddlers they can be hard to detect on symptoms alone. Classical symptoms such as dysuria, frequency, fever, and enuresis may not be present. Often infants present with irritability, not feeding, vomiting, diarrhoea, and failure to thrive.

- The most common organism causing a UTI in children is *Escherichia coli*. However, other organisms such as *Proteus*, *Pseudomonas*, and *Klebsiella* may also be detected.
- UTIs are often caused by vesicoureteric reflux where there is a backflow of urine from the bladder up the ureter.
- Diagnosis is dependent on the urine culture, but a urine dipstick test should be the initial screening test.
  - ⚠ Dipstick tests have poor sensitivity and limited specificity for detecting UTIs. Do **not** rely upon them as the sole means of diagnosis.

Urine collection in children can be problematic.
- In infants a suprapubic aspirate can be a very useful way of obtaining a urine sample. This should be carried out by an experienced clinician using ultrasound as a guide.
- Obtain clean-catch urines by sitting the infant or young child on the parent's lap without a nappy whilst feeding with a sterile collecting utensil. It is very important the child's perineum and genitalia have been cleaned properly to reduce the chance of sample contamination.
- Urine collecting pads can be used in accordance with manufacturer's recommendations. The use of gauze, cotton wool, or sanitary towels is contraindicated and should be avoided.

Management

- Any child less than 3 months of age (this is dependent on local guidelines) or who is systemically unwell should be admitted under the paediatricians for IV antibiotics and further investigations and management.
- Discharge older children on co-trimoxazole for 3 days if they have a lower UTI or cystitis (refer to Children's BNF for guidance about dosages and further advice). They will require follow-up and further investigations. Give advice to parents about encouraging fluids, personal cleansing, and appropriate underwear.
- Refer to the NICE guidelines for the treatment of UTIs.[1]

Reference

1 National Institute for Health and Clinical Excellence (NICE) (2007). *Urinary tract infection: diagnosis, treatment and long-term management of urinary tract infection in children*, Clinical Guideline CG54. NICE, London.

Fitting child

Children commonly present to the ED with seizures or episodes of altered consciousness associated with abnormal posturing, movement, or behaviours. There can be many causes of these seizures or syncopal occurrences (see Box 4.9). A clear history and description of the events and episode can be very useful in establishing the cause.

Box 4.9 Causes of syncope in children

- Epilepsy
- Febrile convulsion
- Hypoglycaemia
- Vasovagal episode
- Lyme's disease
- Breathholding attacks
- Gastro-oesophageal reflux
- Congenital heart condition
- Migraines
- Panic attacks
- Meningitis
- Electrolyte disturbances
- Trauma
- Poisoning

Key history points

- Previous history of convulsions.
- How long has the seizure lasted?
- Obtain an accurate description of the seizure itself. Was it focal or generalized?
- Were they well or unwell prior to the seizure?
- Did any incident precede the event?
- Any family history or developmental abnormalities?

These events can be very frightening to the child's parents or carers. Often, because of the dramatic nature of the episode, they are concerned that the child may be critically ill or die. The parents and carers need constant reassurance and care.

Management

 See Fig. 4.4.

- The immediate management of the fitting child must be to maintain the child's airway and support their breathing with an airway adjunct and high flow oxygen.
- Use anticonvulsants to stop the seizure and check the child's blood sugar. Administer 5mL/kg of 10% glucose if the CBG is < 3mmol/L.
- Insert an IV cannula and take bloods for FBC, U & E, Ca^{2+}, and Mg^{2+}.
- If the child has a temperature > 38°C administer rectal paracetamol.
- A senior clinician must be involved in the child's care.
- Refer all infants presenting with their first fit to the paediatricians for admission and further investigations.

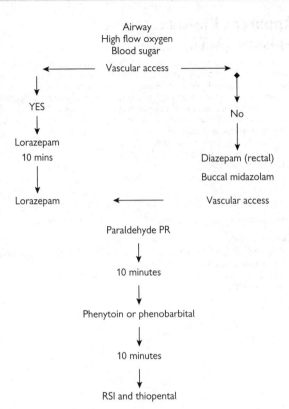

Fig. 4.4 Management of fitting in children. (Reproduced with kind permission of Wiley–Blackwell Publishing from Advanced Life Support Group (2004). *Advanced paediatric life support. The practical approach, 4th edn.* BMJ Books, London.)

Apparent life-threatening episode (ALTE)

Children < 1y who present to the ED following an episode involving one or more of the following symptoms should be admitted under the paediatricians for investigation and observation. On assessment they may be perfectly well and your examination may not reveal any underlying condition. In some cases, there is an obvious diagnosis. Manage children who are obviously unwell as their condition dictates.

- Apnoea (stopping breathing).
- Colour change (cyanosis or pallor).
- Choking (except straightforward choking on a feed).
- Unresponsiveness.
- Hypertonia (stiffening of limbs or neck).
- Floppiness.

It is essential to take a detailed history from all observers.

▶ Ask who was taking care of the infant at the time of the incident.

Examination

- Fully undress the baby and examine thoroughly including a careful look for bruises, petechiae, rash, and injury.
- Examine ears and eyes; the optic fundi should be examined for hemorrhages.

Management of the injured child

The management of the seriously injured child can be extremely challenging, but principles of treatment priorities are identical to those for an adult. Preparation is often the key. Working out the child's treatment variables before arrival speeds up care and reduces much of the stress. The weight of the child is the priority for this. A reasonably accurate way to do this is by [age of the child + 4] x 2 = approximate weight in kg (up to age of 10 y).

The team should be prepared with personal protective equipment and roles should be assigned.

Primary survey

- A (Airway).
  - Assess, clear, and secure airway, while maintaining control of C-spine.
  - Maintain in-line C-spine immobilization until triple point immobilization established. (Do not triply immobilize combative patients.)
- B (Breathing). Assess breathing and oxygenation. Give oxygen.
- C (Circulation).
  - Assess circulation and control haemorrhage.
  - Insert two large-gauge IV cannulae.
  - If evidence of hypovolaemic shock, give bolus of normal saline in 10mL/kg aliquots.
  - Direct pressure to external bleeding sites.
- D (Disability). Carry out a simple neurological assessment using:
  - level of response (AVPU: A, alert; V, responds to vocal stimuli; P, responds to painful stimuli; U, unresponsive);
  - Pupil reaction and equality.
  - ▶ Don't ever forget to take a capillary blood glucose.
- E (Exposure).

Undress the patient completely, taking care to protect the whole of the spine. Remember children lose heat very quickly so they should always be covered.

Once ABC is stabilized, proceed to the secondary survey.

Secondary survey

It is very important to manage the child's pain effectively and ensure the child is comforted throughout. Allow the child's parents to be in attendance at all times. Carry out a full set of observations and monitor the patient accordingly. Take the child off the spinal board as soon as possible and carry out a full assessment for other injuries.

Examine the whole patient systematically

A suggested system is:
- head and face, neck;
- chest;
- abdomen;
- pelvis and perineum;
- back and spine (log roll);

- extremities;
- neurological status;
- pupil reaction;
- Glasgow Coma Score;
- any lateralizing signs.

Paediatric head injury

Head injuries are the most common cause of trauma death in children aged 1–15 years. They are most often caused by falls, road traffic collisions (RTCs), sporting injuries, and non-accidental injury.

First priority is to perform primary survey assessing child's airway and C-spine. Make sure that breathing and circulation are secure and stabilized.

History and examination

Perform an assessment of the child looking specifically at the following.
- Neck and C-spine. Deformity, tenderness, muscle spasm.
- Head. Scalp bruising, lacerations, swelling, tenderness, bruising behind the ear (Battle's sign).
- Eyes. Pupil size, equality, and reactivity; fundoscopy.
- Ears. Blood behind the eardrum, CSF leak.
- Nose. Deformity, swelling, bleeding, CSF leak.
- Mouth. Dental trauma, soft tissue injuries.
- Facial fractures.
- Motor function. Examine limbs for presence of reflexes and any lateralizing weaknesses.
- Perform a full children's coma score.
- Consider the possibility of non-accidental injury.
- Other injuries.

Additional information
- Time, mechanism, and circumstances of injury.
- Loss or impairment of consciousness and duration.
- Nausea and vomiting.
- Clinical course prior to consultation: stable, deteriorating, improving.
- Other injuries sustained.

Management[1]

Minor head injury
- No loss of consciousness.
- One or no episodes of vomiting.
- Stable, alert conscious state.
- May have scalp bruising or laceration.
- Normal examination otherwise.

These children may be discharged from the ED into the care of their parents. Ensure that the child and parents have clear instructions regarding the management of the child at home—especially when they should return to hospital immediately. (Written advice sheet must be provided.)

▶ If there is any doubt as to whether there has been loss of consciousness, assume there has been and treat as moderate head injury.

Moderate head injury
- Brief loss of consciousness at time of injury.
- Currently alert or responds to voice.
- May be drowsy.
- One or more persistent episodes of vomiting.

- Persistent headaches.
- May have a large scalp bruise, haematoma, or laceration.
- Normal examination otherwise.

Assess the child and admit for observations as per local protocol.
- The child may be discharged home if there is improvement to normal conscious levels and no further vomiting. It is important that the child has been observed playing normally during this period of observation and has tolerated fluids and diet.
- Persistent headaches, large haematoma, or possible penetrating wound may need further investigation. If the child is still drowsy or vomiting after a period of observation or there is any deterioration during this time, discuss with a senior as a matter of priority. Consider further investigations and admit child under the inpatient team caring for children with head injuries (⌨ see Box 4.10).

Remember the term 'head injury' is very alarming for parents and carers, it is therefore imperative to offer reassurance and give sound advice, which is reiterated in a written advice leaflet.

Box 4.10 Guidelines for admission of children following head injury

- Patients with new, clinically significant abnormalities on imaging
- Patients who have not returned to GCS 15 after imaging, regardless of the imaging results
- When a patient fulfils the criteria for CT scanning but this cannot be done within the appropriate period, either because CT is not available or because the patient is not sufficiently cooperative to allow scanning
- Continuing worrying signs (e.g. persistent vomiting and severe headaches) of concern to the clinician
- Persistence of symptoms > 4h after the event
- Suspected NAI
- Social. Home situation suspected of being unsuitable for adequate observation
- Mechanism of injury indicative of more severe trauma, e.g. falling from height
- Other medical condition that may involve risk of intracranial complications, e.g. haemophilia, ITP, etc.
- Re-attendance with head injury if there are persisting signs or symptoms
- Bleeding from the ear and nose

Criteria for immediate request for CT scan of the head
- Loss of consciousness lasting more than 5min (witnessed).
- Amnesia (antegrade or retrograde) lasting more than 5min.
- Abnormal drowsiness.
- Three or more discrete episodes of vomiting.
- Clinical suspicion of non-accidental injury.
- Post-traumatic seizure but no history of epilepsy.

- GCS less than 14 or, for a baby under 1 year, GCS (paediatric) less than 15, on assessment in the ED.
- Suspicion of open or depressed skull fracture or tense fontanelle.
- Any sign of basal skull fracture (haemo-tympanum, 'panda' eyes, CSF leakage from the ear or nose, Battle's sign).
- Focal neurological deficit.
- If < 1 year, presence of bruise, swelling, or laceration of more than 5cm on the head.
- Dangerous mechanism of injury (high-speed RTC either as pedestrian, cyclist, or vehicle occupant; fall from a height of greater than 3m; high-speed injury from a projectile or an object).

Reference

1 National Institute for Health and Clinical Excellence (NICE) (2007). *Head injury: triage, assessment, investigation and early management of head injury in infants, children and adults*, NICE Clinical Guideline CG56. NICE, London. Available at ⫐ www.nice.org.uk/cg056

Children's fractures

A fracture is a disruption or a break in the cortex of a bone. Children with fractures often present with swelling, pain, and regional tenderness, lack of movement, angulation, and deformity. However, due to the cartilaginous properties of developing bone, signs and symptoms in young children can be very subtle. Often toddlers will present with symptoms such as not using their arm or crying inconsolably. Children will often find it hard to localize specific areas of pain and this can lead to needless X-rays and investigations. It is important that nurse or clinician spends time examining the limb appropriately and determining where the child's pain is coming from rather than resorting to excessive X-rays. The growth and development of bones in children vary with age and sex.

General guidelines
- All fractures are painful. Give the child regular analgesia.
- All fractures are generally more comfortable immobilized.
- Refer fractures that look clinically deformed to the orthopaedic team.
- Full arm plasters are required on all babies as backslabs tend to slip off.
- All children with grossly deformed limbs require regular neurovascular observations.
- Be alert for children < 2y who present with fractures. Take a very careful history and be mindful of NAI.

Greenstick fractures Greenstick fractures of the forearm are the most common fractures seen in children in the ED. A greenstick fracture (Fig. 4.5) is an incomplete fracture where the cortex of the bone is only disrupted on one side and buckled on the other. Place these fractures in a back slab for support and send to the fracture clinic for further follow-up. Treat greenstick fractures of the proximal end of radius with an above elbow back slab, as there is significant evidence to suggest that they are unstable and become more angulated over time.

Buckle fractures Buckle/torus fractures (📖 see Fig. 4.6) are minimally impacted fractures within an intact periosteum. These occur at the metaphysis. Treat buckle/torus fractures conservatively with splintage. These fractures tend to heal in 2–4 weeks. Follow-up should be arranged as per local guidelines.

Open/compound fractures
Suspect a compound fracture in a child if there is any overlying wound to the fracture.
- These fractures must be properly assessed by an orthopaedic surgeon.
- They require a thorough surgical clean and anti-staphylococcal antibiotic (cefuroxime 25mg/kg via slow infusion).
- It is appropriate for these wounds to be cleaned and dressed.
- A Polaroid or digital picture may be taken of the wound to reduce multiple exposure of the wound.
- Be aware that children may lose a large amount of blood from these injuries. Haemodynamic monitoring is therefore essential.
- Administer IV antibiotic in accordance with local policy and as prescribed.

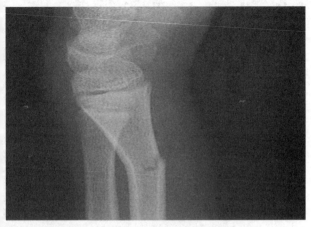

Fig. 4.5 X-ray of a greenstick fracture.

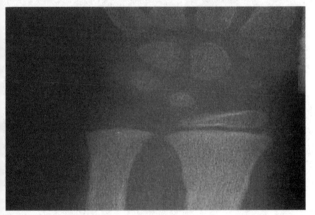

Fig. 4.6 X-ray of a buckle fracture.

Salter–Harris classification of epiphyseal injuries

Epiphyseal/metaphyseal fractures (☐ see Fig. 4.7) are fractures through the growth plate or epiphysis. These can be of particular importance as any disruption of the growth plate in a growing child can have serious implications. Follow-up all of these fractures.

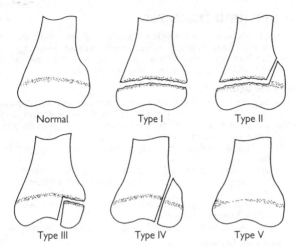

Fig. 4.7 Salter–Harris fracture classifications. (Reproduced with permission from Wyatt, J. et al. (2006). *Oxford Handbook of Emergency Medicine*, 3rd edn, p. 715. Oxford University Press, Oxford.)

Upper limb fractures

Clavicle fractures Most clavicle fractures in children can be treated conservatively. Often they only require simple analgesia, arm sling, and review in a fracture clinic. Occasionally, when there is severe angulation to the clavicle, orthopaedic intervention may be required.

Shoulder injuries

Dislocation of the shoulder in children is extremely rare and often requires a great deal of force. However, some children have some degree of laxity within their rotator cuff and dislocate reasonably easily. As in adults anterior dislocation is more common than posterior.

- Give children with a dislocated shoulder analgesia, and encourage them to relax.
- Numerous techniques are available for the reduction of dislocated shoulders, you are advised to follow local guidance and practised techniques.
- There is evidence to suggest that immobilization of the limb in a collar and cuff for 3 weeks is beneficial.
- Refer the patient to the orthopaedic outpatient clinic for follow-up.

Humeral shaft fractures

- Assess the integrity of the radial nerve. If any deficit or displacement is found refer the child to the orthopaedic team.
- If the fracture is minimally displaced and there is no neurological deficit, place in a collar cuff and refer to the fracture clinic.
- Be suspicious of all spiral fractures in children and investigate for NAI.

Elbow injuries

Supracondylar humeral fracture

This is a relatively common fracture in children, often resulting from a fall on to an outstretched hand. The child normally presents holding the arm rested on their abdomen, with a swollen and tender elbow.

- Assess the neurovascular status of the limb. The integrity of the radial and median nerves as well as of the brachial artery must be given special consideration. Maintain frequent monitoring of radial pulse.
- On initial assessment administer analgesia, place the child in a comfortable position, and request an X-ray.

Management

- ▶ Refer patients for manipulation under anaesthetic (MUA) immediately if:
  - neurovascular deficit is present;
  - > 50% displacement;
  - > 20° angulation of the distal part posteriorly;
  - > 10° medial or lateral angulation.
- Admit patients with a large amount of swelling and pain for analgesia and observation.
- If there is no swelling or angulation give the child analgesia, place in a collar and cuff, and refer to the next fracture clinic.
  - The arm must be placed at 90° in the collar and cuff and kept inside the clothes.

- If the elbow is very painful, use an above elbow back slab for immobilization.
- If concerned at all about the deformity or angulation of the elbow seek senior advice.

Lateral epicondylar epiphyseal injuries often require orthopaedic intervention. Always seek advice if unsure. Children require analgesia and careful positioning. Always assess neurovascular status. If the fracture is undisplaced, treat in an above-elbow back slab, collar, and cuff at 90°, ensure analgesia is given, and arrange fracture clinic for the next day.

Medial epicondylar epiphyseal injury Treat in a collar and cuff at 90° with analgesia and fracture clinic follow-up. Seek orthopaedic opinion if any suggestion of ulnar nerve involvement or excessive displacement of the fracture site.

Elbow injury without obvious fracture Children sometimes present with no obvious fracture on the X-ray but with fat pad signs of injury, i.e. a raised anterior fat pad and the presence of a posterior fat pad (effusion into the elbow joint). Treat in a collar and cuff, give analgesia, and follow up in the fracture clinic.

Radial head fractures Treat in a collar and cuff or broad arm sling, give analgesia, and follow up in fracture clinic. If significant angulation, seek orthopaedic opinion.

Subluxation of the radial head/pulled elbow often results from a sudden pulling of the forearm and only occurs in children < 4 years. The child presents holding the affected arm on one side and not using it. If a good history of a pull and no trauma, no X-ray is necessary. Reduce by flexing the arm to 90° and then place gentle traction on to forearm, supinating the limb at same time. Often a subtle click is felt when it has been successfully reduced. The child will start using the arm again after 10–20min.

Radial/ulna shaft fractures Children often present with significant deformity or angulation to their forearm. These children require immediate assessment and analgesia.
- Place the child in a comfortable position and refer to X-ray.
- Refer these children to an orthopaedic surgeon.
- Always ensure that X-rays are taken of the whole forearm so as not to miss Monteggia and Galeazzi fractures.

Distal radius and ulna fractures

Fractures of the distal radius and ulna are relatively common in children. They are characterized by pain, swelling, and deformity. Often you can feel the haematoma.
- Give the child analgesia and a broad arm sling before sending them to X-ray.
- Treat simple torus/buckle fractures using a torus splint or POP backslab. Follow-up should be arranged as per local guidelines. The nurse should discuss analgesia with the parents and point out that the fracture site often takes at least 2–4 weeks to heal.
- In fractures where there is moderate or severe displacement seek a senior opinion.
- If the wrist is clinically deformed the child will need an MUA.

Scaphoid fractures in children under the age of 12 are rare; this is because the bone only calcifies after age eight. A scaphoid fracture should be suspected in children who have fallen on to outstretched hands and are tender over the anatomical snuffbox. Treat these patients according to the adult protocol. (see p. 273)

Hand injuries Treat as per adult protocols (see p.274).

Lower limb injuries

Hip injuries 📖 see p.108

Femoral shaft fractures

Femoral shaft fractures in children are relatively common and are usually the result of a motor vehicle accident. Be mindful that a significant force is needed to fracture a femur so it is important to assess the child for other injuries. Children can lose up to 40% of the circulating blood volume from the fracture site and thus require a full assessment and ongoing observation.

• If the child is cardiovascularly unstable give 10mL/kg of normal saline and re-evaluate.
• Ensure analgesia, either intranasal diamorphine or IV morphine, is given as prescribed. A femoral nerve block may also be considered.
• Place the child in a traction splint as soon as possible.
• Seek orthopaedic opinion without delay.

Knee injuries

• Most knee injuries in children are due to twisting whilst playing sport, and often consist of a sprain.
• Serious ligamentous injury is rare, due to the laxity of children's ligaments.
• Serious fractures in the knee are very rare, but tibial plateau fractures can occur. Refer all fractures within the knee to the orthopaedic team.
• Otherwise, treat knee injuries with a knee brace, crutches, analgesia, and physiotherapy.

Dislocated patella

A reasonably common presentation especially in teenage girls. The knee will be held in flexion with lateral displacement of the patella and the patient will be in a great deal of pain.

• Reduction is usually achieved using entenox.
• Occasionally IV sedation and analgesia are required (📖 see p.284).
• Once the knee has been reduced, obtain an X-ray and immobilize the knee in a knee brace or cylinder POP. Arrange orthopaedic follow-up.

Tibial shaft fractures

Treat all tibial shaft fractures as you would those in an adult. Always be aware of the potential for compartment syndromes. If you are at all concerned seek a senior opinion.

• These children need analgesia, an above-knee back slab, and regular neurovascular observations.
• Compound fractures should be treated with IV antibiotics.
• Displaced or angulated fractures require orthopaedic intervention, often an MUA.

Toddler fractures

These fractures are seen in children < 4 years, usually caused by a twisting injury and associated with learning to walk. Often the child presents with a reluctance to place their foot on the floor. On examination there is often no swelling or bruising. However, when the foot is twisted pain is elicited.

- An X-ray should be taken. These can be difficult to interpret as the fracture can be very subtle.
- If at all concerned refer for a senior opinion.
- Place child in a below-knee back slab, give analgesia, and refer for an orthopaedic appointment.

Ankle injures

- Treat ankle injuries as in an adult: analgesia, ice, elevation, and rest. A recent study suggests that the Ottawa ankle rules are valid in children > 8y.
- Avulsion Salter–Harris 1 fractures of the distal tibia or fibula may be diagnosed. Give these children a below-knee back slab, analgesia, and crutches and arrange follow-up.
- Nurses must ensure that good advice is given on using crutches as children often find them difficult to use.

Foot injuries Treat as for those in an adult (📖 see Chapter 9, p.300).

The limping child

This is one of the most common reasons for children to attend the ED. For many the causes are obvious from the history, e.g. sprained ankle, foreign body in foot, broken toe, etc. For others the cause is less obvious because:

- the child is too young to say where it hurts;
- the child is too young to say what happened and no one witnessed it, e.g. an accident;
- poor localization of pain, e.g. hip/thigh/knee;
- Pain may be referred from elsewhere, e.g. young children will often complain of knee pain when their hip is the problem.

Toddlers will often continue to limp and play on a tibia that has sustained a greenstick or hairline fracture (toddler fracture). There is often no definable swelling or bruising and apparently no tenderness—only a vague history of the toddler not using that limb or the limb being slightly warmer to touch.

Causes of limp in a child

- Trauma.
- Sepsis: septic arthritis.
- A bleed into a joint due to underlying haematological problem.
- Perthe's disease.
- Slipped femoral epiphysis.
- Viral illness, including rubella.
- Bacterial infection, e.g. meningococcal disease.
- Allergy.
- Recent immunization.
- Rheumatological conditions.
- Leukaemia.

History and examination

In most of these cases it is possible to localize the problem. Look for:
- visible signs, e.g. swelling, bruising, redness;
- the style of the limp;
- local warmth;
- muscle wasting or tenderness;
- pain on movement (but be careful that only one joint is moved).

Investigations:
- X-rays only if able to identify where the problem may be.
- FBC, CRP, ESR if child is systemically unwell or has a temperature.

Treatment If you cannot make a diagnosis and the child is well, it may be appropriate to review the child the following day. By this time the cause may be obvious, or the child may be getting better. Send the child home with appropriate analgesia and advice.

Perthe's disease is a degenerative disorder of the hip joint. It causes avascular necrosis of upper femoral epiphysis. Mainly affects children aged 2–12y (majority 4–8y). Characterized by pain and limping. Interference with vascularity of femoral head but cause of this is still unknown. X-ray appearances are of progressive irregularity, flattening, and increasing density of femoral head; also changes visible in adjacent metaphysis. Detecting

Perthe's is important to ensure femoral head correctly contained within the acetabulum as it reforms with time. This is usually achieved with rest, analgesia, and regular follow-up by the orthopaedic surgeons. If Perthe's suspected, refer to orthopaedic team. Occasionally surgical intervention required.

Slipped upper femoral epiphysis (SUFE) occurs around puberty (8–15y). It is thought to be due to hormonal changes that weaken the epiphyseal plate. It may be gradual in onset (chronic) or sudden (acute), e.g. during a game of netball. Limp or pain predominates depending on chronic or acute history. Pain is often experienced in the knee. Classically, the affected limb is shortened and hip is externally rotated or attempts to flex the hip result in external rotation. Have a high index of suspicion in teenage girls and overweight children. Detection of a slipped femoral epiphysis is important to allow pinning of the epiphysis before further slip occurs. Delay may result in a functionally worse joint position or in an increased risk of avascular necrosis of the femoral head. A frog lateral X-ray of the hips is therefore needed in 8–16 year olds with hip pain. Examination of the contralateral hip is also important as bilateral SUFE is not uncommon.

Irritable hip—transient synovitis, observation hip
- Infective, traumatic, and allergic causes have been suggested.
- Pain caused by inflammation of synovial lining of hip joint, leading to an effusion and distension of capsule. Often bilateral but one side may start a day or two before the other.
- Some children have a lot of pain and are comfortable only when lying down with the affected hip flexed to 30° or 40°. Others may be up and about, but limping a little.
- Recent or current URTIs are common associations. There may have been previous episodes or a family history of irritable hip.
- Look for associated systemic signs such as pyrexia, rash, lymphadenopathy, URTI, etc.

Investigation of the painful hip
- X-ray at presentation if: any significant trauma; any fixed deformity, shortening, or functional deformity; child > 8 years old (look for SUFE).
- FBC, ESR, and CRP if the child is systemically unwell, in severe pain, or on examination there are signs of infection.
- USS. Many consider this examination of choice. Seek senior opinion.

Management
- Ensure appropriate analgesia to children diagnosed with septic arthritis, hip fracture, Perthe's disease, or slipped femoral epiphysis. Refer to orthopaedic team on call. Patients with septic arthritis must commence IV antibiotics as soon as possible.
- Manage children with transient synovitis with simple analgesia and rest. Arrange follow-up within 3 days to ensure they are recovering appropriately and other diagnoses have not been missed.

Surgical emergencies

The assessment of a child presenting to the ED with abdominal pain depends upon the clinician taking an accurate history and carrying out a detailed examination. Often the history given can be very confused and misleading. Clinical findings can mimic other disorders such as gastroenteritis. If unsure always seek senior help.

- Consider appendicitis in all children presenting to the ED with abdominal pain until adequately ruled out.
- Treat any infant or child who presents with bile-stained vomit as a surgical emergency until proven otherwise.

General principles for management of surgical emergencies

- Administer adequate analgesia.
- Administer IV fluids if required.
- Consider taking bloods for U & E, FBC, amylase, and sending for CTS urine.
- Always check the child's blood sugar.
- NG tube insertion if bowel obstruction is suspected.
- Keep the child fasted and seek senior surgical opinion.
- Carry out any specific treatments depending on condition and diagnosis.

Appendicitis

Appendicitis can occur at any age; however, it is very rare in infants. It occurs either when the appendix become obstructed or by lymphatic hyperplasia. Box 4.11 lists general principles for detecting appendicitis.

- The clinical features associated with appendicitis are: mild fever, anorexia, nausea, vomiting, tachycardia, and right iliac fossa pain. Children < 5y often present with atypical features as they are unable to localize the pain.
- Diagnosis is usually made clinically. FBC and CRP may be useful to identify inflammatory markers. However, they can be poor prognostically and should not to be relied upon for diagnosis. Ultrasound can be very useful in diagnosis if carried out by a skilled practitioner. Where there is uncertainty about the diagnosis the child should be seen by a senior clinician and admitted for observation. Usually the diagnosis becomes clear over time.

Management of a suspected appendicitis

- Regular examination.
- Regular analgesia.
- Regular observations of temperature and pulse.
- Chart intake/output.
- IV fluids (if required).
- Appendectomy if required.

Box 4.11 Tips for not missing appendicitis

- Consider the diagnosis in every patient with an appendix and abdominal pain
- Symptoms can progress rapidly over a few hours or slowly over days
- Smaller children are unable to localize pain
- Antibiotics may mask the signs
- Appendicitis may mimic gastroenteritis
- Overweight children mask it
- Children with communication problems and learning difficulties are a high risk group
- If in doubt get an ultrasound

Intussusception

In intussusception one segment of the bowel telescopes into another. Typically seen in children aged 6–12 months.

- Clinical features include vomiting, colicky abdominal pain, red currant jelly stools. Often a sausage-shaped mass can be felt in the abdomen.
- Signs of severe obstruction and shock can develop over 24–48h. Often the child presents as very unwell.
- All children with a suspected intussusception must be referred to a paediatric surgical team for early management.

Pyloric stenosis

Pyloric stenosis is caused by hypertrophy of the pylorus muscle. It usually develops in the first 6 weeks of life.

- Clinical features include projectile vomiting after every feed, weight loss, dehydration, and a hungry cry. Often a walnut-shaped hard mass can be felt in the epigastric area.
- U & E may be helpful as the prolonged vomiting will result in low serum potassium, chloride, and sodium.
- Management includes the correction of any dehydration and electrolyte imbalance and then surgery.

Volvulus is associated with the malrotation of the midgut. Infants present with signs of severe bowel obstruction, bile-stained vomit, and shock. Refer these infants to the paediatric surgical team immediately for surgical management and resuscitation.

Torsion of the testicle The peak age range for presentation with testicular torsion is 15–30y. Clinical features include sudden-onset testicular pain, inability to walk upright, and nausea is often associated with right iliac fossa pain. On examination the testis is riding high, extremely tender, and non-mobile. Refer all patients with suspected torsion of testicle to the urology team immediately. Give analgesia as a supportive measure.

Ear and nose foreign bodies

See p.459 and p.460

Safe guarding children

Types of child abuse
- Physical abuse.
- Sexual abuse.
- Emotional abuse.
- Neglect.
- Fabricated illness.

Suspicion arising from history
Aspects of the history may alert the nurse/health care professional to the possibility of child abuse.
- Frequent attendances.
- Delay in seeking health care.
- Injuries inconsistent with developmental stages.
- Injuries inconsistent with history.
- Third party attendance.
- Vague or poor history.
- Changing, inconsistent history.
- Abnormal parental attitudes.
- Distant relationship between child and parents.
- Child may disclose abuse.
- Child may be abnormally affectionate to strangers.

Physical signs of abuse
- Abnormal bruising.
- Torn frenulum of upper lip.
- Multiple bruising of differing ages.
- Finger imprinting or wounds that may have been caused by a cigarette.
- Long bone fracture in children < 3y, especially humerus and femur.
- Human bite marks.
- Petechiae associated with smothering.
- Scalds in the stocking/glove distribution.
- Perineal wounds or burns.
- Skull fractures.
- Subdural haematoma in an infant or toddler.
- Failure to put on weight.
- Unkempt and dirty (be careful—don't be too judgemental!).

Signs of sexual abuse
- Injuries to the genitalia or anus.
- Inappropriate sexual behaviour.
- Perineal discharge or bleeding.
- Behavioural disturbances, enuresis, encopresis.
- Disclosure of sexual abuse.

If abuse is suspected
Unless you are a specialist in child abuse and protection, your role in suspected child abuse cases is restricted to the detection and referral of children who you suspect may have been abused. If you suspect a child or sibling under your care has been abused, always involve an ED or paediatric

consultant at an early stage. If the child is discharged after examination by the paediatrician make sure the health visitor is aware of the child's attendance at the ED to ensure follow-up. If you still have concerns about the child being discharged make these concerns known to a senior member of the team before the child leaves the department The importance of valuing the views of all team members, however junior, as an essential factor in protecting the child was highlighted by the Laming Report[1] Accurate record-keeping is essential. However, emergency treatment and clinical management of the presenting complaint should not be delayed.

Reference

1 Laming Report (2003). *The Victoria Climbie Inquiry. Report of an Inquiry by Lord Laming*, January 2003. ᗑ www.victoria-climbie-inquiry.org.uk

Obstetric emergencies

Overview

Pregnancy is a natural condition but complications do arise and pregnant patients may attend the ED with medical problems associated with pregnancy, or what the patient perceives as a problem related to pregnancy. Women may also attend in labour. It should be borne in mind that some patients suffering trauma may also be pregnant.

Most emergency nurses are not qualified midwives. They should therefore always refer to specialist staff in the event of an obstetric emergency and not undertake any procedure if they are not competent or qualified to do so. The role of the emergency nurse in obstetric terms is to maintain the safety of the mother and her unborn baby till expert help arrives and also to identify pregnant patients who are vulnerable and potentially at risk. It is therefore important that nurses working in emergency care have a rudimentary knowledge of obstetrics in order to ensure the safety of a pregnant patient and speedy access to specialist care.

This chapter will focus on the conditions of pregnancy that most frequently present as an emergency. It is also important that emergency nurses have an awareness of the patients who are most vulnerable in pregnancy either due to health or socioeconomic reason. A study[1] found a mortality rate in the UK of 13.1 per 100 000 maternities for the period 2000–2002.

- The most common cause of direct maternal death was thromboembolism.
- The most common cause of indirect deaths and the largest overall cause of maternal death was psychiatric illness.
- The report also found that a disproportionate number of women who died were from vulnerable and more excluded groups in our society. Those considered to be at risk included:
  - socially disadvantaged, poor communities
  - some ethnic minorities
  - asylum seekers
  - Black African women
  - women who booked late and whose attendance at antenatal clinics was poor
  - obese women
  - victims of domestic violence
  - substance abusers.

ED nurses are familiar with these vulnerable groups, but it is imperative that they are especially aware of the added vulnerability of pregnant women who are also socially disadvantaged. Ensuring optimum outcomes calls for collaborative working practices between health and social care agencies.

Reference

1 Lewis, G. and Drife, J. (2004). *Why mothers die 2000–2002*: the sixth report of the confidential enquiries into maternal deaths in the United Kingdom. RCOG Press, London.

The pregnant patient

The physiological, anatomical, and biochemical changes that occur in pregnancy are both systemic and local. Most of these changes revert to normal after the birth.

Cardiac output

- To provide the developing fetus and placenta with a greater blood flow, cardiac output (CO) increases in the first trimester of pregnancy by 30–50%. This remains elevated until about the 30th week after which it may decrease as the enlarging uterus obstructs the vena cava.
- ↑ CO causes a heart rate ↑ from the normal 70bpm to 80 or 90bpm; BP ↓ slightly.
- Circulating volume increases proportionally with CO but the increase in plasma is greater initially than RBC mass. This may produce a dilutional anaemia until the 28th week when the increase in RBCs matches the plasma volume increase.
- The WBCs increase from about 9000 to 12 000/mcL.
- Clotting factors are altered during pregnancy. It is essential to understand this and respond with alacrity to patients presenting with more serious complications such as haemorrhage or clotting disorders.

Respiratory changes

Changes in lung function during pregnancy are attributed to the effects of progesterone and to pressure on the diaphragm from an enlarging uterus.

- Tidal volume, respiratory rate, plasma pH, and O_2 consumption increase.
- The ↑ tidal volume causes ↓ of plasma $PaCO_2$ but vital capacity and plasma PaO_2 do not change.

Renal changes

- Glomerular filtration rate (GFR) increases during pregnancy by about 50%, although the volume of urine passed each day is not increased.
- The renal plasma flow rate also increases by 25–50%.
- Glycosuria in pregnancy may be attributed to the ↑ GFR and impaired reabsorption of filtered glucose. Whilst this may not be considered abnormal, ↑ glycosuria may predispose the pregnant woman to UTI.
- Relaxation of ureters due to the ↑ progesterone may lead to urinary stasis and subsequent infection.
- Proteinuria should not be present during pregnancy so any significant rise in proteinuria should raise suspicion of a disease process.
- Pressure on the bladder from the enlarging uterus may cause frequency of micturition.

Gastrointestinal changes

- ↓ gastric motility in pregnancy due to ↑ levels of progesterone.
- Gastric reflux and heartburn are common due to the slower emptying time of the stomach and the relaxation of the cardiac sphincter.
- Constipation is also common due to compression of bowel segments and ↓ gastric motility.

Nursing assessment of the pregnant patient

Pregnant patients presenting with any health problem will understandably be anxious and need reassurance.

- From an emergency perspective patients presenting in the first trimester are regarded as gynaecological and managed in the ED or in an early pregnancy unit.
- In most hospitals patients who are more than 20 weeks pregnant are usually assessed in the labour ward unless delivery is imminent and there is no time to transfer, or the patient's condition is too unstable for transfer.
- If childbirth is imminent and there is no time to transfer the patient, call the paediatrician as well as the obstetrician. Inform the labour ward, and have a neonatal incubator resuscitaire ready.

▶▶ Remember: there are two lives to be considered. Do not delay in calling for specialist help.

History taking

History from a pregnant patient should include:
- last menstrual period (LMP);
- pregnancy test and result;
- number of times pregnant (gravida);
- first pregnancy (primagravida);
- number of viable births (para);
- method of delivery (vaginal/Caesarean);
- number of miscarriages/abortion (abortion is fetal death before 24 weeks' gestation; stillbirth is fetal death after 24 weeks' gestation).

Additional signs and symptoms that must be recorded and include any history of the following:

Vaginal bleeding Bleeding in the first trimester of pregnancy may suggest ectopic pregnancy or threatened abortion. In the second and third trimesters it may be associated with placenta praevia, placental abruption, traumatic injury, or it could be the onset of labour.

Abdominal pain In the first trimester abdominal pain may be associated with ectopic pregnancy especially if the pain radiates to the shoulder. Cramping abdominal pain may also indicate inevitable abortion. Abdominal pain in the third trimester of pregnancy may be associated with placental abruption, or impending labour. It is important to consider other causes of abdominal pain such as UTI or pelvic inflammatory disease (PID).

Nausea and vomiting of varying severity is common: > 50% in the first trimester. Persistent vomiting (hyperemesis gravidarum) can lead to dehydration and weight loss with the patient needing urgent fluid replacement. This can also predispose the patient to greater risk of serious complications such as DVT.

Headaches, visual disturbance, or swelling in the limbs are features that may be associated with pre-eclampsia which usually manifests after 20 weeks' gestation.

Trauma Any recent injury should be recorded. (Nurses should bear in mind that pregnant women are at increased risk of domestic violence.)

Fetal movements A decrease, or change in the normal pattern of fetal movements may be a sign of fetal distress.

Other As with any other history taking any past medical history, current medication, and any known allergy must be recorded.

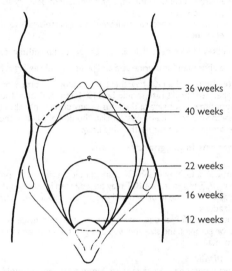

Fig. 5.1 Uterine size in pregnancy (Reproduced with permission from Wyatt, J. et al. (2005). *Oxford Handbook of Accident and Emergency Medicine,* 2nd edn, p. 551. Oxford University Press, Oxford.)

Physical assessment and investigations in pregnancy

Physical assessment

Physical assessment of the pregnant patient includes inspection, palpation, and auscultation.

Inspection
- Observe colour and amount of vaginal loss and inspect any clots or products that have been passed.
- Observe external genitalia for any sign of imminent delivery such as crowning of the head.
- Observe for any cord protrusion from the vagina; this calls for immediate intervention.

▶▶ In all cases of imminent childbirth get expert help without delay.

Palpate the abdomen for uterine size and position (🕮 see Fig 5.1).

Auscultate Listen to the fetal heartbeat with a Doppler probe or a Pinard stethoscope. Fetal heart rate should be 110–160bpm. Where there is any anxiety about the well-being of the fetus or any uncertainty about hearing a fetal heartbeat a midwife or obstetrician should be called without delay to ensure optimum care for mother and baby.

Investigations in pregnancy

Imaging
- As far as possible, X-rays and CT scans should be avoided in pregnancy. If an X-ray/CT is imperative (CT may be indicated in trauma) then the radiographer must be informed and the patient's abdomen covered with a lead apron.
- Ultrasound is useful for determining the location of pregnancy (intra-uterine or ectopic), the size and well-being of the fetus, and the site of the placenta.

Other investigations
- The most common investigations are blood tests, which should include FBC, Group & Save, and coagulation studies.
- Urinalysis and $_\beta$HCG should be carried out.

Nursing interventions

Recording of vital signs and monitoring

This should include blood pressure, pulse rate, pulse oximetry, respiration rate, blood sugar, temperature, and fetal heart rate where indicated. Urinalysis should also be done. Capillary blood glucose should be recorded in patients who are diabetic and when gestational diabetes is suspected.

Venous access Establish venous access for fluid replacement as a priority particularly if the patient is bleeding. Insert a wide bore canulae and infuse normal saline or Hartmann's solution as prescribed. Blood may be obtained at the same time for laboratory investigation. Ensure samples are correctly labelled and sent to the lab as a matter of urgency.

Pain management Ensure the patient receives effective and timely analgesia. Entonox® (50% nitrous oxide, 50% oxygen) can be safely administered to the pregnant patient. The medication prescribed will depend on the presenting condition. Always evaluate effectiveness of the analgesia given.

Pelvic examination Prepare and assist with vaginal examination, ensuring privacy and dignity during the procedure and subsequent comfort.

Psychological support Unforeseen medical problems relating to a pregnancy are likely to cause fear and anxiety for the patient and her family. It is important for staff to understand and acknowledge such distress and offer support and empathy. As far as is reasonable the patient's partner should be allowed to stay with her and nursing staff should involve them both in all decision-making.

Emergency delivery: labour

Childbirth is a natural event that is best managed by midwives and obstetricians. It is not uncommon, however, for a patient to present in the ED in advanced labour.

▶▶ In such situations get specialist help immediately.

Stages of labour

- The first stage of labour is characterized by the onset of regular painful contractions and dilatation of the cervix > 3cm. There may be a 'show' (mucus and blood discharge from the vagina) or the membranes may have ruptured.
- The second stage is from full dilatation of the cervix until the baby is born.
- The third stage is from the birth of the baby until the delivery of the placenta and until the uterus is retracted.

Assessing the patient in labour

- Record maternal vital signs particularly pulse and BP.
- Palpate the abdomen and listen for fetal heart rate using a Doppler probe or Pinard stethoscope.
- Observe rate of contractions.
- Check the perineum and vulva. If the head is crowning or the mother says she wants to push or says 'the baby is coming', call for help urgently (obstetrician/paediatrician /midwife) and prepare to assist delivery. Inform the labour ward and arrange to have a neonatal incubator resuscitaire nearly ready.
- If there is time, transfer the patient to the labour ward.

Assisting delivery (📖 see Fig. 5.2)

The delivery process must be controlled to avoid trauma to the baby from a precipitate birth or tearing of the perineum.

- Sit the mother upright and continue to reassure her and partner if present.
- Offer Entonox® as pain relief.
- Put on sterile gloves to assist delivery from the patient's right side.
- If the head is crowning, instruct the mother to pant and not bear down.
- As the head emerges spread the fingers of the left hand over the baby's head, applying gentle pressure to prevent rapid expulsion of the head.
- The baby's head will then turn to the side and shoulders will rotate into an anterior/posterior position.
- Firmly but gently guide head downwards and deliver anterior shoulder. Give Oxytocin® 10IU as prescribed with the birth of the anterior shoulder.
  - ⚠ Oxytocin® must be prescribed and should not be given by an unqualified or inexperienced person. It is safer to give nothing and keep the cord intact until expert help arrives.
- Then guide head upwards and deliver posterior shoulder.
- The rest of the baby will then deliver immediately.
- Dry and wrap the baby, and place the baby on the mother's abdomen or alongside her facilitating skin to skin contact.

- Clamp the cord in two places and cut between the clamps when the cord has stopped pulsating.
- Use a Hollister crushing clamp 1–2cm from umbilicus.

Delivery of the placenta

- Soon after the infant is delivered the uterus will contract again to detach and expel the placenta. The cord lengthens and there may be a gush of blood from the vagina.
- Apply gentle downward traction on the cord while exerting upward pressure on the abdomen.

Examine the placenta ensuring it is complete. Record findings and retain placenta for further examination by midwife or obstetrician or as per hospital protocol.

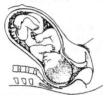

(1)
1st stage of labour. The cervix dilates. After full dilatation the head flexes further and descends further into the pelvis.

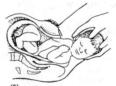

(4)
Birth of the anterior shoulder. The shoulders rotate to lie in the anteroposterior diameter of the pelvic outlet. The head rotates externally. Downward and backward traction of the head by the birth attendant aids delivery of the anterior shoulder.

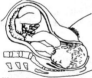

(2)
During the early second stage the head rotates at the level of the ischial spine so the occiput lies in the anterior part of pelvis. In late second stage the head broaches the vulval ring (crowning) and the perineum stretches over the head.

(5)
Birth of the posterior shoulder is aided by lifting the head upwards whilst maintaining traction.

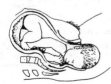

(3)
The head is born. The shoulders still lie transversely in the midpelvis.

Fig. 5.2 Stages of labour. (Reproduced with permission from Wyatt, J. et al. (2005). *Oxford Handbook of Accident and Emergency Medicine*, 2nd edn, p.553. Oxford University Press, Oxford.)

Documenting the birth and postnatal nursing interventions

Documentation
- Record the exact time of birth.
- Calculate the APGAR score (American Paediatric Gross Assessment Record).
- Ensure both mother and baby have identity bracelets.
- Identity bracelet for the baby should include:
  - mother's name/hospital number;
  - sex of baby;
  - date, time, and type of delivery;
  - ward; other information in accordance with local policy.

APGAR score
This is an internationally recognized scoring system (Table 5.1) used to assess the condition of the infant. A score is given for each sign at 1min and 5min after birth. If there are problems with the baby an additional score is given at 10min.
- A score of 7–10 is considered normal.
- A score of 4–7 may require some resuscitative measures.
- Babies with scores of 3 and below require immediate resuscitation.

Immediate postnatal nursing intervention
- Record vital signs, particularly pulse and BP.
- Encourage and assist the mother to breastfeed the infant.
- If indicated prepare for repair of episiotomy.
- Assist patient with washing and make comfortable.
- Ensure baby is wrapped up and kept warm. Transfer mother and child to postnatal ward.

Table 5.1 The APGAR scoring system

		Score		
		2	1	0
A	Activity (muscle tone)	Active movement	Arms & legs flexed	No movement; floppy tone
P	Pulse	Normal	Below 100	Absent
G	Grimace (reflex irritability)	Sneeze, cough, pulls away	Facial movement only; grimace	Absent; no response to stimulation
A	Appearance (skin colour)	Normal over entire body	Normal, except for extremities	Blue-grey, pale all over
R	Respiration	Normal rate & effort; crying	Slow, irregular	Absent; no breathing

Childbirth complications

It is expected that specialist help will be available for an emergency delivery in the ED but, in the event of delivery taking place in another setting, such as a walk-in centre, it is important that nurses can respond in a safe and professional way.

Prolapsed cord

Prolapsed cord occurs after rupture of membranes. It is associated with prematurity, malpresentation, fetal abnormality, and multiparity. Once the cord is out of the uterus the fetal blood supply may become obstructed. Emergency Caesarean section is usually indicated.

- While preparations are being made for the Caesarean delivery, the cord should be pushed back into the vagina and kept in place by a pack or if necessary by hand.
- Positioning the mother and raising the foot of the bed may help further reduce cord compression.
- Supplemental oxygen should be given to the mother.

▶ This is a serious complication and under no circumstances should the patient be left alone.

Breech presentation

This is where the baby's legs or bottom present first. This is more common with a premature labour and is much riskier for the mother and baby.

▶▶ Encourage the mother to pant rather than push and get specialist help immediately.

Postpartum haemorrhage

Blood loss during childbirth is normally about 250–300mL. A loss greater than this is cause for concern. Postpartum haemorrhage may be due to retained placental tissue, laceration to the vagina or perineum, uterine atony, or inversion. These are all obstetric emergencies that must be managed by a specialist.

The nurse's role in these situations is as follows.

- Ensure IV access and collect blood for crossmatching/transfusion.
- Commence IV infusion as prescribed.
- Maintain meticulous recording of vital signs. Support the mother and her partner.
- Assist the obstetrician or midwife in controlling the bleeding.
- If bleeding is due to a tear, apply a sterile dressing and direct pressure while the obstetrician or midwife prepares to suture.
- If it is due to uterine atony the nurse should massage the fundus of the uterus to stimulate a contraction or encourage the mother to breast-feed her infant as this will also stimulate contractions.
- If bleeding is not quickly controlled, operative intervention in theatre may be indicated.
- Prepare patient for theatre.

Vaginal bleeding in pregnancy

Vaginal bleeding in pregnancy is a common presentation in the ED. It is also very worrying for the patient and, in some cases, represents a serious threat to the well-being of mother and baby. It is also important to remember that patients may present with vaginal bleeding and either deny pregnancy or not be aware they are pregnant. Early accurate assessment, intervention and continuous monitoring are essential.

Causes of vaginal bleeding

Causes of bleeding relate to the gestational stage.

First trimester causes include:
• spontaneous abortion (miscarriage);
• ectopic pregnancy;
• trophoblastic disease.

Second trimester causes include:
• spontaneous abortion;
• placenta praevia;
• placental abruption;
• trophoblastic disease;
• cervical erosion/polyp/malignancy.

Third trimester causes include:
• placenta praevia;
• placental abruption;
• early labour 'show'.

Terminology

Spontaneous abortion To the lay person the term 'abortion' implies intention to terminate a pregnancy and therefore seems an inappropriate and insensitive term to a patient experiencing a spontaneous abortion. Miscarriage is a more acceptable and more widely understood term to use when caring for patients in the ED.

Miscarriage refers to the loss of the pregnancy before 24 weeks' gestation. There are different forms of miscarriage including the following.
• Threatened abortion: bleeding per vagina but cervical os is closed. Pregnancy may be viable.
• Inevitable abortion: bleeding per vagina; os open; crampy abdominal pain. Pregnancy cannot continue.
• Incomplete abortion: cervical os is open; tissue visible in vagina. Pregnancy not viable.
• Complete abortion: os is closed; tissue has passed. Pregnancy has ended.

Missed abortion Cervical os open; no products have been passed; fetus not viable. On rare occasions patients may present in the ED long after fetal death being unaware of what has occurred.

Septic abortion Infection may complicate abortion once cervix starts to dilate or instruments are introduced into the uterine cavity. Sepsis may follow spontaneous or surgical abortion, particularly an illegal abortion.
• There is vaginal bleeding and an offensive discharge.

- Os is open; tissue may have been passed or is in the cervix or vagina.
- Temperature ↑; BP ↓.
- Abdominal and vaginal tenderness on examination.
- Generally very unwell.

Trophoblastic disease occurs when fertilized ovum forms abnormal trophoblastic tissue but no fetus. Abnormality ranges from benign hydatidiform mole to invasive choriocarcinoma requiring chemotherapy.

Choriocarcinoma is a rare occurrence—81 in 40 000 pregnancies—but nonetheless devastating for the patient The patient may present with per vagina bleeding at 12–16 weeks' gestation The patient may also present with abdominal pain and hyperemesis gravidarum, which may be due to very high HCG levels. Diagnosis is by ultrasound and serum HCG. These patients will need very skilled emotional as well as physical care.

Patient assessment Signs and symptoms will depend on type of miscarriage. Assessment follows the principles outlined in this chapter, see 📖 Physical assessment and investigations in pregnancy, p.122. Treatment is directed towards managing pain, controlling blood loss to prevent shock, and, in septic abortion, treating infection.

- Observe for signs of shock. Record vital signs especially pulse, blood pressure, respiration rate, and temperature.
- Undress patient and assess blood loss (how long has patient been bleeding? have any clots been passed? and how many pads are being used?).
- Assess pain and offer analgesia as prescribed.

Investigations include blood tests, FBC, coagulation studies, cross-match, ultrasound scan. If septic abortion is suspected, blood cultures and vaginal swabs should be taken prior to commencement of antibiotic therapy.

Nursing interventions

Ensure early assessment of patient.

- Reassure and comfort patient and partner.
- Regular recording of vital signs, fluid balance, and blood loss.
- Establish venous access using wide bore cannulae if blood loss is moderate or severe.
- Blood samples. Send urgently for FBC, clotting screen, group and save.
- Administer appropriate pain relief and evaluate effectiveness.
- Initiate infusion of normal saline or Hartmann's solution as prescribed.
- Enquire about the need for anti-D immunoglobulin1g if mother is rhesus negative and miscarriage has occurred or is inevitable.
- Assist with gynaecological examination. Keep patient nil by mouth in case emergency surgery is indicated.
- Accompany patient to scanning room. Prepare for theatre if indicated.

Do not leave patients unattended or alone: they can deteriorate rapidly and will also be very anxious and frightened. Document all interventions.

Discharge If miscarriage threatened or complete and patient is allowed to go home from the ED give follow -up advice.

- Rest, avoid sexual intercourse, use sanitary towels not tampons. Patient should see own doctor or return to ED if condition/bleeding does not settle or if she develops crampy abdominal pain.

Ectopic pregnancy

Ectopic pregnancy has ↑ in recent years to about 1 in 100 pregnancies. It occurs when the products of conception implant outside the uterine cavity, most commonly in the Fallopian tube. Risk factors include:

- previous history of salpingitis or pelvic inflammatory disease
- previous ectopic pregnancy
- intrauterine contraceptive devices
- abnormal tubal structure or tubal surgery
- fertility treatment
- no known cause.

An ectopic pregnancy is a gynaecological emergency. Rupture will lead to profound hypovolaemic shock and can be fatal if not diagnosed and treated swiftly. Treatment is aimed at preventing shock, terminating the pregnancy and preserving the Fallopian tube where possible.

▶ Where there is any suspicion of an ectopic pregnancy, close monitoring and early assessment by the gynaecologist is essential.

Patient assessment

Patients with an ectopic pregnancy may not be aware that they are pregnant or may deny pregnancy. For this reason, ectopic pregnancy must always be considered as a possible diagnosis in any female of a childbearing age with abdominal pain or vaginal bleeding, or in young women who collapse for no obvious reason.

Presenting symptoms may include:

- abdominal pain;
- pain referred to the shoulder;
- possible vaginal bleeding (there may also be no bleeding);
- one or two missed menstrual periods;
- feeling dizzy, weak, or faint.

Signs

- Observe for signs of shock.
- Vaginal examination may be painful and blood may be visible around the cervix.
- Positive pregnancy test.
- Pain in the abdomen may vary from mild discomfort to severe pain with rebound tenderness and peritonism.

Investigations

- Recording and monitoring vital signs, especially BP and pulse, is imperative from arrival in the ED.
- Record CBG.
- Urinalysis is important to exclude urinary infection as a cause of abdominal pain.
- Pregnancy test is usually positive but serum B-HCG may be below normal.
- Bloods must be taken for FBC, coagulation studies, group and save. Crossmatch ~ 6 units of blood.
- Transvaginal ultrasound is usually done to confirm ectopic pregnancy.

Nursing intervention

- Commence regular monitoring and documentation of vital signs.
  - ⚠ Do not be lulled into a false security by normal vital signs on initial assessment, although it is likely that the patient will have a tachycardia.
- ▶ Remember that these patients are otherwise healthy young women who will initially compensate despite shock and then rapidly deteriorate.
- Give O_2.
- Establish venous access as a priority and obtain blood samples.
- Ensure samples are sent to the lab without delay.
- Initiate infusion of normal saline or Hartmann's solution as prescribed.
- Administer appropriate analgesia as prescribed and monitor effect.
- Assist with pelvic examination.
- Prepare patient for theatre.
- Give anti-D IG if prescribed.

Antepartum haemorrhage

Antepartum haemorrhage is bleeding from the genital tract after the 24th week of pregnancy and before the birth. Causes include placental abruption and placenta praevia.

Placental abruption

Abruptio placenta is a premature separation of the placenta from the uterine wall before the delivery of the fetus. It usually occurs after 20 weeks' gestation Risk factors include multiparity, diabetes, smoking, pre-eclampsia, and trauma.

Fetal distress and death may occur and maternal haemorrhage may lead to disseminated intravascular coagulation (DIC).

Placenta praevia

Placenta praevia occurs where the placenta is implanted low in the uterus, either partially or completely covering the os. The patient may present during the 2nd or 3rd trimester with fresh painless bleeding per vagina. As the uterus grows the placenta praevia may move upwards away from the cervix, and bleeding ceases. If this does not happen bleeding will increase in the 3rd trimester particularly when the cervix begins to dilate in labour. If placenta praevia is suspected a vaginal examination with a speculum should be avoided.

Nursing intervention

Antepartum haemorrhage is an obstetrical emergency that threatens the well-being of the mother and baby. It is a terrifying experience for the patient and partner. It is therefore essential that the emergency nurse (who may be the first person to assess the patient) acts swiftly while maintaining a sense of calm.

- Call for an obstetrician and paediatrician immediately.
- Commence regular monitoring and documentation of vital signs.
- Monitor fetal heart rate.
- Give O_2.
- Establish venous access as a priority using wide bore cannulae and obtain blood samples: FBC; U & E; glucose; clotting screen; G & S cross-match; rhesus; and antibody status.
- Ensure samples are sent to the lab without delay.
- Initiate infusion of normal saline or Hartmann's solution as prescribed.
- Administer appropriate analgesia as prescribed and monitor effect.
- Prepare patient for emergency Caesarean section.

Other causes of abdominal pain in pregnancy

Any abdominal pain may be a chance happening and unrelated to pregnancy but nonetheless very frightening for the patient. It is therefore advisable to involve the obstetrician from the outset.

Urinary tract infection The main causes are stasis of the urine and increased susceptibility to ascending infection.

Gallstones Biliary colic may present for the first time in pregnancy; Treatment is usually conservative.

Appendicitis In early pregnancy appendicitis may be difficult to differentiate from ectopic pregnancy. In later pregnancy the pain may be located in the right hypochrondrium.

Assessment

Nurses should follow the same assessment guidelines as for pregnant patients mindful that there are two lives to be considered.
- Call for specialist help early.
- Referral to the surgeons as well as the obstetrician may be indicated.

Medical problems in pregnancy

Diabetes

Pregnancy will affect established and otherwise stable diabetes and also may precipitate impaired glucose tolerance in non-diabetic patients. Hyperglycaemia is a common presentation in pregnancy. Diabetic patients often find their condition more difficult to manage as insulin requirement ↑ and diabetic ketoacidosis (DKA) may occur more frequently.

It is good practice to record a CBG reading on any patient presenting in the 2nd or 3rd trimester of pregnancy and at any stage in established diabetic patients.

Pre-eclampsia and eclampsia

Pre-eclampsia is a disease of the second half of pregnancy characterized by proteinuria, hypertension, and oedema. It occurs in ~ 7% of primigravid pregnancies. In previously well patients, it is regarded as 'primary' pre-eclampsia. In patients with pre-existing hypertension or renal disease it is regarded as secondary pre-eclampsia.

• Pre-eclampsia is diagnosed when the patient exhibits 2 or more of: hypertension (BP > 140/90); proteinuria; or oedema.
• Pre-eclampsia causes an alteration in the placental circulation that may adversely affect the fetus.
• Risk factors for pre-eclampsia include diabetes, multiple pregnancies, pre-existing renal disease, and substance misuse.

Eclampsia and HEELP syndrome

Pre-eclampsia is a disease of signs but no symptoms. If it is not detected it can escalate to eclampsia where the patient may complain of:
• headache;
• visual disturbance;
• abdominal pain.

The patient may appear restless/agitated/hyper-reflexive. Other symptoms include:
• ↑ BP
• tremor
• confusion
• an epileptic-type seizure may occur.

A related variant of pre-eclampsia is HEELP syndrome (haemolysis, elevated liver enzymes, low platelet count). Immediate treatment is crucial to prevent disseminated intravascular coagulation (DIC). Eclampsia and HEELP, while relatively rare (< 1/1000), are dangerous complications of pregnancy.
• Maternal mortality from eclampsia is 2%.
• Perinatal mortality is 15%.
• Nurses must be aware of these signs and symptoms in a pregnant patient and respond urgently.

▶▶ Get help!

Trauma in pregnancy

Pregnant patients are more vulnerable to trauma than non-pregnant patients, especially during the 2nd and 3rd trimesters because of the increasing size and change in position of the uterus. Trauma may be due to all the usual causes, i.e. falls, RTCs, or assault. Emergency nurses need to be vigilant and aware of the evidence that suggests that pregnant women are more prone to domestic violence. Injuries that are inconsistent with the history should be regarded with suspicion and reported to the midwife caring for the patient.

- While there are 2 lives to be considered, give priority to resuscitating and stabilizing the mother as this offers the best chance for both.
- In assessing the patient it is essential to bear in mind the physiological changes in pregnancy (☐ see p.118).
- ▶▶ Get specialist obstetric and paediatric help at the outset.
- The type of injury will determine treatment but in the first instance adhere to ATLS principles in assessing the patient.
- Determine the stage of pregnancy (☐ see Fig 5.2).
- Establish and maintain an airway. Remember there is ↑ risk of regurgitation and vomiting in pregnancy; have suction at hand. Early anaesthetic help may be required.
- Give O_2 100%. Remember O_2 consumption ↑ in pregnancy.
- Establish venous access and collect blood for FBC, U & E, clotting, cross-match. Send to lab as matter of urgency.
- Administer crystalloid fluids or blood products as prescribed.
- Relieve pressure on the inferior vena cava by raising the mother's right hip with a (Cardiff) wedge or pillow or manually displace the uterus
- Once C-spine injury has been excluded, nurse patient in the left lateral position to prevent compression of the inferior vena cava.
- Record vital signs, CBG, and neurological observations.
- Establish the presence of a fetal heart and rate (use Pinard stethoscope or Doppler probe).
  - Consider continuous monitoring if fetal heart rate abnormal.
- Palpate fundal height and mark skin. Feel for fetal movement and document.
- Observe for any bleeding per vagina or rupture of membranes. Collect any evidence of blood loss such as towels/clothing/clots.
- Insert urinary catheter and record fluid intake /output.
- Insert nasogastric tube to minimize vomiting or aspiration. Consider orogastric tube in head trauma.
- Administer pain relief as prescribed.
- Consider anti-D 1g if the patient is rhesus negative.
- Consider tetanus prophylaxis if appropriate (pregnancy is not a contra-indication).
- Assist with investigations and diagnostic procedures indicated by the injury.
- Prepare patient for possible surgery or emergency Caesarean section.
- Stay with the patient throughout offering consistent support and realistic assurances.
- Keep partner and family informed of proceedings.
- Keep meticulous records of all interventions.

Neurological emergencies

Overview

Altered consciousness or coma are common reasons for presentation to the ED. 'Coma', which comes from the Greek word for deep sleep, is defined as a prolonged period of unconsciousness. This is an acute life-threatening situation and early recognition and swift intervention by nursing and medical staff is essential to prevent or minimize further neurological damage. Active resuscitation may be indicated to maintain and support the cardiovascular and respiratory systems. Coma is caused by bilateral hemisphere damage failure of the reticular activating system or both.

Impaired level of consciousness may be due to:
- haemorrhage or structural lesions that compromise the CNS, e.g. stroke, subdural/subarachnoid haemorrhage, fits, infection, or space-occupying lesions (tumours);
- decreased supply of oxygen or glucose to the brain, e.g. hypoxia due to respiratory conditions; hypoglycaemia as a symptom of diabetes;
- ingestion or exposure to substances that adversely affect the CNS, e.g. drugs or alcohol ingestion (increasingly common);
- psychogenic, e.g. psychiatric disorders (very rare).

Some knowledge of functional anatomy will aid the nurse in making an informed assessment.
- lesions in the left hemisphere of the brain will cause right sensory and motor deficits.
- lesions in the right hemisphere will produce left sensory and motor deficits.
- occipital lobe injury will affect visual interpretation and interpretation of written language.
- parietal lobe injury will affect sensation and recognition of body parts.
- frontal lobe injury will affect personality, humour, motor movement, spatial awareness, and perceptual information.
- temporal lobe injury will affect hearing, long-term memory, and understanding of speech and written language.

The role of intracranial pressure

The brain, spinal cord, and spinal fluid are encased in a rigid bony enclosure. The volume of blood, spinal fluid, and brain in the cranium must remain constant in order to maintain a normal ICP of 7–15mmHg (Munro–Kellie doctrine). Thus any increase in volume from a swelling or a haematoma results in a rise in ICP. As ICP rises cerebral perfusion pressure decreases as:

Cerebral perfusion pressure = mean arterial pressure − ICP.

Once cerebral perfusion pressure falls to < 70mmHg, significant 2° brain injury may occur. ↑ in ICP leads to a reflex ↑ in systemic arterial BP and an associated bradycardia.

▶ It is imperative for nurses caring for patients with any neurological injury to understand this process.

Neurological assessment

The assessment of a patient with actual or potential neurological deficit should follow the same format irrespective of the cause. The aim of assessment is to:
- establish baseline vital signs;
- identify any deviations from the baseline;
- recognize significant neurological changes.

One quick and simple tool to use in initial assessment is AVPU:
- **A**lert;
- responsive to **V**oice;
- responsive only to **P**ain
- **U**nresponsive.

▶ Any patient who is not alert on AVPU assessment requires senior intervention.

History-taking

In cases of altered level of consciousness gaining a history from the patient can be unreliable. A history is more likely to be obtained from family, friend, carer, or paramedic. In most emergency situations history-taking and initial management occur simultaneously. Where a history can be obtained questions must be asked about any trauma, any exposure to environmental hazards, chemical or substance misuse, as well as routine questions about the presenting complaint and past medical history. It is important to establish whether there is any history of seizures or psychiatric illness.

Physical examination

This should focus on determining the depth of coma or any obvious signs that may give a clue to the cause of altered consciousness.

Inspect the patient using the Glasgow Coma Scale (GCS) to assess level of consciousness (📖 see Table 6.1). When assessing, record best motor, best verbal, etc. Record as, for example, E4, M6, V5 =15.

⚠ Tracheotomy/intubation or oral/facial injuries invalidate verbal assessment.

Coma is defined as GCS of E2, M4, V2, or less.

The British Society of Rehabilitation Medicine defines the scale of head injuries as:
• mild (GCS 13–15);
• moderate (GCS 9–12);
• severe (GCS < 9).

Pupillary response

Assess pupil size and reaction to light. If pupils are equal and reacting to light and accomodation record as 'PERLA'.

Proper assessment of pupils requires a bright light. Ocular injury will affect responses as will the use of miotic eye drops. Bear in mind that drugs such as atropine and dopamine also have an effect on pupillary reactions. Unequal pupils with sluggish reaction may be due to compression of the oculomotor nerve (III cranial nerve) as a result of ↑ ICP. Pinpoint pupils may be caused by opiate overdose.

Eye movements The presence of purposeful eye movements in a patient who in every other way is unresponsive, may indicate a psychogenic cause, e.g. catatonia or locked-in syndrome.

General observation and assessment

Observe for any of the following.
• Facial droop (cranial XII) as this may indicate a stroke.
• Look in the patient's ears—any bleeding or leaking of CSF may indicate a fracture of the base of the skull.
• Periorbital bruising ('racoon eyes') and bruising around the mastoid process (Battle's sign) may also be indications of a basilar skull fracture.
• Any palpable depression of the skull may indicate a depressed skull fracture.
• Observe skin colour and sensation. Clammy skin may indicate hypoglycaemia. Hot dry skin may indicate fever.
• Observe for needle marks, which may indicate recent drug use.
• Observe for any sign of trauma, bruising to the face or skull. Look for any lacerations and consider the need for tetanus prophylaxis.
• Incontinence is a common presentation in stroke or seizure.
• Observe for smell of alcohol but never assume that ↓ GCS is due to alcohol.
• Observe for the smell of acetone as this may indicate ketosis.

Palpation

Assess the patient's reflexes and motor responses.

- Note any abnormal motor activity such as Babinski reflex (great toe moves upwards while other toes curl downwards when the sole of the foot is stimulated) indicating damage to the CNS.
- Unequal strength may occur in stroke. Flaccid responses and decerebrate (adduction, extension, and hyperpronation of the arms) or decorticate movement (flexion of arms at elbows, wrists, and fingers) indicate severe injury and poor prognosis.

Table 6.1 Glasgow Coma Scale*

	Score
Eye opening (E)	
Nil	E1
In response to pain	E2
In response to verbal cue	E3
Spontaneous	E4
Motor response (M)	
Nil	M1
Abnormal extension	M2
Abnormal flexion	M3
Weak flexion	M4
Localizing	M5
Obeys commands	M6
Verbal response (V)	
Nil	V1
Incomprehensible	V2
Inappropriate	V3
Confused	V4
Orientated fully	V5

* Adapted from Teasdale, G. and Jennett, D.B. (1974). Assessment of coma and impaired consciousness. A practical scale. *Lancet* **2**, 81–4 with permission.

Initial nursing interventions

Airway/breathing

- Establish and protect airway.
- Airway adjuncts or intubation may be necessary.
- If GCS is < 8 the patient needs intubating.
- Intubated patients will require capnography (☐ see Capnography, p.590).
- Gently suction to remove any secretions and remove dentures.
- If patient's gag reflex is reduced or absent they will need intubating.
  ▶▶ Call for the anaesthetist.
- If there is any suggestion of trauma, immobilize the C-spine. Remember that up to 10% of patients with a head injury also have an associated neck injury.
- Once the airway has been secured, administer high flow oxygen.
▶ Remember that inadequate resuscitation may lead to the development of a secondary brain injury.

Circulation

- Establish venous access using wide bore cannula and collect blood samples for FBC, group and save, U & E, coagulation studies, toxicology screening, and, if appropriate, prescribed medication screening.
- Capillary blood glucose should be established on arrival in the ED and, corrected accordingly .
- Attach the patient to a monitor and commence meticulous recordings of vital signs.
- Record a 12 lead ECG.
- If patient is hypotensive give IV fluids as prescribed.
  - ▶ Be careful as fluid overload can exacerbate cerebral oedema. However, this has to be balanced with the need to maintain adequate cerebral perfusion pressure.
  - A urinary catheter may be necessary to ensure accurate monitoring of fluid balance.
- A gastric tube may be indicated to empty the stomach, but the nasal route is contraindicated if there is any suggestion of facial or base of skull fractures.

⚠ Do not underestimate the potential for massive haemorrhage (some of which may not be immediately obvious) from a scalp laceration.

Neurological monitoring

Record GCS and make sure neurological status is frequently re-assessed. Meticulous monitoring and frequent re-assessment are crucial to detecting any further deterioration in conscious level (□ see p.642).

▶ Remember that changes in the GCS may be more significant than the overall score. If the GCS is < 8 the patient needs intubating.

Investigations
- Blood tests.
  - Immediate checking of blood glucose when patient arrives in the ED is imperative.
  - Other blood tests such as FBC, U & E, cross-matching, and clotting screen if patient is on anticoagulants or perceived as vulnerable to bleeding, e.g. alcohol.
  - Blood cultures should be considered where the patient is pyrexial.
- Following the NICE guidelines, traditional X-rays are now increasingly being replaced by CT scanning. CT scanning is used to identify brain injury, especially conditions such as haematomas that may be responsive to surgical intervention and treatment.
- In a patient with ↓ conscious level, localizing neurological signs, or papilloedema, a CT should precede a lumbar puncture. Lumbar puncture may be performed where there is suspicion of infection of the CSF, e.g. in meningitis, and to conclusively rule out subarachnoid haemorrhage following a negative CT, but this procedure should take place on the ward.

Skull fractures

The brain is well protected by the skull, spinal fluid and the meninges and it takes a significant trauma to cause a skull fracture and cerebral contusion. Skull fractures are usually classified as linear, depressed, or base of skull.

- A linear fracture is a simple fracture that may be seen in the occipital, temporal–parietal, or midline areas of the skull. These fractures are caused by a significant trauma to the skull and may cause a space-occupying haematoma.
- A depressed skull fracture is more complicated and may be associated with a scalp laceration. The depressed segment may be evident on examination and neurosurgical intervention may be required to elevate the segment to prevent further damage to neural tissue.
- A fracture of the basilar bone of the skull occurs in the floor of the skull. Fractures in this bone can cause tears in the sac compartments that hold the brain, resulting in a leakage of the CSF and thus exposing the cranial vault to the outside environment and potential infection. Prophylactic antibiotics may be considered.

Signs of basilar skull fracture may include:
- eye bruising (racoon eyes);
- bruising over mastoid (Battle's sign);
- blood in the ear canals.

Patients may complain of:
- visual disturbance;
- facial muscle weakness;
- loss of hearing;
- balance problems;
- altered facial sensation;
- loss of smell;
- nasal drip from leaking CSF.

Nursing assessment/management of traumatic brain injury

Serious head injury may be obvious from initial examination or from the history, but the possibility must always be considered where there is altered conscious level or coma, and in vulnerable groups such as alcoholics, epileptics, or the elderly. Injury to the brain encompasses both the primary injury and any secondary damage that develops during the first few hours or days after injury.

⚠ Nurses need to be mindful that the two main contributing factors to increased mortality and morbidity are failure to correct hypoxaemia and hypotension and delay in appropriate surgical management.[1]

Identify patients who have a serious injury from:
- information given by paramedics;
- the mechanism of injury;
- assessment of vital signs including GCS and a capillary blood glucose;
- motor responses.

Summon senior clinical help without delay and proceed with full neurological assessment (🕮 see Neurological assessment, p.642 and Physical examination, p.142). When assessing patients with traumatic brain injury also consider the following.
- Consider an associated C-spine injury and immobilize C-spine.
- Give analgesia as prescribed and monitor its effectiveness.
- Give IV antibiotics as prescribed if there is an open skull fracture.
- Check tetanus status.
- Clean and suture any head/facial wound as necessary. This should not take priority over resuscitation or a CT scan except when controlling haemorrhage is necessary.
- Prepare patient and accompany him/her to CT scanning room.
- Assist medical staff in examining the patient.
- Escort patient on any transfer to a neurosurgical unit.
- Provide emotional support and explanations to relatives and carers.

Indications for neurosurgical referral[2]
- CT shows a recent intracranial lesion.
- Patient meets criteria for CT but facilities not available locally.
- Persisting coma after initial resuscitation.
- Confusion that persists > 4h.
- Deterioration in conscious level.
- Progressive focal neurological signs.
- Seizure without full recovery.
- Depressed skull fracture.
- Definite or suspected penetrating injury.
- CSF leak or other sign of basal skull fracture

Checklist to ensure patient stable for transport
- Airway safe or secured by intubation
  - Tracheal tube position confirmed by X-ray.

- Breathing
  - Sedation, analgesia, and muscle relaxant.
  - Ventilation established on transport ventilator.
  - Adequate gas exchange confirmed by ABG.
- Circulation
  - Heart rate/BP stable.
  - Tissue and organ perfusion adequate.
  - Any obvious blood loss controlled.
  - Circulating volume restored.
  - Haemoglobin adequate.
  - Minimum of two routes of venous access.
  - Arterial line and central venous access.
- Neurology
  - Seizures controlled; metabolic causes excluded.
  - Raised ICP appropriately managed.
  - Pupil checks to be maintained throughout the journey.
- Trauma
  - C-spine protected.
  - Pneumothoraces drained.
  - Intra-thoracic and intra-abdominal bleed controlled.
  - Intra-abdominal injuries investigated and appropriately managed.
  - Long-bone/pelvic fractures stabilized.
- Metabolic
  - Blood glucose >3mmol/L.
  - Potassium 3.5–6mmol/L.; ionized calcium > 1mmol/L.
  - Acid–base balance acceptable.
  - Temperature maintained within normal limits.
- Monitoring
  - ECG.
  - Blood pressure—arterial and non-invasive.
  - Oxygen saturation; $EtCO_2$.
  - Temperature.
  - Pupils.
- Documentation
  - Patient records.
  - CT scans. All X-rays.
  - Blood results and blood products if available.
  - Referral letter, observation charts, and all nursing records.
  - Intertransfer observation chart.
  - Details of neurosurgical unit, telephone number, accepting consultant name, mobile phone number of receiving specialist registrar.

In addition to this checklist clear instructions must be given to any family or carers who wish to follow the patient by car (📖 also see Transporting the critically ill p.672).

References

1 Acute management of adults with traumatic brain injury University College London Hospitals.
2 National Institute for Health and Clinical Excellence (NICE) (2007). *Head injury: triage, assessment, investigation and early management of head injury in infants, children and adults*, NICE Clinical Guideline 56. NICE, London.

Complications of head injury

Intracranial haematoma

- Deteriorating consciousness after head injury may be due to an intracranial haematoma.
- Accurate observation and monitoring is essential in identifying such developments early as surgical intervention may be life-saving.
- Increased agitation or confusion, increasingly severe headache, or persistent vomiting require re-assessment by a senior clinician.
- ⚠ Patients on anticoagulants or those with bleeding disorders are at increased risk of developing intracranial haematoma after head injury.

Extradural haematoma

Extradural haematoma results from rupture of one of the meningeal arteries that run between the dura and the skull. The most common cause is a linear fracture of the temporo-parietal bone with associated injury to the middle meningeal artery.

Injury/laceration of this artery may result in a rapidly expanding haematoma that, if not evacuated, may be fatal. These patients may be difficult to assess as initial injury will often be relatively minor. More than half of cases occur in persons < 20 years old. The patient may report a period of unconsciousness followed by full coherence and as subsequent ↓ GCS.

Signs and symptoms will be due to rising ICP. Nurse's role with these patients is accurate neurological assessment and consistent monitoring.

Subdural haematoma

A subdural haematoma is a blood clot that forms beneath the dura mater. This type of venous bleed is usually caused by trauma such as a fall, an assault, or acceleration/deceleration patterns associated with an RTC.

There are two main types of subdural haematoma:

- acute—develops within 24h of initial trauma and is associated with severe brain insult;
- chronic—develops over several days after the initial trauma and often occurs in the elderly and alcoholics. The patient may present with a fluctuating level of consciousness and there may be a vague or, sometimes, no history of trauma.

A poor prognosis is likely if the subdural haematoma is bilateral, accumulates rapidly, or if there is > 4h delay in achieving definitive neurosurgical management.

Diffuse axonal injury

This is a severe brain injury often due to rapid deceleration and the commonest cause of coma and subsequent disability. Patients with diffuse axonal injury are often in a deep coma immediately after injury despite an initially normal ICP and normal CT scan.

Minor head injury

⚠ Never assume a patient is drunk or attribute ↓ GCS to alcohol alone; consider other possible causes

Most patients who present with minor head injury can be safely discharged from the ED. However, assessment of these patients is far from straightforward and caution should be exercised where the patient is elderly, epileptic, or there is a history of substance or alcohol misuse.

- Although these patients may not have a severe head injury it is important to obtain a clear history, especially any history of unconsciousness, and assess the GCS.
- Patients with significant neurological symptoms, e.g. vomiting, dizziness, visual disturbance, or severe headache, or a history of unconsciousness may need admission for observation. Ensure frequent reassessment and monitoring in the ED. Report any deteriorating symptoms.
- If the patient is being discharged ensure that there is a responsible adult to stay with the patient overnight and that they are given comprehensive head injury instructions and advice about analgesia.

Cerebral concussion

The number of people who sustain a mild head injury and experience subsequent post-concussion symptoms is very high. In Great Britain each year, 250–300 hospital admissions per 100 000 of the population involve head injuries, of which only a small minority (~ 8%) are severe.

Concussion is an injury to the brain that usually occurs following a blow or jolt to the head. In most instances, consciousness is not lost. Common causes include head injury from an RTC, a fall, a sports injury, or an assault.

- People who fall often—because of difficulties with walking or balance, for example—and those involved in contact sports are most at risk.

Symptoms of post-concussion include:
- headaches (which may be severe and persistent);
- dizziness;
- nausea;
- vision disturbance;
- poor balance;
- confusion;
- amnesia (retrograde or post-traumatic);
- poor concentration;
- tiredness;
- irritability;
- anxiety;
- low mood.

Post-concussion syndrome may occur with symptoms persisting weeks or months after the initial injury. These patients need reassurance that this condition will eventually resolve spontaneously but that it can last for up to 6 months.

Stroke

Stroke is the third most common cause of death in the UK. It is also the single most common cause of severe disability. 70% of strokes occur in those > 65y but stroke can occur at any age. 80% of strokes are due to occlusion of an artery that carries blood to the brain. Stroke may be caused by:

- a cerebral thrombosis, as a result of atherosclerosis or hypertension;
- cerebral embolism, as a result of atrial fibrillation, myocardial infarction, or valve disease.

20% of strokes are caused by haemorrhage into the brain. This may be due to:

- an intracerebral haemorrhage, when a blood vessel ruptures within the brain;
- a subarachnoid haemorrhage, when a blood vessel on the surface of the brain bleeds into the subarachnoid space;
- carotid dissection.

Risk factors for stroke

- Hypertension.
- Age > 70 years.
- Trauma.
- Hyper/hypocoagulable state.
- Smoking.
- Atrial fibrillation/myocardial infarction.
- Diabetes.
- Oral contraceptives.

Signs and symptoms of stroke

- Varying levels of consciousness.
- Motor weakness (opposite side of CVA).
- Incontinence.
- Speech deficits.
- Loss of tongue control/facial drooping.
- Cranial nerve involvement (same side as CVA).

The Newcastle 'face arm speech test' (FAST)

The FAST was developed in Newcastle UK in 1998 and consists of 3 key elements (facial weakness, arm weakness, and speech disturbances). FAST was designed for assessment of a seated subject and so does not assess leg weakness. It is considered a reliable tool for paramedics identifying stroke in the community, optimizing the potential for thrombolysis.

Nursing assessment and intervention

- Assess and resuscitate as needed. Call for senior help and do a full neurological assessment.
- Position the patient to avoid aspiration and establish IV access.
- Collect blood samples and ensure these are sent to the lab.
- Record capillary blood glucose and correct blood glucose if < 4mmol/L.
- Record an ECG and request a CXR. Keep patient NBM until swallow assessment has been performed.

- An NG tube may be indicated but a urinary catheter should not be routinely sited.
- Assist medical staff in a full examination of the patient and provide reassurance to the patient throughout any procedure.
- Ensure personal hygiene and pressure area care and keep the patient's mouth clean and moist.
- Provide emotional support for patient and relatives who will be very anxious and upset. If the patient has lost his speech or is having difficulty communicating, advise relatives that he/she may still understand what is being said.
- If the patient is restless or agitated ensure the cot sides are kept in place on the trolley to prevent further injury. Make every effort to establish the cause of restlessness and remedy it where possible.

Thrombolysis in 'brain attack'

Thrombolysis using recombinant tissue plasminogen activator (r-tPA) within 3h of stroke onset is increasingly being adopted as best practice. While there is no age limit to the use of thrombolytic therapy at present, only a small minority of patients fit the narrow time window and other strict criteria such as mandatory CT prior to initiation of thrombolysis. However, the rise of specialized stroke units and the rapid recognition of stroke in the community and by paramedic and emergency clinicians will lead to more patients benefiting from this therapy.

Inclusion criteria
- Significant neurological deficit (more than minimal weakness, isolated ataxia, isolated sensory deficits, or dysarthria).
- Time of onset < 3h.
- No scan evidence of intracranial haemorrhage.

Contradictions to thrombolysis
- Time of symptom onset unknown or symptoms that began > 3h ago.
- Minor neurological deficit or symptoms that are improving.
- Seizure at onset of stroke.
- Symptoms suggestive of subarachnoid haemorrhage even if CT normal.
- Stroke or serious head injury in last 3 months.
- Major surgery or serious trauma within 2 weeks.
- Previous stroke and diabetes.
- Intracranial tumour.
- GI haemorrhage in last 3 weeks
- On anticoagulation (INR > 1.7) therapy.

Following physical examination, these patients also not be suitable for thrombolysis are those with:
- rapidly improving neurological signs (no benefit; manage as TIA);
- systolic BP > 185mmHg or diastolic BP > 110mmHg or aggressive continuous treatment required to lower BP to this range;
- platelet count < 100 000/mm^3;
- INR > 1.7;
- glucose < 50mg/dL or > 400mg/dL;
- positive pregnancy test.

Blood should be sent for group and cross-match in case transfusion is required.

Investigations
- A CT or MRI scan is mandatory to differentiate the type of stroke before commencing treatment.
- Access to these investigations should be available 24h a day. Even if the window for thrombolysis has passed the Royal College of Physicians still states that all patients should have CT or MRI within 24h.[1]
- An ECG should be recorded as it is useful in diagnosing pericarditis and possible causes of stroke including MI and AF.

Reference

1 Royal College of Physicians (2003). *National Clinical Guideline for Stroke* ⊕ www.rcplondon.ac.uk

Subarachnoid haemorrhage

Subarachnoid haemorrhage is the sudden rupture of a blood vessel over the surface of the brain. A subarachnoid haemorrhage occurs under the arachnoid membrane. It is another form of stroke. Most bleeds follow rupture of a (berry) aneurysm in the circle of Willis. A subarachnoid haemorrhage also can occur because blood leaks from an abnormal tangle of blood vessels called an arteriovenous malformation (AVM). Subarachnoid haemorrhage occurs more often in people with hypertension and people who smoke. It is more common in women and in older people.

Signs and symptoms

The headache usually starts very suddenly (like a 'blow to the head') and within seconds becomes the most intense headache the patient has ever felt. After minutes to hours the headache spreads to the back of the head, neck, and back as blood tracks down the spinal subarachnoid space.

Up to 70% of patients present with a severe 'worst ever' headache, often at the back of the head, which eases off followed by nausea and vomiting. Neck stiffness is a feature but is not always evident in the ED. A rising BP and a bradycardia is indicative of raised ICP. In the most severe cases (30–40%) the person may lose consciousness, and some (10%) may have a seizure.

Nursing assessment/intervention

- Immediate resuscitation may be indicated if the patient is unconscious.
- ▶▶ If the patient is conscious and gives a history of the 'worst ever' headache, get senior help.
- Perform complete neurological assessment and nursing interventions (⊞ see Neurological assessment, p.642 and Initial nursing interventions, p.144). Record all observations meticulously.
- If unconscious or GCS < 8 and agitated and restless, intubate to secure the airway.
- Ensure blood samples are obtained and sent urgently.
- Request a CXR.
- Ensure the patient is given appropriate analgesia and monitor effect.
- Prepare to accompany patient to CT. If CT is normal, lumbar puncture should be considered. This procedure should be undertaken on the ward rather than the ED.
- Reassure and comfort relatives and carers who will be very anxious. Keep them informed and where appropriate, allow them to stay with the patient.

Meningitis

- Meningitis is an infection of the covering layers of the brain (the pia mater and the arachnoid mater) collectively known as the meninges.
- Meningitis also involves the CSF and the ventricles. The cause of the infection can be bacterial, viral, and occasionally fungal.
- Viral meningitis is usually considered to be benign and is a fairly common complication of viral infection. There is no specific treatment, but initial assessment and management are the same as for suspected bacterial meningitis.
- Fungal meningitis occurs in patients who are immunosuppressed (AIDS, lymphoma, or those on steroid therapy).
- The three main causes of bacterial meningitis have been:
  - *Haemophilus influenzae* type b (Hib);
  - *Meningococcus*;
  - *Pneumococcus*.
- In recent years the introduction of a Hib vaccination has led to a virtual eradication of Hib meningitis, which leaves *Meningococcus* and *Pneumococcus* as the major causes of bacterial meningitis.

Symptoms
- Malaise.
- Fever.
- Neck and back stiffness.
- Oversensitivity to light (photophobia).
- Severe headache.
- Drowsiness.
- Nausea/vomiting.

Signs
Meningitis may start like a flu-like illness and may be difficult to diagnose. It should be considered in any febrile patient with the above symptoms, any neurological signs, and any ↓ conscious level and/or irritability. In addition, there will be varying degrees of pyrexia as high as 41°C. A very specific meningeal sign is a positive Kernig's sign (straightening the knee while the hip is flexed produces ↑ discomfort in the presence of meningeal irritation). Meningococcal meningitis has a rapid onset and can result in septicaemia and death within a few hours. Diarrhoea and/or a rash may be evident. Sometimes a seziure may occur.

The rash If there is a rash it is worth trying the 'glass test'. This involves pressing a glass tumbler against the rash to see if the red/purple lesions disappear under pressure. The rash of meningococcal meningitis does not disappear on application of pressure.

Nursing assessment and intervention
- Assess ABCs and administer O_2.
- Get help.
- Establish IV access as a priority and if the patient is shocked and deteriorating and/or there is a suspicion of meningococcal infection, administer IV antibiotics as prescribed.
- Give IV fluids as prescribed.

- Ensure patient is given analgesia and an anti-emetic if vomiting.
- Collect blood for FBCs, U & E, blood cultures, and glucose screen. A sample should also be taken for polymerase chain reaction (PCR) as well as a clotting sample that can be used for meningococcal serology. Ensure these samples are expedited to the laboratory.
- In addition to assessing and monitoring the patient in terms of GCS, BP, pulse, SpO_2, and temperature, evaluate the effect of analgesia given.
- Prepare for and assist medical staff with a lumbar puncture. Make sure samples of CSF are conveyed to the lab. A CT should be done before a lumbar puncture if there are focal neurological signs or evidence of papilloedema.
- Ensure pressure area care and personal hygiene.
- As far as possible the same nurse should care for the patient and accompany them to X-ray/CT or, if indicated, on transfer.
- Remember patients with meningitis are frequently young and parents and carers will be very worried. Make sure they are kept fully informed and involved where appropriate.
- ▶ In caring for the patient, nursing and medical staff should be diligent in their efforts to prevent further spread of infection.

Prophylaxis for meningococcal infection

Prophylactic antibiotics may be needed by the patient's family and those who have had close contact with the patient. Hospital and paramedic staff may also need prophylactic treatment depending on the degree of contact they have had with the patient and in accordance with local policy.

▶ Meningococcal infection is a notifiable disease and the local public health department needs to be informed.

Encephalitis

Encephalitis is an inflammation of the brain, which is frequently caused by a virus. It is a rare disease that occurs most commonly in children, the elderly, and people who are immunosuppressed.

In mild cases of encephalitis, signs and symptoms may mimic flu or even go unnoticed. In more severe cases, a person is more likely to experience high fever and have symptoms that relate to the CNS including:
- severe headache
- nausea and vomiting
- neck stiffness
- drowsiness
- personality changes
- seizures
- problems with speech or hearing
- hallucinations
- amnesia
- confusion
- coma.

Because encephalitis can follow or accompany common viral illnesses, there are sometimes characteristic signs and symptoms of these illnesses beforehand. Often, however, the encephalitis occurs spontaneously.

Causes

- Encephalitis can be caused by many types of organisms. One of the most dangerous of these is the herpes simplex virus (HSV). Fortunately, HSV encephalitis is very rare.
- Encephalitis can be a complication of Lyme's disease, which is transmitted by ticks, or of rabies, which is spread by rabid animals.
- Nursing assessment and management of encephalitis will be the same as for meningitis but treatment may differ depending on the causative organism.

Seizures

A seizure occurs as a result of a sudden surplus of electrical activity in the brain producing an abnormal neuronal discharge within cerebral tissue. The type of seizure a person has depends on the area of the brain where this activity occurs. Grand mal seizures that produce repetitive tonic/clonic movements are those most frequently seen in the emergency setting. Epileptic seizures are classed as partial or generalized. Partial seizures involve part of the brain, while generalized seizures involve the whole brain. It is possible for partial seizures to become generalized seizures if the epileptic activity spreads to the whole brain.

- After a seizure, a post-ictal state follows with muscle relaxation and deep respiration. This may last from a few minutes to several hours.
- In 'status epilepticus' there are multiple seizures without respite or recovery between seizures. This is an emergency condition and can result in respiratory difficulties or irreversible cerebral damage if not treated immediately. Nurses must remember that seizures are a manifestation of an underlying condition.

Disorders that give rise to seizures include:
- epilepsy
- stroke
- metabolic disorders
- pregnancy-induced hypertension
- alcohol withdrawal
- overdose of barbiturates, cocaine, benzodiazepines, and previous neurological trauma.

Symptoms
- Aura: taste, smell, or sounds preceding seizure.
- Fever/tremors.

Signs
- Active seizure; tonic/clonic seizure.
- Deep respiration.
- Possible cyanosis.
- Raised temperature.
- Incontinence.

Nursing assessment and intervention
The immediate aim of treatment is to stop the seizure and protect the patient during the seizure.
- Position the patient in recovery position.
- Check ABCs and give high flow O_2.
- Use suction if necessary; keep cot sides up on trolley.
- Get IV access, check capillary blood glucose, and administer anticonvulsant medication as prescribed (IV, or PR if no IV access) or as per local policy.
- Record vital signs as soon as seizure ceases and maintain frequent observation while patient is post-ictal.
- Continuously reassure the patient who may feel very confused and frightened after a fit.

- Other investigations that may be indicated if this is a first fit include FBC, U & E, blood glucose, ECG, and chest X-ray.

Nurses must remember that any disorder of the CNS is very frightening for the patient and, in caring for the patient, they must be calm and reassuring.

Useful websites

⤻ www.stroke.org

⤻ www.nice.org.uk

Respiratory emergencies

Overview

A significant proportion of patients attending the ED will have a respiratory problem. Breathlessness as a presenting complaint is extremely common and can indicate a physiological problem in any system not just the respiratory system. For example, an increase in the respiratory rate is a compensatory mechanism in diabetic ketoacidosis (DKA). Classically, deep sighing respirations are seen in an attempt to increase the elimination of CO_2. Conversely, a reduced respiratory rate is often seen in CNS depression or opiate drug overdose.

⚠ A change in respiratory rate indicates either a physiological or psychological problem. The respiratory system is usually the first system to respond to altered homeostasis and changes to rate and depth of respirations happen within seconds of a problem that may be remote from the respiratory system.

The measurement of respiratory rate in clinical practice continues to be omitted or, if recorded at all, serial measurements are often absent.

▶ *Always* record respiratory rates on ED patients other than those with the most minor of injuries.

The respiratory system

The respiratory system (Fig. 7.1) can be divided into the upper airway, which consists of the nose, pharynx, and larynx, and the lower airway, consisting of the trachea, bronchus, bronchioles, and alveoli.

Other structures crucial to normal ventilation are the ribs, intercostal muscles, and diaphragm. If any of these are injured, respiratory function can be adversely effected.

Respiration is a collective term that refers to several functions: ventilation; gas exchange; and cellular respiration.

Ventilation

Ventilation is the term used to describe the mechanical element of breathing. Ventilation consists of two phases; inspiration and expiration.

Inspiration begins with the stimulation of the diaphragm by the phrenic nerve. The diaphragm contracts and flattens, which increases the longitudinal dimension of the thorax. The external intercostal muscles pull the chest wall out, which increases the diameter of the thoracic cavity. As the lung capacity increases, intrathoracic pressure becomes lower than atmospheric pressure and air is drawn into the lungs until the pressures are equal.

Expiration occurs passively. The diaphragm relaxes and moves upwards, the intercostal muscles compress the chest, and the lungs recoil passively. Intrathoracic pressure becomes greater than atmospheric pressure and air is forced out of the lungs.

Gas exchange occurs at the interface between the alveoli and the pulmonary capillaries. Oxygen in the alveoli is exchanged for CO_2 and oxygen-rich blood is then transported to the tissues for cellular metabolism.

Arterial blood gas (ABG) sampling measures the O_2 and CO_2 concentrations in arterial blood and assesses the effectiveness of lung function 📖 see Arterial blood gas sampling, p.576).

Cellular respiration is the use of O_2 and production of CO_2 by the mitochondria of the cells.

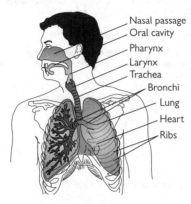

Nasal passage
Oral cavity
Pharynx
Larynx
Trachea
Bronchi
Lung
Heart
Ribs

Fig. 7.1 The human respiratory system.

Nursing assessment: overview and history

▶▶ Some patients with respiratory problems require immediate resuscitative interventions. Always undertake an ABC assessment. This will identify those patients with actual or impending airway obstruction or those with absent or ineffective respirations (📖 see Box 7.1).

Box 7.1 Respiratory distress/difficulty

Patients with any number of respiratory problems may present acutely short of breath and exhibit some or all of the following signs and symptoms that require immediate intervention
- Marked tachypnoea (RR >30)
- Altered conscious level, agitated, confused, moribund
- Marked accessory muscle use
- Inability to speak due to breathlessness
- Cyanosis
- Exhaustion

History

Any of the following features should be recorded in the nursing documentation.
- When the difficulty breathing started.
- Breathlessness on exertion.
- Nocturnal dyspnoea.
- Orthopnoea.
- Cough.
- Sputum (colour, amount, presence of blood).
- Breathlessness or inability to take a deep breath. Patients with a chest injury often state that they are breathless but questioning may reveal that they are unable to take a deep breath due to pain.
- Chest pain: site and quality. Differentiate between pleuritic and cardiac type pain if possible—this can often be difficult. If in doubt consider that the pain could be cardiac and manage appropriately.
- Any trauma: elicit a clear mechanism if the patient has been injured.
- Fever, rigors.
- Smoking.
- Exercise tolerance: how many stairs can be climbed or how far can the patient walk on the flat without breathlessness?
- Treatment at home/pre-hospital. Patients with asthma or COPD may have increased their own medication prior to attending the ED. No improvement after increasing their own inhaled therapy is significant.

For patients with existing respiratory disease it is important to document:
- medication;
- recent admissions;
- any ICU admissions/intubation/ventilation;
- non-invasive ventilation;
- annual flu vaccination;
- previous pneumothoraces.

Physical assessment

Inspection

- Observe for nasal flaring or pursed lip breathing.
- ▶▶ Drooling indicates an upper airway problem that requires immediate attention
- ▶▶ Cyanosis; central or peripheral, requires immediate intervention.
- Ability to talk in complete sentences. Inability to complete a sentence indicates a severe problem.
- Record the respiratory rate, depth, and pattern.
- Note the patient's posture. Patients with partial or impending upper airway obstruction will adopt a posture that maximizes ventilation. Usually they lean forward (Fig. 7.2).
- Observe chest rise and fall, noting any asymmetry or paradoxical movement. Following trauma, paradoxical chest rise and fall may indicate a flail segment.
- Inspect the chest wall for any signs of surface trauma: abrasions; bruises; wounds; foreign bodies; scars.
- Observe for accessory muscle usage, which indicates ↑ work of breathing.
- Observe and document the patient's conscious level and degree of agitation, confusion, and restlessness.

Palpation

- ▶▶ Feel the position of the trachea to check it is midline. A deviated trachea is a late clinical sign and indicates a tension pneumothorax, which is a life-threatening emergency and requires immediate treatment.
- Palpate the clavicles, sternum, and ribs in patients with a chest injury. This may reveal crepitus, surgical emphysema, or tenderness.

▶ Patients with a lower chest injury may also have sustained a significant upper abdominal or retroperitoneal injury as well.

Auscultation and percussion

Listening to breath sounds and percussing the chest is increasingly being undertaken by RNs in the ED. Auscultation in particular is a relatively simple and useful skill to acquire and can be mastered with practice and supervision.

- Listen for breath sounds: are they equal and clear bilaterally? Are there any added sounds: wheeze or crepitations? 📖 See Fig. 7.3 for landmarks for anterior and posterior chest auscultations.
- ▶▶ A silent chest in an asthmatic is life-threatening and requires immediate action. Get senior help.
- Is there any stridor or audible wheeze?
- Is the percussion note normal? Dullness indicates fluid or consolidation. Hyperresonance indicates air in the pleural cavity.

Vital signs

Record vital signs to include:

- pulse;
- respiratory rate;
- blood pressure;
- oxygen saturations;
- temperature;
- peak flow (in patients with asthma).

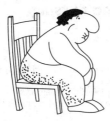

Fig. 7.2 Position that facilitates respiration.

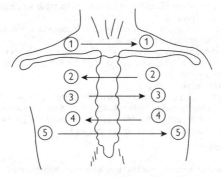

Fig. 7.3 Landmarks for chest auscultation.

Investigations and nursing interventions

Investigations
- Arterial or venous blood gases in patients with SpO_2 < 93% on air.
- Sputum for culture and sensitivity.
- FBC if clinical indication, e.g. infection, anaemia.
- U & E if signs of dehydration (may be seen in asthma through insensible losses).
- Pain score.
- CXR.
- ECG if indicated.

Nursing interventions
- Positioning. Patients should be nursed in an upright position. Patients with severe respiratory distress often want to sit with their legs over the side/edge of the ED trolley. It can be comfortable for patients to be supported in this position by a bedside trolley.
- Venous access. Some patients will require IV steroids and/or broncho-dilators. Not all patients will require IV access.
- Oxygen therapy. All patients who are unable to maintain normal oxygen saturations on air will require oxygen therapy. ▶▶ 📖 See following section on oxygen therapy.
- Inhaled therapies.
- Psychological support. It can be extremely distressing to be breathless. A calm, reassuring manner will help to reduce a patient's anxiety.
- Analgesia. Pleuritic chest pain can respond well to NSAIDs. Patients with severe pain may require opiate analgesia.

Oxygen therapy

⚠ All patients with respiratory problems must be protected from the dangerous effects of hypoxia and hypercarbia
▶▶ Only premature infants and COPD patients with a hypoxic drive require controlled oxygen therapy. *All* other patients should receive enough supplemental oxygen to maintain a normal saturation

There continues to be much controversy over delivering oxygen to patients with COPD. Normally, respiratory drive is stimulated by an increase in CO_2 levels. For example, in health, a rise in CO_2 will stimulate an ↑ respiratory rate to remove the excess CO_2. In a small group of patients with COPD, CO_2 levels are chronically elevated and this drive is lost. These patients depend on hypoxia to drive respiration (hypoxic respiratory drive). For this group of patients (remember *not all* patients with COPD have a hypoxic respiratory drive), increased levels of O_2, which may be given in an emergency, switch off their hypoxic drive to breathe and they will develop worsening respiratory depression, hypercapnic acidosis, reduced conscious level, and will require ventiltion.
- Give supplemental O_2 by mask to all patients with SpO_2 < 95%.

- In patients with known or suspected COPD give a controlled amount of O_2 by mask starting at 24–28% gradually increasing if saturations fall below 90%. Oxygen concentrations should be reduced if the patient becomes drowsy or saturations ≥ 93%. Obtain an ABG *as soon as possible* as oxygen therapy should be titrated to ABGs not saturations.
- If patient is found to have type II respiratory failure, which is defined as a $PaCO_2$ > 6kPa, the cause should be sought and treated.

Asthma: introduction

Asthma is a reversible disease of the airways which still causes in excess of 1500 preventable deaths per year. Recent evidence suggests patients with a combination of severe asthma and adverse behavioural or psychosocial features are more likely to die.

Asthma means 'panting' and is characterized by acute exacerbations interspersed by symptom-free periods. The airways become inflamed, narrow, and hyperresponsive. Wheeze tends to be regarded as the principal symptom of asthma. Other symptoms are cough, breathlessness, chest tightness, and accessory muscle usage. These symptoms are variable, intermittent, and often worse at night. When patients are symptom-free all objective signs of asthma are absent.

Intrinsic asthma has no known allergic cause and tends to occur later in life. Extrinsic asthma has allergic triggers—pollen, animal hair (use of), food, drugs. Emotion and exercise can also trigger an exacerbation.

The British Thoracic Society (BTS) and Scottish Intercollegiate Guidelines Network (SIGN) *British guideline on the management of asthma* details the assessment of severity and treatment required for acute exacerbations in the ED (📖 see Box 7.2).

Box 7.2 BTS/SIGN levels of severity of acute asthma exacerbations*

Brittle asthma
- Type I: wide PEF variability (>40% diurnal variation for >50% of the time over a period >150 days) despite intensive therapy
- Type 2: sudden severe attacks on a background of apparently well controlled asthma

Moderate exacerbation
- Increasing symptoms
- PEF >50–75% best or predicted
- No features of acute severe asthma

Acute severe exacerbation
Any one of the following
- PEF 33–50% best or predicted
- Respiratory rate ≥25/min
- Heart rate ≥110/min
- Inability to complete sentences in one breath

Life-threatening exacerbation
Any one of the following in a patient with severe asthma
- PEF <33% best or predicted
- SpO_2 <92%
- PaO_2 <8kPa
- Normal $PaCO_2$ (4.6–6.0kPa)
- Silent chest
- Cyanosis
- Feeble respiratory effort
- Bradycardia
- Arrhythmia
- Hypotension
- Exhaustion
- Confusion
- Coma

Near-fatal exacerbation
Raised $PaCO_2$ and/or requiring mechanical ventilation with raised inflation pressures

* Reproduced from British Thoracic Society (2003). British guideline on the management of asthma. Thorax **58**, 1–121.

Assessment of the asthmatic patient

Despite already identifying the general assessment approach for the breathless patient (☐ see p.166, p.168, p.170), it is worth reinforcing the importance of the following observations. These assist in establishing the severity of asthma on arrival to the ED and also enable the success of treatment interventions to be evaluated.

- Pulse.
- Respiratory rate.
- SpO_2.
- ABG if $SpO_2 \leq 92\%$.
- Temperature.
- Blood pressure.
- CXR if pneumothorax or consolidation suspected or if life-threatening asthma or failure to respond to treatment.
- Peak expiratory flow rate (PEF).
- Pain score.
- AVPU/GCS.

▶ PEF is the only objective measurement of lung function available in the ED. It *must* be measured on arrival and the % of best or predicted calculated and recorded. Fig. 7.4 can be used to compare the PEF recorded in the ED with the expected best for sex and height.

Following assessment of the patient with asthma, identifying how severe the asthma is (☐ see Box 7.2, p.173) is crucial as this guides treatment and the need for admission for in-patient treatment.

▶▶ If any features of severe or life-threatening asthma are present, get help *immediately*. Give high flow oxygen and commence inhaled bronchodilator therapy as per BTS guideline.[1]

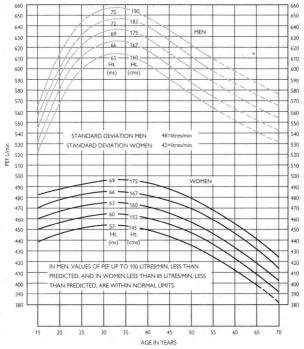

Nunn AJ, Gregg I. (1989). New regression equations for predicting peak expiratory flow in adults. BMJ **298**: 1068–70.

Fig. 7.4 Peak expiratory flow in normal adults (Reproduced with permission from Wyatt, J., et al. (2006). *Oxford Handbook of Emergency Medicine*, 3rd edn, p. 105. Oxford University Press, Oxford.)

Nursing interventions for the asthmatic patient

Once the severity of the asthma exacerbation is diagnosed some or all of the interventions listed below may be required (see Fig. 7.5). Management priorities depend on the severity of asthma.

- Nurse upright.
- Continuous SpO_2 and HR monitoring.
- RR should be recorded half-hourly as a minimum until stable.
- Supplemental high flow O_2 to maintain saturations > 95%.
- Nebulized bronchodilators (may be required 'back-to-back').
- Oral/IV steroids.
- IV bronchodilators.
- IV magnesium.
- ABG.
- CXR if pneumonia or pneumothorax is suspected.
- PEF should be recorded 30min post-nebulization.
- Analgesia.

Asthma severity may improve rapidly with treatment or worsen significantly despite treatment. It is important to reassess severity following any intervention that is given and treat any change in condition accordingly.

Admission

- Patients who show any features of life-threatening or near-fatal asthma **must not** be discharged from the ED. Any patients with a persistent symptom of a severe attack despite treatment should not be discharged. Admission **must** be considered for those with psychosocial risk factors, e.g. the socially isolated.
- HDU/ICU admission is indicated in type II respiratory failure or if near-fatal/life-threatening features fail to respond to treatment.

Discharge BTS guidelines provide details of those patients who may be suitable for discharge; see Fig. 7.5.

Smoking cessation

The opportunity to give smoking cessation advice/brief intervention should not be dismissed because of current pressures to move people out of the ED. Nurses are increasingly becoming the treating and assessing clinician and may enter into discussions with patients about various lifestyle choices during the consultation. Equally there may be opportunities during your time caring for a patient when discussion about smoking arises. There is evidence that patients are more receptive to lifestyle changes during periods when their behaviours have contributed to a health problem, the so-called 'teachable moment'. All patients who smoke should be advised to stop and offered referral/information about the local stop smoking support programme.

Reference

1 British Thoracic Society/Scottish Intercollegiate Guidelines Network (2008). British guideline on the management of asthma. *Thorax* **58** (Suppl. IV): 1–121.

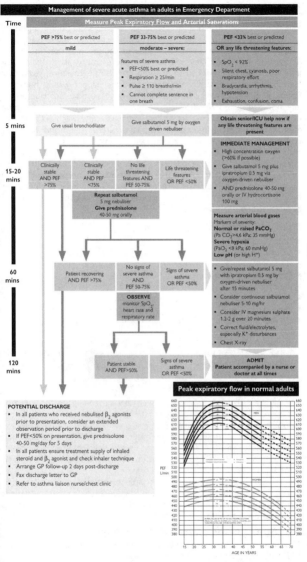

Fig. 7.5 Management of acute severe asthma in adults in the ED. (Reproduced with kind permission from British Thoracic Society/Scottish Intercollegiate Guidelines Network (2008). British guideline on the management of asthma. *Thorax* **58** (Suppl. IV), Annex 3, p.97.)

Pneumonia

Infection of the substance of the lungs is most commonly caused by bacteria. The terms pneumonia and chest infection are often used interchangeably. Use the term pneumonia with caution when discussing the illness with patients/relatives. This term causes more alarm than chest infection. Community-acquired pneumonia (CAP) is the term given to a chest infection that was contracted whilst the patient was at home, as opposed to 'hospital-acquired pneumonia', which is used to describe a chest infection contracted within 48h of hospital admission. The most common causative agent of CAP is *Streptococcus pneumoniae* which accounts for approximately 1/3 of infections. Hospital-acquired pneumonia is usually contracted by patients already vulnerable to infection, e.g. immunocompromised, critical illness, intubation, and ventilation. Hospital-acquired pneumonias usually have a different bacterial origin and tend to be more resistant to standard antibiotic therapy. Patients may present to ED with signs of a chest infection after a recent admission and this is worth noting. Mortality from all pneumonias continues to be significant in the elderly population and those with HIV.

Signs and symptoms

- Breathlessness.
- Cough.
- Purulent sputum.
- Fever, shivers, aches, and pains.
- Pleurisy.
- Haemoptysis.
- Hypoxia.
- Signs of consolidation either on CXR or on auscultation/percussion of the chest.

⚠ The elderly can often present 'atypically' with a chest infection or UTI and may attend the ED with acute confusion or reports of being 'off their legs'

The patient's signs and symptoms will vary depending on the infecting pathogen. As *S. pneumoniae* is the most common cause of bacterial pneumonia, it is worth mentioning its typical onset. There is often a precipitating viral infection followed by a temperature > 39.5°C, dry cough, and pleuritic chest pain. The elderly do not usually develop a pyrexia. Several days later there is rusty coloured sputum, breathlessness, and reduced chest wall movement on the affected side.

In the ED initial management of the patient with pneumonia is based on an assessment of its severity. A decision is made as to whether the patient can be discharged on oral antibiotics or admitted for oral or IV treatment. Once the infecting pathogen is isolated treatment can be adjusted.

Assessment of the patient with pneumonia

As well as the standard respiratory assessment (📖 see p.166, p.168, and p.170), note should be made of the following:

- Any immunocompromise.
- Recent hospital admission.

- Signs of dehydration.
- Signs of hypoxia.
- Social circumstances.
- Acute confusion.

Investigations
- Sputum for C & S.
- CXR.
- ABG if SpO_2 < 93% on air.
- Blood cultures if pyrexial.
- FBC, U & E if symptoms are severe.

Nursing interventions for patient with pneumonia

Scoring the severity of pneumonia

Patients with pneumonia should be scored using the validated CURB-65 score to assess severity, risk of death, and risk of ICU admission. Scoring in this way can also guide subsequent treatment ± the need for hospital admission.[1]

One point is given for each of the following.

- **C**onfusion.
- **U**rea > 7mmol/L.
- **R**espiratory rate ≥ 30/min.
- **B**P low (systolic < 90mmHg or diastolic ≤ 60mmHg).
- Age ≥ 65y.

Patients with relatively mild symptoms (CURB-65 score 0 or 1) with good social circumstances and no other significant health problems can usually be discharged home. Patients with more severe symptoms (CURB-65 score 2) are at increased risk and should be admitted. Patients with a CURB-65 score ≥ 3 are at most risk—a score of 3 has a 17% risk of death.

Discharge

- Oral antibiotics.
- Analgesia for pleuritic chest pain—vital for deep breathing exercises and expectoration.
- GP follow-up in 48h to assess for improvement/deterioration.
- Advice to rest, take on regular oral fluids, and not to smoke.

Admission

Patients who require hospital admission will need the following interventions.

- Nurse upright.
- Supplemental oxygen to maintain saturations > 93% (careful administration if COPD) (📖 see Investigations and nursing interventions, p.170).
- IV fluids if dehydrated.
- IV antibiotics.
- Analgesia.
- Antipyretic.

Antibiotics The hospital formulary/local antibiotic guidelines should be followed to ensure that the right empirical treatment is commenced.

Sepsis The elderly are particularly vulnerable to developing sepsis from pneumonia and general assessment of the breathless patients should identify those with signs of sepsis (📖 see p.246).

Reference

1 See ⏷ www.brit-thoracic.org.uk.

Tuberculosis

Mycobacterium tuberculosis infects 1.5 billion people worldwide and in the UK 8000 new cases are reported each year, mostly in major cities especially London. TB is a notifiable disease and contact tracing is usually done through chest clinics. There are increasing strains of multiple drug resistant (MDR) TB.

Primary TB is the initial infection. It usually infects the lungs. TB is spread by inhaling droplets containing the bacteria coughed or sneezed by an infected person. TB can infect any organ but is usually only infectious when it infects the lungs. Because TB can infect many sites the symptoms can be varied and diagnosis difficult. However, pulmonary TB infection is by far the commonest and should be considered in patients who have the following risk factors.

- Ethnic minority communities.
- Immunocompromised.
- Poor health and nutrition; homeless; drug or alcohol use.
- Overcrowded living accomodation.
- Close household contact with an infected person.
- Travel to countries where TB is common.

And consider it in those who present with the following signs and symptoms.

- Cough.
- Fever.
- Night sweats.
- Haemoptysis.
- Weight loss.

TB should be considered as a possible diagnosis in anyone with fever, weight loss. and other unexplained symptoms.

Investigations

- Specific investigations include CXR, which shows classical changes.
- Culturing the TB bacteria from sputum or other samples confirms the diagnosis.

Nursing interventions for the patient with suspected TB

Not all patients will require admission—only those who are ill, highly infectious, or where the diagnosis is uncertain. Consider isolation measures whilst the patient is in the ED.

Treatment The most important factor in treatment is continuous antibiotic therapy for 6 months. The homeless/transient population may need special consideration in relation to maintenance of therapy and follow-up.

Chronic obstructive pulmonary disease (COPD)

COPD is an umbrella term used to describe various diseases, e.g. chronic bronchitis, emphysema, and chronic asthma. COPD is a slowly progressive and irreversible disease, although some patients may show a degree of reversibility with bronchodilators. COPD usually occurs in people > 50y with smoking as a major factor in the development of the disease.

Assessment of the breathless patient with COPD

Useful information can be gained from the patient's history as to the severity of the disease. In mild disease a 'smoker's' cough is the only abnormal sign. In moderate disease, there is breathlessness/wheeze on moderate exertion, cough, and generalized reduction in breath sounds. In severe disease there is breathlessness at rest, cyanosis, prominent wheeze/cough, and lung overinflation. Also consider and record:
- current treatment: inhalers, nebulizers, antibiotics, steroids, oxygen, and theophyllines;
- exercise tolerance;
- previous admissions: especially intensive care or treatment with non-invasive ventilations (NIV);
- reason for ED attendance. It is important to identify if the exacerbation has been accompanied by an increase in the amount or type of sputum produced. A recent fall/chest injury may be the cause of the symptoms.

In the ED assess for the following.
- Cough.
- Cyanosis.
- Sputum: colour and amount.
- Wheeze.
- Tachypnoea.
- Accessory muscle usage.
- Lip pursing on expiration.
- Chest expansion (which is often poor).
- Fever.
- Dehydration.
- Confusion/reduction in conscious level.
- Pain.

Investigations
- Continuous monitoring; HR, RR, SpO_2.
- CXR.
- ECG.
- ABG *as soon as possible*.
- FBC, U & E, theophylline level if on a theophylline.
- Sputum for C & S if purulent.
- Blood cultures if pyrexial.

Nursing interventions
- Reassurance.
- Nurse upright.

- Oxygen therapy to keep saturations above 90% (📖 see, p.170).
- Nebulizers (may need to be continuous).
- Steroids.
- IV theophyllines (for patients who do not respond to nebulizers).
- Assessment for NIV.
- Mouth care.
- IV fluids if dehydrated.
- Analgesia.
- AVPU/GCS.

NIV is increasingly used in ED resuscitation rooms for the treatment of patients with COPD or heart failure. Evidence suggests that using NIV in patients with COPD reduces mortality and the need for invasive ventilation. NIV should be considered in patients who fit the following criteria.[1] (📖 see p.678.)

- Respiratory acidosis (pH < 7.35 $paCO_2$ > 6kPa) that persists despite maximal medical therapy.
- Not moribund, GCS > 8.
- Able to protect airway.
- Cooperative and conscious.
- Few co-morbidities.
- Haemodynamically stable.
- No excess respiratory secretions.
- Potential for recovery to a quality of life acceptable to the patient.

Ideally, patients should have an anaesthetic assessment prior to the commencement of NIV to assess suitability and to outline what the ceiling treatment should be. A DNAR order may be completed at this time if the patient is not suitable for invasive ventilation (see 'Intensive care').

Intensive care Patients with exacerbations of COPD should not be automatically excluded from invasive ventilation if all other treatments are failing. The assessing anaesthetist will consider the following.

- Quality of life, ideally involving the family in the discussion.
- Oxygen requirements when stable.
- Co-morbidities.
- FEV1.
- BMI.

Hospital at home schemes Increasing numbers of schemes are available to manage patients with exacerbations of COPD in their own home, avoiding admission completely or reducing the length of hospital stay. Patients may know of a 'COPD community nurse' who will be able to give useful clinical information about the patient and their treatments. If there is a local community scheme it would be worth identifying how the ED can become involved in identifying suitable patients.

Reference

1 ⁂ www.brit-thoracic.org.uk.

Pulmonary embolism

Pulmonary embolism (PE) occurs when a thrombus, which has usually travelled from a distant site (the deep veins), lodges in the pulmonary vasculature. Less commonly, fat (from long bone fracture), air, or amniotic fluid can cause PE. There is an incidence of 60–70 per 100 000 annually. Half of these cases are in hospitalized patients or those in some form of long-term care. Death arising from untreated PE is ~ 30%. PE is the most common cause of death following elective surgery and the commonest cause of maternal death.

❶ PE is notoriously difficult to diagnose—only about 10% of patients who are suspected of having a PE actually have one. Hypoxia is common but young healthy patients can have normal saturations and PaO_2. PE should be considered in cases of sudden collapse or cardiac arrest.

Signs and symptoms
- Tachypnoea (> 20/min)—often the only symptom.
- Tachycardia.
- Pleuritic chest pain.
- Haemoptysis.
- Hypotension

Massive PE causes sudden circulatory collapse with hypotension. This is rare—only about 5% of PEs present in this way.

Small/medium PE presents more classically with breathlessness, pleuritic chest pain, and haemoptysis.

Multiple recurrent PE presents as increased breathlessness over weeks or months with associated lethargy, exertional syncope, and occasional angina.

Nursing assessment for patients with possible PE
A careful history may reveal a known significant risk factor; abdominal or orthopaedic surgery; late pregnancy; Caesarean section; pre-eclampsia; malignancy; lower leg fracture; or varicose veins. Sedentary travel, which is a often a reason for patients presenting concerned about DVT, is only a minor risk factor. Some patients have no obvious risk factors. Assess for:
- tachypnoea;
- tachycardia;
- chest pain: site, quality, and severity;
- pyrexia (low grade fever may be a response to the inflammatory changes in infarcted lung tissue);
- hypotension (can be suggestive of massive PE);
- haemoptysis;
- AVPU/GCS.

Investigations
- ECG sinus tachycardia or AF may be present. Signs of RV strain or rSR in Lead V1.
- CXR to rule out other causes.
- SpO_2.

- ABG.
- FBC, U & E.
- D dimer (but see following paragraph).
- CTPA (computerized tomographic pulmonary angiography).

D dimer testing

The inappropriate requesting of D dimer sometimes done by ED nurses in an attempt to reduce a patient's wait for blood results can lead to incorrect interpretation of the results and may falsely exclude PE. There are various clinical probability scoring systems available and the ED nurse should work in conjunction with the assessing clinician to ensure that patients with a higher probability **do not** have a D dimer requested and are commenced on LMWH while imaging is arranged.

❶ D dimer is useful *only* in excluding PE and should *only* be used in conjunction with clinical pre-test probability scoring. If D dimer is not detectable or below a threshold pre-set by your laboratory, PE can be excluded.

Nursing interventions for the stable patient with a high probability of PE

- Continuous monitoring.
- Oxygen.
- Analgesia.
- LMWH.
- Imaging.

Interventions for patients with massive PE

Massive PE is highly likely if there is collapse/hypotension, unexplained hypoxia, and engorged neck veins.

- Thrombolysis. Alteplase 10mg over 1–2min followed by an infusion of 90mg over 2h. See BNF for further information.
- In cardiac arrest a bolus dose of 50mg alteplase can be considered and CPR should be continued for at least 30min.
- If stable (alert, RR 10–30, systolic BP > 100, sats < 92% on air), heparin.
- Urgent echocardiography or CTPA. If PE is confirmed give alteplase 10mg over 1–2min followed by an infusion of 90mg over 2h. See BNF for further information.

Heart failure

Patients with mild, moderate, or severe heart failure may present to the ED with breathlessness. The incidence of heart failure increases with age and, despite advances in treatment, mortality remains high. 50% of patients die within 5 years. Acute heart failure can result from myocardial infarction arrhythmia, anaemia, infection, medication changes, or patients reducing their diuretic therapy.

Features within the history that may point to heart failure as the cause of dyspnoea are:
• fatigue;
• breathlessness on exertion;
• nocturnal breathlessness;
• orthopnoea (breathlessness when laying flat).

Patients with acute heart failure often present to the ED in the early morning and are severely breathless with pulmonary oedema. For more details on the assessment and interventions for heart failure see p.206

Simple/spontaneous pneumothorax

A pneumothorax is the collection of air in the pleural space that surrounds the lungs (☐ see Fig. 7.6). A tear in the lung tissue causes inspired air to pass though it into the pleural space. It can occur following trauma, as a consequence of lung disease, e.g. COPD, asthma, cystic fibrosis, or bullous lung disease, or it can occur spontaneously (usually in tall, thin young men).

Spontaneous pneumothorax (SP)

The phenomenon of SP in tall, thin young men is interesting. The male to female ratio of SP is 6:1. It is thought that tall, thin men are more prone to the rupture of bullae (blisters on the pleura that arise from a rupture in the alveoli wall) in the apex because they are subject to more distending pressure as the thorax is longer.

There is also a significant relationship between smoking and the development of SP. This should be emphasized to patients in an attempt to discourage them from smoking. The lifetime risk of SP in smoking men is 12% as opposed to 0.1% in non-smokers.

Signs and symptoms

- Breathlessness.
- Unilateral pleuritic chest pain.
- Cough.
- Reduced or absent breath sounds on the affected side.
- Hyperresonance on percussion of the affected side.
- Decreased chest wall movement on the affected side.

Nursing assessment

- Past medical history.
- Previous SP. Patients may already have had a SP and know their symptoms well.
- Lung disease. Patients with underlying lung disease are more likely to need admission for observation even with a small pneumothorax or one that has successfully been re-inflated with needle aspiration.
- Pulse.
- Respiratory rate.
- Blood pressure.
- SpO_2.
- Temperature.
- Pain score.
- AVPU/GCS.

Investigations CXR. Relatively asymptomatic patients can often be sent directly to X-ray following a brief assessment. Those with abnormal observations will require further assessment or intervention prior to CXR.

Nursing interventions

- Reassurance—chest pain and breathlessness can be very frightening. If patients have had a previous SP they may be anxious about needle aspiration or chest drain insertion.
- Nurse upright.

- Oxygen—to maintain saturations > 93%.
- Analgesia.

Management (📖 see Fig 7.6)

Mildly symptomatic patients with a small SP (📖 see Box 7.3) and no underlying lung disease can be discharged home with clear written and verbal advice to return if breathlessness increases. Early follow-up should be arranged. Patients with underlying lung disease require observation and high flow oxygen (improves the rate of re-inflation 4-fold) if not contra-indicated in COPD. These patients are more likely to require active intervention with aspiration or a chest drain.

Symptomatic patients with small SPs will require needle aspiration. If this is unsuccessful a chest drain is usually indicated (📖 see p.604). Patients with underlying lung disease are more likely to require active intervention. For patients with large SPs and no underlying lung disease, needle aspiration is still the treatment of choice. However, patients with underlying lung disease (particularly those > 50 years old) usually need a chest drain.

Box 7.3 Classification by size of an SP

Small SP has a visible rim of < 2cm between the lung edge and the chest wall

Large SP has a visible rim ≥ 2cm between the lung edge and the chest wall

---

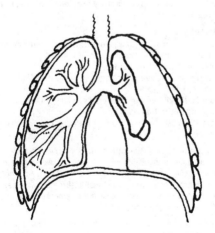

Fig. 7.6 Pneumothorax.

Chest trauma

In addition to patients presenting with respiratory problems arising from medical causes many patients will present to an ED each year following chest injury. The majority of these patients will have suffered minor chest wall trauma from contact sports or falls. However, a small number will have sustained significant chest wall trauma with underlying damage to the lungs, heart, great vessels, and/or abdominal organs.

Mechanism of injury Minor mechanisms tend to be falling over (often landing on an arm bent across the chest wall) or receiving a punch or elbow to the chest wall during sports or an assault. However, just because a mechanism appears minor, a significant underlying lung injury cannot be reliably excluded. More significant mechanisms involve considerable blunt mechanical forces applied to the chest, e.g. falls from heights, RTCs, pedestrian RTCs. Penetrating chest wall trauma can also cause significant injury even though the surface wound may appear insignificant.

Nursing assessment

- History of injury. A clearly documented mechanism of injury is a crucial part of assessing the patient's risk of having underlying pulmonary or other organ damage. Generally speaking, the more force involved, the more the risk of underlying damage. However, in the elderly population a relatively minor mechanism can result in significant chest injuries.
- Past medical history.
- Patients who smoke or those with pre-existing respiratory problems are more likely to develop respiratory problems from even the most minor of mechanisms.

Signs and symptoms

Assessing for the following signs/symptoms can identify patients who require further assessment or intervention.
- Pain—ascertain the site and nature.
- Breathlessness. Is the patient tachypnoeic or do they find it difficult to breathe due to pain?
- Hypovolaemic shock—in significant chest injury 1500mL of blood can be sequestered in the thoracic cavity.
- Respiratory distress. Hypoxia and the resultant agitation can indicate a significant underlying injury.

Inspection Signs of surface trauma to the anterior and/or posterior chest wall can include bruising, lacerations, abrasions (these may have characteristic markings for example from a seatbelt). An impaled object is an obvious sign of penetrating chest wall trauma. Look for asymmetrical chest wall movement and/or paradoxical movements these are significant and can indicate a pneumothorax flail segment.

Auscultation Breath sounds should be equal and clear bilaterally. Any abnormality (reduction or absence) will usually require further evaluation with a CXR except where they is a strong suspicion of a tension pneumothorax; this should be treated immediately with needle decompression (📖 see p.640).

Palpation The clavicles, ribs, and sternum should be palpated. Crepitus may indicate an underlying fracture. Surgical emphysema detected clinically or on a CXR indicates an 'air leak' somewhere in the pulmonary tree. Pain on palpation is often present and can sometimes be pinpointed to a specific rib/s. However, pain on laughing, coughing, movement, changing position when in bed, or deep inspiration may be present without any chest wall tenderness.

Percussion of part of the chest wall may be hyperesonant (dull), which indicates fluid. In an acute chest injury this dullness is likely to be blood. Hyper-resonance on percussion indicates air in the pleural cavity and may indicate pneumothorax.

Nursing interventions

All patients should have a full set of vital signs recorded regardless of how minor the mechanism.
- Pulse and temperature.
- Respiratory rate, BP, and oxygen saturations.
- Pain score.
- GCS/AVPU

Further interventions include the following.
- Analgesia.
- CXR (Box 7.4) is indicated if the assessing clinician cannot confidently exclude pneumothorax/underlying pulmonary injury from history and examination.
- Arterial blood gas if SpO_2 < 93% on air.
- ECG if there has been blunt anterior chest wall trauma.
- FBC, U & E, and G & S/cross-match if significant injury suspected.

Box 7.4 CXR in chest trauma

- A CXR is a standard X-ray in a multiply injured patient
- 50% of isolated rib fractures do not show up on a standard CXR
- In patients with minor chest injuries, a CXR is usually not required
- CXRs are indicated in patients where the clinician suspects an underlying injury to the lungs or mediastinum from either the history or clinical examination
- If a tension pneumothorax is suspected treat it first. Do CXR afterwards

Minor chest wall injuries

Patients with a relatively minor mechanism of injury, no overt signs of respiratory distress/difficulty, and normal observations are usually discharged from the ED. The diagnosis is clinical and the rationale for not X-raying this group of patients may need to be explained ([] see Box 7.4).

Discharge planning Patients will require analgesia appropriate to their pain score, advice about deep breathing exercises (to prevent the secondary development of a chest infection), and the knowledge that their symptoms may persist for up to 4 weeks. Patients should also be advised to seek further medical advice if any additional symptoms develop.

Multiple rib and sternal fractures

Multiple rib fractures

Patients with multiple rib fractures (2 or more ribs) are diagnosed clinically and often have them confirmed by CXR.

Previously fit, healthy patients with no pre-existing respiratory problems or other injuries can often be discharged home (📖 see p.190, 191) Give patients clear written and verbal advice about when to return to the ED. Review several days later is often useful to ensure that no secondary problems such as a small haemothorax/effusion have developed.

- The elderly or those with underlying lung disease may need a short period of hospital admission or intermediate care to ensure adequate pain management and the monitoring of any complications such as chest infection.
- Admission may also be indicated in some patients with multiple rib fractures if an underlying pulmonary contusion is suspected or severe pain requires well controlled analgesia and/or an intercostal nerve block.

Sternal fracture

Fractures to the sternum are usually caused in RTCs from blunt trauma to the anterior chest wall from either the seatbelt or steering wheel. The sternum is acutely painful and underlying cardiac or great vessel injury must be ruled out prior to discharge.

Specifically, patients require the following.

- ECG to exclude arrhythmias, MI, or contusion which may be evidenced by ST segment changes.
- Echocardiogram may be undertaken in the resuscitation room in symptomatic patients.
- Cardiac troponins. These can identify myocardial damage.
- Sternal X-ray usually shows a transverse fracture (± CXR if associated injuries are suspected).

Admission Patients should be admitted if there are any signs of myocardial contusion.

Discharge Patients should only be discharged if they have an isolated sternal fracture with no other injuries and no pre-existing cardiorespiratory problems. Discharged patients require analgesia and advice (📖 see discharge advice in this chapter, 'Chest trauma', 'Minor chest wall injuries', p.191).

Traumatic pneumothorax

Mechanisms ranging from relatively minor, e.g. elbow to the chest while playing rugby, to major trauma can cause a traumatic pneumothorax. Treatment for all but the smallest pneumothorax is with a chest drain (📖 see p.604).

Tension pneumothorax

A tension pneumothorax can result from chest trauma or as a consequence of underlying lung disease (📖 see Fig. 7.7). Although rare, its early detection and prompt treatment is critical to the survival of the patient. Patients with tension pneumothorax rapidly deteriorate and it is a well recognized cause of PEA cardiac arrest.

A tension pneumothorax is a pneumothorax that ↑ in size with every breath. A tear in the lung tissue creates direct communication with the pleural space and the flap of injured tissue acts like a one-way valve. On inspiration the flap of tissue is forced open and inspired air passes through it into the pleural space. On expiration the flap closes and the air that has passed into the pleural space is trapped. Consequently, with every breath more air passes through the flap and the pneumothorax is under 'tension'. It continues to increase in size until the lung on the affected side has completely collapsed. The pneumothorax continues to expand putting pressure on the mediastinum, causing it to shift towards the uninjured side. Pressure on the mediastinum causes compression of the heart and great vessels, which leads to impaired cardiac output, hypotension, and cardiovascular collapse. The larger the tension pneumothorax, the more extreme the patient's symptoms and the greater the chance of cardiorespiratory collapse.

Signs and symptoms
- Profound tachypnoea; gasping for breath.
- Tachycardia.
- Acute respiratory distress.
- Altered conscious level: agitated, confused, uncooperative.
- Cyanosis.
- Decreased or absent breath sounds on the affected side.
- Hyper-resonance on the affected side.
- Hypotension.
- Surface trauma to the chest.
- Bony crepitus may be present in injury.
- Decreased chest wall movement on the affected side.
- Engorged neck veins, due to impaired cardiac emptying.
- Tracheal deviation, as the mediastinum shifts towards the uninjured side.
  - ⚠ This is a late sign.

Nursing assessment
▶▶ It is critical that patients in acute respiratory distress are assessed immediately and managed in an appropriate resuscitation area.
- Pulse.
- Respiratory rate.
- Blood pressure.
- SpO_2.
- Temperature.
- Cardiac monitoring.
- AVPU/GCS.

Nursing intervention
- High flow oxygen.
- Continuous monitoring.
- Preparation for needle decompression.

Management Immediate needle decompression (📖 see p.640) followed by chest drain insertion (📖 see p.604).

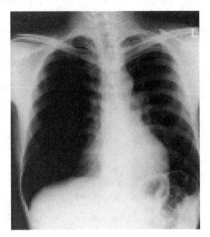

Fig. 7.7 A tension pneumothorax. (Reproduced with permission from Warrell, D.A., et al. (2005). *Oxford Textbook of Medicine*, 4th edn, vol. 2, p. 1519. Oxford University Press, Oxford.)

Haemothorax

A haemothorax is almost always a consequence of blunt or penetrating trauma, although occasionally it can arise from the erosion of a pulmonary vessel by a tumour.

- In penetrating trauma an intercostal, pulmonary, or great vessel is lacerated and the thoracic cavity fills with blood.
- In blunt chest trauma a fractured rib can be the cause of the lacerated vessel.

As well as the obvious respiratory compromise a thorax full of blood can cause, there may be profound hypovolaemic shock and therefore two life-threatening situations to deal with. One side of the thorax can hold 30–40% of the total circulating volume and, as the thorax fills, compression on the mediastinum and shift can occur. A haemothorax causing hypovolaemic shock is termed a 'massive haemothorax'. A 'haemopneumothorax' is the collection of blood and air in the pleural cavity.

Signs and symptoms
- Tachypnoea.
- Tachycardia.
- Respiratory distress.
- Pleuritic chest pain.
- Surface trauma to the chest wall or signs of a penetrating wound.
- Bony crepitus may be present in injury.
- Altered conscious level: agitated, confused, uncooperative.
- Cyanosis.
- Narrowed pulse pressure (see Box 7.6, p.197) as a consequence of shock.
- Decreased or absent breath sounds on the affected side.
- Dullness to percussion on the affected side.
- Hypotension.
- Decreased chest wall movement on the affected side.
- Flattened neck veins if shocked.
- Tracheal deviation as the mediastinum shifts towards the uninjured side. This is only present if the haemothorax is massive.

Investigations
- CXR: shows diffuse hyperdensity on the affected side.
- Blood for FBC, U & E, and urgent cross-match.
- Consider O neg/positive blood in massive haemothorax.

Nursing assessment
▶▶ It is critical that patients in respiratory distress are assessed immediately and managed in an appropriate resuscitation area.
- Pulse.
- Respiratory rate.
- Blood pressure, noting if the pulse pressure (see Box 7.6) is narrowing.
- SpO$_2$.
- Temperature.
- Cardiac monitoring.
- AVPU/GCS.
- Pain score.

Nursing intervention
- High flow oxygen.
- Continuous monitoring.
- Analgesia.
- IV access, two large bore lines in the antecubital fossa with IV fluid bolus if signs of hypovolaemic shock.
- Ensure blood has been sent for cross-match.
- Provide continuous support and reassurance as the insertion of a drains can be very frightening for the patient and stressful for the relatives.
- Assist with chest drain insertion (□ see p.604).

Management
A large bore intercostal drain should be inserted (□ see Box 7.5). A large drain helps to ensure that blood clots do not block the tube.

Box 7.5 Monitoring intercostal drainage

This drain requires close monitoring. If the drain collects 1000mL of blood following insertion or subsequently drains 200mL/h, an urgent cardiothoracic opinion is required and the patient may need urgent transfer for an open thoracotomy

---

Box 7.6 Pulse pressure

Pulse pressure is the difference between the systolic and diastolic pressure. Trends in pulse pressure are most easily detected when serial measurements are documented on a TPR chart. Changes in pulse pressure reflect physiological changes in the cardiovascular system. Systolic blood pressure reflects cardiac output, therefore if the systolic falls, cardiac output is lower. Diastolic blood pressure reflects systemic vascular resistance (SVR), therefore as the pressure that the blood exerts within the vessels falls, so does the diastolic.

A narrow pulse pressure occurs in the early stages of shock as peripheral vasoconstriction causes pressure in the vessels to increase causing a rise in the diastolic. A small elevation in systolic may arise as a consequence of this as 'squeeze' in the vessels increase cardiac pre-load and therefore cardiac output.

Flail chest

A flail chest arises when two or more ribs are fractured in two or more places . A segment of rib(s) is now no longer attached and the integrity of the chest wall is compromised (📖 see Fig. 7.8). Following blunt trauma a flail segment affects the patient's ability to adequately ventilate as the chest wall is no longer intact. There may also be an underlying pneumothorax, haemothorax, or pulmonary contusion. Significant alterations in oxygenation are more likely to be caused by underlying pulmonary contusions than the disruption to the mechanics of ventilation. Significant forces need to be applied to the chest wall to create a flail segment, e.g. high speed RTC or a fall from a height. However, with advancing age, osteoporosis, or bony metastases a simple fall can cause multiple fractures and a flail segment.

Signs and symptoms
- Tachypnoea.
- Tachycardia.
- Respiratory distress.
- Pleuritic chest pain, usually severe.
- Surface trauma to the chest wall: bruising; swelling; bony crepitus.
- Cyanosis.
- Decreased or absent breath sounds on the affected side.
- Decreased chest wall movement on the affected side.
- Paradoxical chest wall movement—the flail segment moves in the opposite direction to the rest of the chest wall with respiration (Fig. 7.9). This is not always apparent clinically as the intercostal muscles can splint the segment during the initial phase following injury.

Nursing assessment
- Pulse.
- Respiratory rate.
- Blood pressure.
- SpO_2.
- Arterial blood gas.
- Temperature.
- Cardiac monitoring.
- AVPU/GCS.
- Pain score.

Nursing intervention
- High flow oxygen.
- Continuous vital signs monitoring.
- IV access.
- Analgesia.
- Assist with chest drain insertion if indicated (📖 see p.604).
- Assist with intercostal nerve block if required.
- Assist with intubation (📖 see p.570) and ventilation if required (📖 see p.580).

Management Most patients can be managed with adequate pain control, which may require a thoracic epidural or intercostal nerve block. These patients are usually transferred to a high dependency area to enable their respiratory status to be closely monitored. A small number of patients will require intubation and ventilation. This is usually reserved for those who have persisting respiratory inadequacy or secondary complications despite the above management.

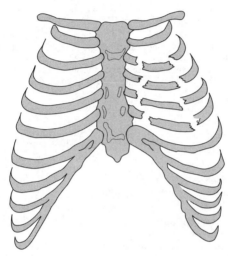

Fig. 7.8 Flail chest.

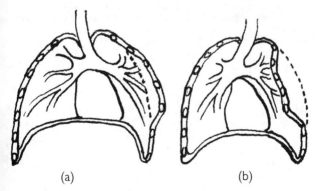

Fig. 7.9 Flail chest on (a) inspiration and (b) expiration.

Pulmonary contusion

When significant forces are applied to the chest wall these can be transmitted to the lung tissue and cause haemorrhage into the lung tissue. Pulmonary contusions vary in size. The clinical signs and symptoms listed range from mild to severe depending on size of the affected area.

Signs and symptoms

- Tachypnoea.
- Tachycardia.
- Respiratory distress.
- Pleuritic chest pain.
- Surface trauma to the chest wall: bruising; swelling; bony crepitus.
- Cyanosis.
- Decreased or absent breath sounds on the affected side.
- Decreased chest wall movement on the affected side.

Nursing assessment

- Pulse.
- Respiratory rate.
- Blood pressure.
- SpO$_2$.
- ABG.
- Temperature.
- Cardiac monitoring.
- AVPU/GCS.
- Pain score.

Nursing interventions

- High flow oxygen.
- Continuous vital signs monitoring.
- IV access.
- Analgesia.
- Assist with chest drain insertion if indicated (☐ see p.604).
- Assist with intubation (☐ see p.570) and ventilation (☐ see p.580) if required.
- Mechanical ventilation

Open chest injury

Open chest injuries develop as a result of penetrating trauma to the chest wall. An impaling object may still be present—do not attempt to remove this. In the case of gun crime an entrance ± an exit wound may be visible on the chest or abdominal wall or the over flanks. As well as damage to the thoracic content, the abdominal and retroperitoneal organs may also be damaged. Open chest injuries can cause haemothorax, haemopneumothorax, pneumothorax, diaphragmatic rupture, open haemopneumothorax, pulmonary contusion, and rib fracture. Signs and symptoms of respiratory difficulty ± hypovolaemic shock depend on the site and size of the injury and the involvement of other organs.

Nursing assessment

- Pulse.
- Respiratory rate.
- Blood pressure, noting if the pulse pressure (☐ see Box 7.6) is narrowing.
- SpO$_2$.
- ABG.
- Temperature.
- Cardiac monitoring.
- AVPU/GCS.
- Pain score.

▶▶ Observe the patient closely for the development of a tension pneumothorax.

Nursing interventions

- High flow oxygen.
- Continuous vital signs monitoring.
- IV access ensuring blood has been sent for cross-match.
- Analgesia.
- Temporary dressing.
- Assisting with chest drain insertion if indicated (☐ see p.604).
- Assist with intubation (☐ see p.570) and ventilation (☐ see p.580) if required.
- Mechanical ventilation.
- Prepare for urgent thoracotomy.

Cardiovascular emergencies

The heart

A basic understanding of cardiac anatomy and physiology is an essential pre-requisite for nurses assessing patients with cardiac-type symptoms. The adult heart is about the size of a fist and sits in the anterior thorax on the left side of the chest in front of the lungs. It is a muscular pump with four chambers:

• right atrium (RA);
• right ventricle (RV);
• left atrium (LA);
• left ventricle (LV).

The atria are the smaller, upper chambers of the heart and the two ventricles are the larger, lower chambers of the heart.

The heart is rotated about 30° to the left lateral side making the right ventricle the most anterior structure of the heart. The left ventricle is about twice as thick as the right ventricle because it needs greater force to push blood into the aorta and around the body while the right ventricle only needs to push blood through the lungs.

The heart has four valves.

• The tricuspid valve lies between the right atrium and right ventricles.
• The pulmonary valve lies between the right ventricle and the pulmonary artery.
• The mitral valve lies between the left atrium and the left ventricle.
• The aortic valve lies between the left ventricle and the aorta.

Healthy valves ensure that blood only flows in one direction.

Beating of the heart

Heartbeats follow a sequential pattern. Contraction of the atria (atrial systole) is followed by contraction of the ventricles (ventricular systole). All chambers then relax during diastole. Simultaneous pressure characteristics occur in the aorta, left atrium, and left ventricle through one cardiac cycle. The cardiac conduction system arises at the SA (sinoatrial) node and depolarizes through the atrioventricular node, the bundle of His, and the Purkinje system. Depolarization of the myocardium through this route generates a pulsed beat shown on an ECG as a sinus rhythm (📖 see Fig. 8.3).

The cardiovascular system

The function of the cardiovascular system is to transport oxygen and nutrients to the cells and remove carbon dioxide and metabolic waste products from the body. The right side of the heart pumps deoxygenated blood to the lungs where gas exchange takes place and then returns the oxygenated blood to the left atrium through the pulmonary veins (PV). The left side of the heart pumps blood to the rest of the body through the aorta, arteries, arterioles and systemic capillaries, and then returns blood to the right atrium through the venules and great veins.

The heart has its own blood supply via the coronary arteries. The left and right coronary arteries, which originate in the aortic valve annulus, branch into a network of arteries that supply both the right and left side of the heart. It is worth noting that the coronary arteries fill during diastole. Disease processes that affect the cardiovascular system can interfere with the body's ability to maintain tissue oxygenation and cardiac output.

The cardiovascular patient

Cardiovascular emergencies are a common presentation in the ED and the number of deaths from heart disease remains high. Most patients with chest pain arrive by ambulance but a significant number arrive by public and private transport. Any patient presenting with chest pain that appears to have a cardiac origin should have an ECG recorded without delay to ensure that a cardiac cause is either identified in a timely way or ruled out.

Typically, patients with chest pain of cardiac origin present with anterior wall pressure/discomfort, which can radiate to left arm and shoulder/neck and be associated with nausea and vomiting. (► Patients can present with pain radiating to either their left or right arm). ED nurses need to be mindful that patients who are having a cardiac event may present with atypical symptoms such as nausea and vomiting, shortness of breath, or generally feeling unwell. Equally, patients presenting with a cardiac event may complain of pain in the left side of neck, jaw, shoulder, or arm but no chest pain. These are not uncommon presentations of cardiovascular problems, particularly in diabetic patients, and failure to recognize a cardiac cause may result in possible treatment delay.

Cardiac problems are very frightening for the patient and family as mortality in this area is still high. Nurses need to demonstrate not only competence and speed but also empathy and understanding when caring for this group. Walk-in centres and minor injury unit must have the capability to respond to common cardiovascular emergencies whilst waiting additional emergency assistance. Equally, the ED may be requested to respond to an emergency in non-clinical areas, e.g. car parks, and as such portable equipment should be ready and accessible for such a response.

Preparation for cardiovascular emergencies

Being prepared is essential. Ensure all equipment necessary to assess the patient is ready and in working order. If the patient is being brought in by ambulance, a nurse and doctor should meet the ambulance as it arrives. Not only can they help the paramedics convey the patient into the ED while listening to the history, but it is also very reassuring for the patient and family to be met by medical staff.

Careful listening to the crew's hand over ensuring you understand their provisional diagnosis, treatment given, social circumstances, and, if available, the patient's pharmacological history is essential Do not be dismissive of the ambulance crew as you can miss vital information but also don't get sidelined by either a GP or ambulance provisional diagnosis—things change.

Assessment of the cardiovascular system

Use a systematic approach—follow ABCDE.

- A. Ensure a patent airway. If at risk summon help immediately.
- B. Record respiratory rate, rhythm, and depth. Note use of accessory muscles and abnormal noises. Record SpO_2 and administer O_2 therapy as indicated.
- C. Record BP, attach to cardiac monitor, and manually record pulse. Note pulse pressure—avoid recording rate directly from cardiac monitor. Obtain 12-lead ECG.
- D. Assess conscious status—consider AVPU or GCS. Note any limb weakness or altered sensation.
- E. Ensure the patient is undressed to enable a full assessment (remember to keep the patient warm). Record temperature. Don't forget to record blood sugar and correct any abnormality.

Obtain an 'AMPLE' at the same time as assessing the patient.

- **A**llergies.
- **M**edication—prescribed/over-the-counter/herbal/supplements.
- **P**ast (relevant) medical history.
- **L**ast meal.
- **E**vents leading up to admission; duration of pain.

Assess pain 'PQRST'.

- Provokes. What causes the pain/makes it better or worse?
- Quality. What does it feel like, e.g. sharp/dull?
- Radiates. Does it radiate/is it only in one place/did it start in one place and then move location?
- Severity. How severe on a scale of 0 (no pain) to 10 (worse pain ever)? Remember to assess how the pain was at its worst compared to now. (□ see p.648)
- Time. Time it started/how long did it last/when was it at its worse?

Nursing intervention

- Attach cardiac monitoring and record 12 lead ECG.
- Establish IV access and collect blood for FBC, U & E, clotting, and cardiac markers.
- Ensure pain relief.
- For acute coronary syndrome (ACS) consider aspirin and clopidogrel (unless contraindicated).
- Request chest X-ray if indicated.
- Reassure and offer support and comfort to the patient and family minimizing anxiety as much as possible.

ECG

ECG interpretation by pattern recognition is acceptable, but all ECGs must be reviewed by a clinician empowered to commence treatment within 10min of the patient arriving in the ED. Remember that the ECG cannot be interpreted in isolation—the key is always in the history. Ensure ECG leads are correctly placed and electrodes are attached to the bare chest—sweaty and hairy patients can cause difficulties. Dry, then clean the skin with an alcohol wipes. If required shave chest hair.

Precordial or chest leads

Attach the chest leads, which are labelled V1–V6. The correct positions for the chest leads are as follows (☐ see Fig. 8.1).

- V1. 4th intercostal space (ICS) right sternal border.
- V2. 4th ICS left sternal border.
- V3. Midway between V2 and V4.
- V4. 5th ICS left mid-clavicular line.
- V5. Left anterior anxillary line at the same horizontal* level as V4.
- V6. Left mid-axillary line at the same horizontal* level as V4 and V5.

* at right angles to the mid-clavicular line.

When recording an ECG on a female patient it is conventional to place electrodes V4–V6 under the left breast. Although it is acknowledged that attenuation of the signal does not change when electrodes are placed over the breast, there is insufficient published evidence to support this.

For further information see ☐ p.614.

Limb leads Fig. 8.2 shows the placement of the limb leads, which are either colour-coded or labelled:

- red lead—right arm (RA);
- yellow lead—left arm (LA);
- green lead—left leg (LL);
- black lead—right leg (RL).

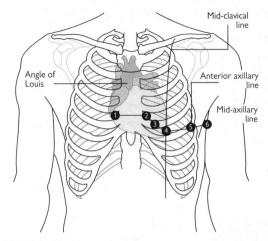

Fig. 8.1 ECG chest lead placement.

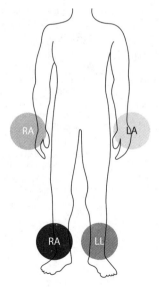

Fig. 8.2 ECG limb lead placement.

Interpreting the ECG

A systematic approach will enable the practitioner to identify normal ECG parameters and over time recognize abnormalities and their clinical significance (📖 see Table 8.1 and Fig. 8.3).[1]

- Is there any electrical activity?
- What is the ventricular (QRS) rate?
- Is the QRS rhythm regular or irregular?
- Is the QRS complex width normal or prolonged?
- Is atrial activity present?
- Is atrial activity related to ventricular activity and, if so, how?

▶ Remember: **all** ST segment deviation is abnormal until proven otherwise!

Reference

1 Nolan, J. (ed.) (2006). *Advanced life support*, 5th edn. The Resuscitation Council, London.

Table 8.1 Common ECG changes

ECG change	Possible cause
ST segment elevation	Possible STEMI I, II, III, aVL, aVF (1mm or 1 small square) and V1–V6 (2mm or 2 small squares) (NB. 2 contiguous leads required)
T-wave inversion	ACS (NB. 2 contiguous leads required)
ST segment depression	ACS (NB. 2 contiguous lead required)
Tachycardia (HR > 100bpm)	Numerous. Significance depends on haemodynamics and clinical history
Bradycardia (HR < 60bpm)	Numerous. Significance depends on haemodynamics and clinical history
Narrow complex tachycardia (HR > 100bpm)	Numerous. Significance depends on haemodynamics and clinical history
Broad complex tachycardia	Possible VT
AF (HR > 120bpm, irregularly irregular)	Numerous. Significance depends on haemodynamics and clilnical history. Consider infection, shock, dehydration, etc.
Irregular	Numerous. Significance depends on haemodynamics and clinical history
LBBB	Nearly always pathological in origin. Possible AMI
RBBB	May be normal. Significance depends on haemodynamics and clinical history (e.g. PE)

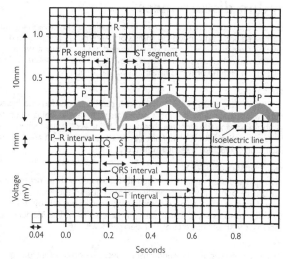

Fig. 8.3 Pulsed beat displayed on ECG (Reproduced with permission from Wyatt, J., et al. (2005). *Oxford Handbook of Accident and Emergency Medicine, 2nd edn*, p. 65. Oxford University Press, Oxford.)

Rhythm disturbances

These are commonly treated in the ED. Not all are life-threatening but they may require intervention or admission. Arrythmias are classified as originating from the atria or the ventricles and, while usually a symptom of more chronic cardiovascular disease, they may also present acutely in a young person with no previous history of cardiac problems.

Tachycardia

By definition tachycardia = HR > 100bpm. It can be subdivided into broad or narrow complex with the most common tachycardias being sinus or atrial fibrillation and the most life-threatening being ventricular tachycardia. Patients presenting with arrhythimias should be assessed in an area where resuscitation equipment is readily available.

Atrial fibrillation (AF)

AF is a rapid and disorganized atrial activity associated with an inconsistent ventricular response. It is increasingly common due to the ageing population. By definition it is a narrow complex tachycardia but it is often incorrectly referred to as supraventricular tachycardia (SVT). The incidence of AF increases with age but that of SVT decreases with age.

Acute causes

Acute AF may be triggered by underlying disease pathologies including:
- heart disease (failure, ACS);
- structural abnormalities (including mitral valve disease);
- substance abuse (alcohol, drugs);
- dehydration;
- medication-induced (e.g. 2° to digoxin toxicity);
- hypoxia;
- infection;
- pulmonary embolus;
- endocrine abnormalities (e.g. thyrotoxicosis);
- post cardiac surgery.

Chronic AF has numerous causes ranging from alcohol to thyroid malfunction although it is often idiopathic/age-related.

ECG diagnosis The ECG is irregularly irregular without organized atrial activity. Fibrillation waves are best seen in V1 (also V2 and II).

Treatment is designed to either slow the ventricular rate or to cardiovert the rhythm. The decision is based on the clinical condition (☐ see Fig. 8.4) and the duration of AF (< 48h or > 48h). Patients may spontaneously revert, particularly if underlying conditions such as dehydration, infection, or hypoxia are treated.

Nursing intervention

Utilize the ABCDE approach.
- Vital signs: temperature; BP; pulse; RR; SpO$_2$.
- Attach the patient to a cardiac monitor with defibrillator nearby and ensure serial ECGs.
- Assess pain and give analgesia and anti-emetic as prescribed.

- Request CXR.
- Establish IV access and collect blood for FBC, U & E (Mg priority), CK, troponin-I/T, coagulation screen, and thyroid function.
- Patients on digoxin: check digoxin levels.
- Consider the need for IV fluids (in absence of cardiac failure) to hydrate and correct electrolyte imbalance.
- Ensure the administration of other drugs as prescribed.

► Remember the patient may feel unwell and anxious—the need for empathy and reassurance to reduce anxiety is paramount

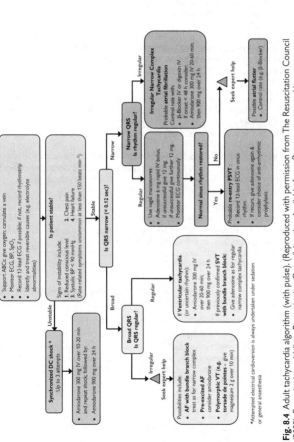

Fig. 8.4 Adult tachycardia algorithm (with pulse). (Reproduced with permission from The Resuscitation Council (2005). *Resuscitation guidelines*. Resuscitation Council. London. Available from ⏁ www.resus.org.uk)

Ventricular and narrow complex tachycardias

Ventricular tachycardia (VT)

VT is a clinical emergency requiring immediate medical review. Its causes are variable, but an acute cardiac cause must be considered in all patients. Treatment will be dictated by haemodynamic compromise (📖 see Fig. 8.4) and may require immediate cardioversion.

Diagnosing VT on an ECG

The following are common features of VT.
- Wide QRS > 3 small squares.
- Rate > 100bpm.
- Capture beats (a normal QRS within the VT) or fusion beat, which is a single bizarre beat not resembling the previous broad complex (the underlying rhythm and the VT are 'fused together').
- V lead concordance: all pointing the same direction (↑ or ↓).

Nursing intervention

These patients are very unstable as sudden deterioration is a risk with VT. The monitoring of BP/pulse is mandatory. If patient is compromised immediate cardioversion is required.
- A defibrillator must be immediately available and the patient should not be left unattended.
- All patients with VT should be admitted to a monitored area (typically CCU or cardiology ward) for ongoing management and close observation.
- During transfer the ED nurse must ensure immediate access to a defibrillator.

Common drugs used

Amiodarone is a commonly used anti-arrhythmic.
- Ideally amiodarone should be administered via a large vein as opposed to a peripheral line as thrombophlebitis can occur.
- Amiodarone may induce hypotension/bradycardia/heartblock. This risk is increased if administered fast or administered with other anti-arrhythmic agents.

⚠ Complex arrhythmias may be induced following an overdose. Specific management is required. There is **no** role for generic anti-arrhythmic therapy.

Narrow complex tachycardia

The term supraventricular tachycardia (SVT) has been superseded by 'narrow complex tachycardia'. Assessment and basic treatment is as for AF/VT—specific treatment is in accordance with local policy and the tachycardia treatment protocol (📖 see Fig. 8.4, p.213).

Treatment options

Vagal stimulation
- Should only be undertaken following specific training and with monitoring/IV access.
- Ask the patient if a specific manoeuvre has worked in the past.

- The most effective treatment is the Valsalva manoeuvre (raising intra-thoracic pressure) this can be performed by instructing the patient to attempt to blow out the plunger of a 20mL syringe. The rhythm will not change until *after* the stimulus has stopped.
- Carotid sinus massage is the least effective manoeuvre and is potentially dangerous (increased risk of embolic stroke) in the elderly. Record rhythm strip for at least 1min post-manoeuvre.

Adenosine

- Blocks the AV-node inducing temporary AV-block
- Adenosine has a very short half-life and must be rapidly administered and followed by a saline bolus.
- A rhythm strip of any rhythm change must be recorded.
- Adenosine can make patients feel unwell and may induce bronchospasm.

▶ Be careful to warn patients that they may feel unwell after adenosine but that this will pass quickly.

Cardioversion

Defibrillation and cardioversion share common processes especially regarding operator safety and paddle/pad position. The principal differences in cardioversion are lower DC energy selection, mandatory use of the synchronized function on the defibrillator, and patient sedation. For more information see p.594.

Bradycardia

Bradycardia is defined as a ventricular rate < 60bpm. Treatment is directed by adverse clinical signs (🕮 see Fig. 8.5). Remember that bradycardia may be normal in people who are physically fit.

Causes

- SA or AV node ischaemia, e.g. cardiac disease.
- Raised ICP.
- Pre-terminal hypovolaemia.
- Hypoxia.
- Vagal stimulus, e.g. vasovagal/faint.
- Drugs, e.g. beta-blockers.

Atrioventricular block

1st degree AV block is demonstrated by a prolonged PR interval (> 5 small squares/> 0.2sec). It doesn't require treatment but may indicate pathological disease. It can also be 2° to medication (e.g. beta-blockers and some calcium channel antagonist

2nd degree AV block is subdivided into Möbitz type 1 (Wenckebach) and Möbitz type 2. Both indicate AV node disease.
- Type 1 is demonstrated by increasingly lengthening PR interval until a QRS complex is dropped. It can be remembered by saying 'going, going, gone, and welcome [Wenckebach] back'.
- Type 2 is demonstrated by the loss of a QRS complex non-conducted P wave. This can be predicted (e.g. 2:1 block (2 atrial contractions to 1 ventricular contraction), etc.) or can be unpredictable. It indicates an increased risk of 3rd degree AV block or asystole.

3rd degree AV is demonstrated by disassociation between the atria (P waves) and the ventricles (QRS complexes). Ventricular rate is generated at the AV node or below. The width of the QRS complexes will be dependent on the site of the ventricular stimulus. Within the bundle of His, they will be narrow; below the bundle of His they will be broad. Generally, the broader the complex, the more unstable.

Treatment

Follow the Resuscitation Council treatment guidelines (Fig. 8.5) and treat the underlying cause.
- Atropine remains the most commonly used drug. It is particularly effective for narrow bradycardias but is unlikely to work in 3rd degree AV block.
- AMI can present with 3rd degree AV block either due to AV ischaemia (inferior AMI) or destruction of the bundle branch (anterior AMI). Prompt reperfusion is required to reperfuse ischaemic tissue and shouldn't be delayed in an attempt to introduce a pacing wire.
- External pacing is an emergency technique that can stabilize haemodynamically unstable patients. Patients will need to be informed that the procedure is uncomfortable even with sedation. (🕮 See p.592.)

If appropriate give oxygen, cannulate a vein, and record of 12-lead ECG

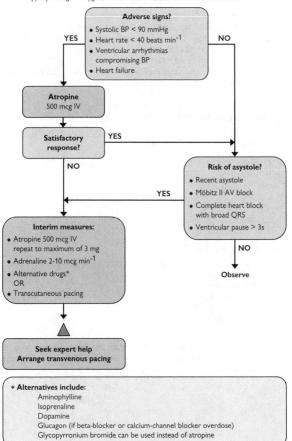

Adverse signs?
- Systolic BP < 90 mmHg
- Heart rate < 40 beats min⁻¹
- Ventricular arrhythmias compromising BP
- Heart failure

YES

NO

Atropine
500 mcg IV

Satisfactory response?

YES

NO

Risk of asystole?
- Recent asystole
- Möbitz II AV block
- Complete heart block with broad QRS
- Ventricular pause > 3s

YES

NO

Interim measures:
- Atropine 500 mcg IV repeat to maximum of 3 mg
- Adrenaline 2-10 mcg min⁻¹
- Alternative drugs*
OR
- Transcutaneous pacing

Observe

**Seek expert help
Arrange transvenous pacing**

* **Alternatives include:**
 Aminophylline
 Isoprenaline
 Dopamine
 Glucagon (if beta-blocker or calcium-channel blocker overdose)
 Glycopyrronium bromide can be used instead of atropine

Fig. 8.5 Adult bradycardia algorithm (includes rates inappropriately slow for haemodynamic state) (Reproduced with permission from The Resuscitation Council (2005). *Resuscitation guidelines*. Resuscitation Council, London. Available from ⌁ www.resus. org.uk)

Adult basic life support

ED nurses may be called to perform resuscitation procedures within the ED or within the community—the principles are the same.

- Cardiac arrest may happen anywhere in the ED. Resuscitate patient where they arrest; do **not** move to the resuscitation room.
- The ED may be summoned to emergencies outside (e.g. hospital car park). The priority is to instigate effective resuscitation. Do **not** delay moving to the ED.

(📖 See p.582.)

Receipt of a prehospital cardiac arrest

Confirm who is going to 'run' the arrest, e.g. the cardiac arrest team or run 'in-house' (according to local policy).

Nominated roles

- Team leader.
- Compressions/CPR
- IV access.
- Airway management.
- Defibrillation and/or drugs.
- Care of next-of-kin.

Ambulance crew handover

- Time of arrest/estimated downtime (this can be unreliable).
- Any bystander CPR.
- Drugs administered.
- Defibrillator shocks given.
- Any return of circulation.
- Special circumstances (e.g. overdose).
- Known past medical history

Transfer the patient to the ED trolley while the team leader takes the history. Compressions should not be interrupted. Attach monitor/confirm ETT placement or assist anaesthetist in intubation.

Advanced life support

 See Chapter 20, Defibrillation, p.608. Fig. 8.6 gives the adult advanced life support algorithm.

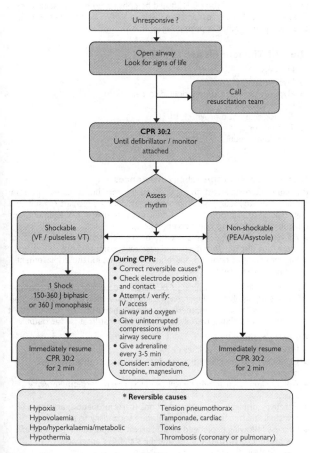

Fig. 8.6 Adult advanced life support algorithm (Reproduced with permission from The Resuscitation Council (2005). *Resuscitation guidelines.* Resuscitation Council, London. Available from ⌁ www.resus.org.uk)

Cardiac arrest

Causes of cardiac arrest

The most common cause of adult cardiac arrest is thromboemboli (AMI/PE) but the '4 Hs and Ts' (Box 8.1) should be considered in all cardiac arrests. These cause cardiac arrest and not just non-VT/VF as it's possible to have a tension pneumothorax presenting in VF.

Box 8.1 The four Hs and four Ts

- Hypoxia
- Hypovolaemia
- Hyper/hypokalaemia/metabolic disorders
- Hypothermia
- Tension pneumothorax
- Tamponade
- Toxic/therapeutic
- Thromboemboli

Cardiac arrest in special circumstances

Pregnancy Cardiac arrest during pregnancy is rare but requires significant modification to BLS. Physiological changes during pregnancy result in a high risk of aspiration, increased difficulties in airway management, and difficulty in performing chest compressions.

- All visibly pregnant patients need to be resuscitated whilst tilted 15° to the left to displace the uterus and ease caval compression.
- Higher hand positions may be required to adjust for the displacement of the internal organs.

ALS remains the same including ABCDE/early defibrillation with consideration of early intubation. Emergency Caesarean section ideally within 5min (> 23 weeks to maximize mother/fetal survival) should also be considered. At < 20 weeks the uterus is unlikely to compromise maternal cardiac output.

Poisoning/overdose

- May be accidental or deliberate.
- Consider the agent. Some are toxic to the rescuer (e.g. cyanides, organophosphates).
- ABCDE approach should be followed to prevent cardiopulmonary arrest.
- Effective compressions and ventilations (early intubation) are the principal treatments during resuscitation secondary to poisoning.
- Success following prolonged cardiac arrest is reported, regardless of the presenting rhythm, utilizing the 4 Hs and 4Ts approach.
- Identification of the poison may enable the use of an appropriate antidote (e.g. naloxone for opioids).

Trauma Cardiac arrest secondary to trauma has a poor outcome.

- Use normal ABCDE approach with aggressive and prompt treatment of injuries. These may encompass intubation, bilateral needle decompression, and bilateral chest drain placement, fluid bolus (± O negative blood) with compressions supported by adrenaline.

- Thoracotomy should be considered where there is a history of penetrating trauma. It is not advocated in blunt trauma.

Electrocution Relatively infrequent but potentially devastating multisystem injury.
- The normal ABCDE approach should be utilized with early defibrillation as required.
- Removal of clothing will reduce further burns and allow full inspection for tissue damage/burns/compartment syndrome and secondary injuries from falls, etc.
- Consider IV fluids if extensive tissue damage.

Asthma Cardiac arrest as the result of an severe asthma attack is often a terminal event. It is linked to bronchospasm, mucous plugging, tension pneumothorax and arrhythmias. Dehydration is also common.
- The ABCDE/early defibrillation approach should be followed using the 4 Hs and 4 Ts to guide management.
- Ventilation/compressions may be ineffective due to ↑ airway pressures.
- Early intubation assists with oxygenation.
- In tension pneumothorax needle decompression, if required, should be followed with a definitive chest drain.

Anaphylaxis 📖 See Shock, p.246.

Electrolyte imbalance 📖 See Table 8.2.

Drowning Standard ABCDE approach. Common cause of accidental death, typically due to hypoxia. ↑ survival if linked to hypothermia.
- Prolonged CPR should be considered.
- If possible, ascertain history (e.g. intoxication, head injury, chest pain whilst swimming, fell from a height) that led them to be in the water. (📖 see p.504)
- Consider ARDS for up to 72h.

Hypothermia Defined as a core temperature < 35°C.
- Standard ABCDE approach but pulse checks should be at 1min intervals and defibrillation is less effective with body temp < 30°C.
- Give initial shock then review strategy.
- Survival after prolonged CPR is possible.
- Rewarming required, ideally by cardiopulmonary bypass. If unavailable, warmed fluids, air, oxygen and bladder/gastric irrigation, or warmed peritoneal/pleural lavage can be used. Administer all fluids at 40°C.
  - During rewarming vasodilatation occurs requiring large volumes of IV fluids (📖 see p.504).
  - Active rewarming should be reviewed once body temp 32–34°C as active hypothermia may be beneficial in the comatose patient.

Massive PE is common cause of cardiac arrest (typically PEA)—diagnosis is difficult. Treat with bolus thrombolysis and heparin (at least 30 mins of CPR is required). (📖 see p.184.)

Table 8.2 Electrolyte imbalance in cardiac arrest

Possible causes	Likely presentation	Potential ECG changes	Treatment considerations
Hyperkalaemia Renal failure Drugs (ACE, ARB, potassium-sparing diuretics) Rhabdomyolysis Metabolic acidosis Endocrine disorders (Addison's disease) Diet	Weakness Flaccid paralysis Paraesthesia Bradycardia Ventricular tachycardia Cardiac arrest	Prolonged PR interval Flat/absent P waves Peaked T waves T wave greater than R wave ST segment depression Prolonged QRS Bradycardia Ventricular tachycardia Cardiac arrest	IV furosemide Calcium resonium IV dextrose/insulin Nebulized salbutamol Calcium chloride (protects the heart but does not lower K^+) Haemodialysis
Hypokalaemia GI loss Drugs (diuretics, laxatives) Renal dysfunction (tubular disorders, diabetes) Dialysis Endocrine disorders (Cushing's disease) Magnesium depletion Decreased dietary intake Treatment of hyperkalaemia	Fatigue Weakness Leg cramps Constipation Rhabdomyolysis Ascending paralysis Respiratory difficulties	U waves evident T wave flattening ST segment elevation Arrhythmias Cardiorespiratory arrest	IV potassium IV magnesium (replenishment of magnesium facilitates uptake of potassium)
Hypercalcaemia Hyperparathyroidism Malignancy Sarcoidosis Drugs	Confusion Weakness Abdominal pain Hypotension	Short QT interval Prolonged QRS Flat T waves AV block	IV fluids IV furosemide IV hydrocortisone IV pamidronate

	Clinical features	ECG / Cardiac	Management
	Arrhythmias Cardiac arrest	Cardiac arrest	IM calcitonin Review medications Haemodialysis
Hypocalcaemia Chronic renal failure Acute pancreatitis Calcium channel blocker overdose Toxic shock syndrome Rhabdomyolysis	Paraesthesia Tetany Seizures AV block Cardiac arrest	Prolonged QT interval T wave inversion Heart block Cardiac arrest	IV calcium chloride IV magnesium sulphate
Hypermagnesaemia Renal failure Iatrogenic	Confusion Weakness Respiratory depression AV block Cardiac arrest	Prolonged PR interval Prolonged QT interval Peaked T waves AV block Cardiac arrest	IV calcium chloride IV furosemide Ventilatory support Haemodialysis
Hypomagnesaemia GI loss Polyuria Starvation Alcoholism Malabsorption Drugs (diuretics)	Tremor Ataxia Nystagmus Seizures Arrhythmias (torsade de pointes) Cardiac arrest	Prolonged PR interval Prolonged QT interval ST segment depression T wave inversion Flat P waves Prolonged QRS Torsade de pointes	IV magnesium sulphate

Drugs for cardiac arrest and post-resuscitation nursing care

Drugs for cardiac arrest
📖 See Table 8.3.

Post-resuscitation nursing care
- Maintain airway. If not intubated nurse in left lateral position.
- Administer high flow O_2.
- Maintain neurological monitoring (If GCS < 8 patient needs intubation).
- Observe for any seizures as this may indicate cerebral hypoxia and possible raised ICP (an indication for intubation).
- Monitor rhythm/BP/pulse/respiratory rate/O_2 saturations, blood glucose, and temperature (haemodynamic instability may indicate need for inotropic support).
- Repeat ECG (changes to ECG must be immediately reported). Initial ECG may be undiagnostic. CPR is not a contraindication for thrombolysis.
- CXR
- Check U & E (to include magnesium), FBC, and clotting.
- ABG.
- Maintain accurate fluid balance and observe urine output.
- Cooling to a body temp of 32–34°C for neuroprotection.
- Confirm admission area/bed.
- Debrief the resuscitation team.
- Keep family informed and involved.

Cooling
- For 12–24h to minimize hypoxic brain damage (should be instigated in the ED).
- External cooling blankets, cold fluid bolus (4°C), ice packs to groin/axilla/forehead are initially effective.

Table 8.3 Drugs that may be used in cardiac arrest

Drug	Dose & rationale	Comments
Adrenaline	1mg every 3–5min. ↑ systemic vascular resistance during CPR, resulting in relative ↑ of cerebral & coronary perfusion	↑ cardiac oxygen demand; can be arrhythmogenic; avoid iin cardiac arrest; 2° to solvent abuse
Atropine	3mg (once only) for asystole or PEA pulse < 60bpm. Titrate 0.5mg–3mg for symptomatic bradycardia	Blocks effect of vagus nerve on SA & AV nodes. Side effects dose-related
Amiodarone	300mg for VF/pulseless VT. 300mg over 20–60min (use local protocols); then 900mg infusion over 24h. Use for haemodynamically unstable SVT/VT/ tachycardias (broad & narrow). Cell membrane stabilizer	Can be arrhythmogenic. Can cause hypotension/bradycardia. ↑ warfarin & digoxin plasma levels. Avoid using more than 1 anti-arrhythmic
Sodium bicarbonate	1mL/kg of 8.4%: typically 50mL. Use for tricyclic overdose; hyperkalaemia; correction of severe acidosis	ABG monitoring. Exacerbates intracellular acidosis. Requires ↑ ventilation. Has limited role—limit to special circumstances
Calcium chloride	10mL 10%. Use for hypomagnesia, hyperkalaemia, hypocalcaemia, & calcium channel blocker overdose. Has role in mechanisms linked to myocardial contraction	Has limited role—limit to special circumstances
Thrombolysis	As for AMI. Used if PE or AMI is suspected. Both have a thromboembolic component	CPR for minimum of 60–90min post-treatment

Chest pain: common causes

This is a common condition representing the largest patient group requiring medical admission. Diagnosis may be cardiac, non-cardiac, or benign. Chest pain is a very frightening experience for the patient and any patient presenting with this condition should be classed as urgent. Box 8.2 describes cardiovascular emergencies that may present with chest pain and Box 8.3 gives other possible causes of chest pain.

The type and nature of chest pain support diagnosis plus associated risk factors—beware of the atypical presenter. Triage nurses need to be alert to the atypical presenter as failure to consider a cardiac cause can delay treatment; Patients at greatest risk of being missed are the elderly, females, diabetics, patients with poor command of English, and alcoholics.

Box 8.2 Cardiovascular emergencies presenting with chest pain

Myocardial infarction
- Pain gradual onset although may suddenly become worse
- Band-like pain, tight/crushing/pressure
- Indigestion/epigastric ache
- Commonly associated with nausea and vomiting
- May radiate to arm/neck/back/shoulder
- May be associated with SOB
- Beware of atypical presentation plus isolated epigastric/back pain—inferior AMI.

Acute coronary syndrome Presentation as for AMI

Dissecting thoracic aneurysm
- Immediate onset of pain
- Severe and/or tearing
- Predominantly located in or radiating to the back and/or shoulder blades
- Disparity between left and right BP > 20mmHg

Pulmonary embolism
- Pleuritic in nature
- Tachycardic and hypotensive
- Dyspnoea, tachypnoea, and hypoxia
- Fever, cough, and haemoptosis
- ECG showing signs of RV strain or rSR in lead V1

Common pitfalls
- Pain relief with GTN does not exclude AMI.
- Normal ECG at initial assessment.
- Pain relief with antacids.
- Thinking that the patient is 'too young'.

Patients can describe cardiac pain as sharp (indicating intensity—not nature of pain), play down their symptoms, and present without chest pain but with confusion, collapse/stroke, back pain, isolated jaw/neck/arm/epigastric pain, and belching. Many patients perceive it as discomfort rather than pain. Some patients may deny chest pain but cite SOB as their reason for coming to the ED. SOB/confusion/collapse all indicate the need for an immediate ECG.

Box 8.3 Other causes of chest pain

Pericarditis
- Sharp in nature
- Aggravated by lying down, turning, coughing, and deep inspiration
- Associated with a fever, cough, and sputum
- Diminished by sitting up and leaning forward
- ECG shows saddle-shaped ST segments, often globally

Pleurisy
- Sharp in nature; worse on inspiration and coughing
- Can be precisely localized by the patient
- Anterior wall localization may be accompanied by tenderness of a costochondral juction

Pneumothorax
- May be acute/chronic
- COPD
- Tearing; increased by breathing
- Dyspnoea, tachycardia, agitated
- Decreased breath sounds, chest wall movement. Sudden onset of pleuritic pain

Musculoskeletal
- History of trauma
- Localized tenderness and worse on movement. (Pain of AMI can also increase with application of pressure!)

Oesophagitis/spasm
- Central chest pain/burning
- Possibly associated with belching (beware of atypical cardiac patient!)

Costochondritis
- Localized pain worse over costochondral junction and with 'springing' of the chest—beware cardiac pain reproducible with chest palpation

Shingles
- Intense pain—rash often not initially present
- Dermatome distribution

Chest pain: assessment and nursing interventions

Patient assessment

Patients presenting with chest pain should be assessed in an area where resuscitation equipment is easily accessible.

- Rapid assessment ABCDE/AMPLE/PQRST.
- Attach the patient to a cardiac monitor
- Record BP and HR every 15min in the 1st hour; then reduce to hourly if stable.
- 1st ECG <10min after arrival and reviewed by a clinician empowered to treat.
- Repeat every 15min in the 1st hour—each ECG is reviewed in its correct sequence. If ACS suspected repeat an ECG every 15min and if patient develops additional pain.
- Summon help if ST segment deviation is detected.
- Record temperature.

Nursing intervention

- GTN (according to local PGD) or as prescribed.
- Aspirin 300mg (unless known allergy) via PGD or as prescribed.
- Establish IV access and collect blood for U & E (including magnesium), FBC, cardiac enzymes, troponin I/T (according to local policy), blood glucose, clotting, lipids (for risk stratification). If tachycardic request thyroid function.
- Request CXR.
- Assist the assessing clinician in examination and assessment of patient.
- Reassure patient and keep the relatives informed.

Angina

Angina can be defined as pain or chest discomfort due to inadequate coronary blood supply to the myocardium. It usually brought on by exertion and the patient presents with central chest pain sometimes radiating to the jaw neck or back. Its onset may be rapid or gradual. Patients presenting to the ED may be experiencing their first episode of angina and be very fearful. Consider myocardial infarction in pain lasting >15min. Immediate ECG/cardiac monitoring is indicated.

Acute coronary syndrome (ACS)

The term ACS covers a spectrum of conditions including unstable angina, non ST elevation myocardial infarction (NSTEMI), and ST elevation myocardial infarction (STEMI). Predictable angina is *not* an ACS.

The most common cause of an ACS is the rupture of a lipid-rich atheromatous plaque within a coronary artery causing local coronary artery spasm and activation of platelets and fibrin to heal the local damage resulting in the formation of a thrombus.

This healing process results in total or partial occlusion of the coronary artery leading to myocardial cell death. The end diagnosis depends on the degree of damage confirmed with serial ECG and cardiac markers.

Unstable angina: diagnosis

Any condition that affects myocardial oxygen demand can worsen existing stable angina leading to unstable angina (□ see Box 8.4).

Unstable angina and myocardial infarction may be hard to differentiate initially so the assessment and early management is similar. Unstable angina is a medical emergency with a high 30 day mortality.

> ### Box 8.4 Conditions that can cause stable angina to worsen to form unstable angina
>
> - Anaemia. Hb affects O_2 delivery. Obtain FBC
> - Tachycardia, e.g. AF. ↑ myocardial O_2 demand
> - Hypoxia. ↓ O_2 delivery
> - Hypotension. Significant hypotension ↓ coronary artery perfusion
> - Pyrexia. ↑ myocardial O_2 demand—typically by increasing vasodilatation and thus HR
> - Valve disease. Aortic stenosis ↑ myocardial O_2 demand/workload. All valve disease increases the risk of AF
> - Multiple pathologies. A combination of systemic illness (e.g. pneumonia), pyrexia, ↓ oxygenation, and ↑ HR can combine to produce unstable angina

Symptoms
- Pain at rest.
- Pain lasting > 15min.
- Pain greater than patient's normal angina.
- Pain increasing in frequency/severity/duration.
- Associated SOB, nausea and vomiting, or other new symptoms.
- Arrhythmia or LVF.

Diagnosis
The initial diagnosis is based on clinical history confirmed by ECG changes and troponin I/T. A normal ECG doesn't exclude an ACS and traditional cardiac enzymes (CK or CKMB-mass) may be normal.

ECG changes in ACS/unstable angina (□ see Figs. 8.7 and 8.8)
- ST segment changes > 0.5mm =1/2 small square.
- T wave depression/inversion or flattened T wave.
- Significant T wave inversion can be indicative of a NSTEMI.

Normal lead II

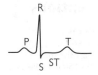

Ischaemic changes in lead II

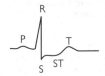

Fig. 8.7 ECG changes in ACS unstable angina (Reproduced with permission from Wyatt, J., et al. (2005). *Oxford Handbook of Accident and Emergency Medicine*, 2nd edn, p.67. Oxford University Press, Oxford.)

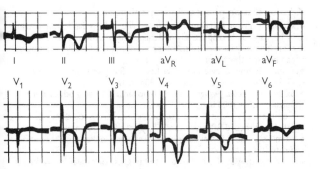

Fig. 8.8 ECG of NSTEMI (subendocardial infarct). (Reproduced with permission from Wyatt, J., et al. (2005). *Oxford Handbook of Accident and Emergency Medicine*, 2nd edn, p.73. Oxford University Press, Oxford.)

Unstable angina: management and nursing interventions

Immediate management
- Rapid assessment ABCDE/AMPLE/PQRST.
- Attach the patient to a cardiac monitor.
- Record BP and HR every 15min in the 1st hour; then reduce to hourly if stable.
- After repeating every 15min in the 1st hour, if patient develops additional pain this is an indication of potential instability.
- Review ECGs in their correct sequence.
- Summon help if ST segment deviation is detected.

Nursing intervention
- Supplementary as indicated.
- GTN (according to local PGD) or as prescribed.
- Aspirin 300mg (unless known allergy) by PGD or as prescribed
- Establish IV access and collect blood for U & E (including magnesium), FBC, cardiac enzymes, troponin I/T (according to local policy), blood glucose, clotting, lipids (for risk stratification). If tachycardic request thyroid function.
- Request CXR.
- Assist the doctor in examination and assessment of patient.
- Reassure patient and keep the relatives informed.

Administration of prescribed medications
- Opiate analgesia (draw up 10mg morphine or 5mg diamorphine, dilute in 10m and 5mL, respectively, and saline flush). Upwards of 15–20mg of morphine may be required. Anti-emetic if required (avoid cyclizine as can be arrhythmogenic).
- Aspirin 300mg (chewed then swallowed). Still give if on warfarin.
- GTN 400mcg unless systolic BP < 90mmHg.
- SC low molecular weight heparin (enoxaparin 1mg/kg bd) or heparin infusion (800–1000 units/h aPTT × 2 control).
- Commence IV nitrates as prescribed, increase rate to achieve pain relief, and record BP every 15min if systolic BP ≥100mmHg.
- Administer clopidogrel 300mg and oral beta-blocker (unless contra-indicated)
- Patient with ACS should be admitted to CCU or similar environment for ongoing monitoring/pain management and to ensure prompt response to clinical deterioration—arrhythmia or conversion to AMI.

Acute myocardial infarction: types and presentation

The different types of AMI are shown in Table 8.4.

NSTEMI The initial diagnosis, management, and admission are the same as for unstable angina. Formal diagnosis is made at 24h following ECG review and assessment of cardiac enzymes (e.g. troponin T/I, CK, CKMB). This type of infarct is becoming more common and care is required to ensure early identification and admission to CCU.

STEMI remains the single largest cause of death associated with CHD within the developed world. It is the end of a spectrum of disease following the same process as other ACS but involves total occlusion of a coronary artery. Initial management remains the same for STEMI as for ACS but the use of reperfusion therapy is a priority. Symptoms are the same as for other ACS but beware of atypical presentation.

Atypical/painfree AMI presentation

Symptoms of AMI do not have to include pain. Careful consideration should be given to patients who do not fit the classical AMI picture. Early ECG will help in making the correct diagnosis. There is an increase in mortality and morbidity associated with late diagnosis of atypical AMI. Patients can describe cardiac pain as sharp (indicating intensity not nature of pain), play down their symptoms, and present without chest pain but with confusion, collapse/stroke, back pain, isolated jaw/neck/arm/epigastric pain and belching. Many patients perceive it as discomfort rather than pain. Some patients may deny chest pain but cite SOB as their reason for coming to the ED.

Table 8.4 Types of AMI

ECG changes	Coronary artery	Comments
Inferior AMI ST elevation (≥ 1mm/1 small square) II, III, & aVF	Right coronary	Bradycardia, heart block, & AF. High risk for RV infarction & rupture of papillary muscle
Anterior lateral AMI ST elevation: I, aVL (≥ 1mm/1 small square); V1–V6 (≥ 2mm/2 small squares)	Left main stem or anterior descending	High risk for LV dysfunction
Anterior AMI ST elevation: V1–V6 (≥ 2mm/2 small squares)	Anterior descending or sub branch	High risk for LV dysfunction
Lateral AMI ST elevation: I, aVL (≥ 1mm/1 small square); V5–V6 (≥ 2mm/2 small squares)	Circumflex	ST elevation can be limited to I & V6
Posterior AMI (Fig. 8.9) ST depression: V1–V3 with associated ↑ R wave height. ST elevation V7–9 (≥ 1mm/1 small square)	Right coronary ± posterior descending	Record posterior ECG leads in all patients with ST depression V1–V3 regardless of presence of ↑ R wave height
Right ventricular Isolated ST elevation in V1	Right coronary	Record V3–5 (right-sided ECG) in all inferior AMI & hypotensive AMI patients

ST elevation in V1–6 can be diagnostic of an AMI at 1mm/1 small square particularly in V4–6 but the evidence base for treatment supports 2mm/2 small squares.

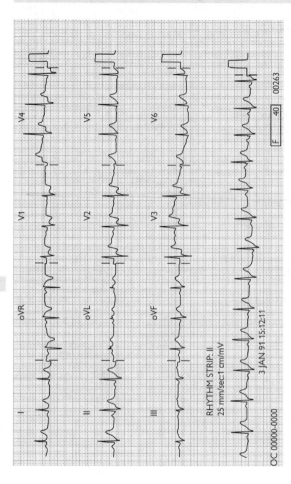

Fig. 8.9 Posterior AMI.

Acute myocardial infarction: diagnosis and management

Diagnosis

Diagnosis is based on the triad of:

- ECG changes (ST-segment/LBBB) in two contiguous leads ± reciprocal changes (□ see Figs. 8.9 (p.235), 8.10, and 8.11).
- Clinical presentation.
- Changes to cardiac markers.

Immediate interventions

Patients with a myocardial infarction can be extremely anxious, are likely to be in pain, and may have a sense of impending doom. They will need a calm and competent response from the nurse caring for them.

▶ Local policies and procedures should be followed in all instances.

- Opiate analgesia (draw up 10mg morphine or 5mg diamorphine dilute in 10mL or 5mL, respectively, and saline flush). Upwards of 15–20mg of morphine may be required. Anti-emetic if required (avoid cyclizine as it can be arrhythmogenic).
- Aspirin 300mg (chewed then swallowed). Still give if on warfarin.
- GTN 400–800mcg sublingually unless systolic BP < 90mmHg.
- SC low molecular weight heparin (enoxaparin 1mg/kg bd) or heparin infusion (800–1000 units/h aPTT × 2 control). *Note*. Heparin use will depend on choice of lytic (generally not used with streptokinase).
- Commence IV nitrates, ↑ rate to achieve pain relief, and record BP every 15min if systolic BP ≥100mmHg.
- Administer clopidogrel 300mg (unless contraindicated).
- Start oral beta-blocker (unless contraindicated).

Treatment

Primary percutaneous coronary intervention (PCI) or primary angioplasty

Primary angioplasty is increasingly the main or first treatment for patients suffering a myocardial infarction as it is the most effective way of re-establishing coronary artery flow, thus limiting damage to the heart muscle. It re-establishes coronary flow in more cases than thrombolysis but it needs to be delivered quickly or it may lose lose some of the advantages. There is also evidence of the longer-term benefits of primary angioplasty over thrombolysis but primary angioplasty facilities are still restricted to some areas due to resources. Where there is local/regional agreement patients suffering a myocardial infarction will be conveyed to the nearest PCI facility as opposed to the nearest ED. However, it should always be considered for patients in cardiogenic shock or for those for whom thrombolytics are contraindicated.

Preparation for PCI

Pre-treatment with clopidogrel 300–600mg and use of glycoprotein IIb/IIIa inhibitors may be requested prior to transfer. In addition, IV beta-blockers have additional proven benefit for reducing mortality.

During transfer, ongoing cardiac monitoring and access to a defibrillator and resuscitation equipment is essential. Analgesia may be required (IV nitrates and possible opiates). ∴ a suitable escort must go with the patient to ensure continuity of care and to offer constant reassurance to the patient. The family and significant others must also be kept informed of progress as this can be a stressful event for them as well.

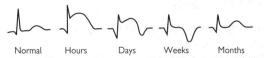

Normal   Hours   Days   Weeks   Months

Fig. 8.10 ECG changes following MI (Reproduced with permission from Wyatt, J., et al. (2005). *Oxford Handbook of Accident and Emergency Medicine*, 2nd edn, p. 70. Oxford University Press, Oxford.)

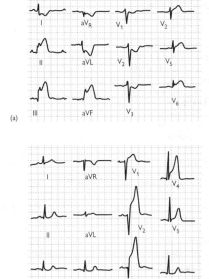

Fig. 8.11 (a) Acute inferolateral infarction with 'reciprocal' ST changes in I, aVL, and V₂–V₃. (b) Acute anteroseptal infarction with minimal 'reciprocal' ST changes in III and aVF. (Reproduced with permission from Wyatt, J., et al. (2005). *Oxford Handbook of Accident and Emergency Medicine*, 2nd edn, p. 71. Oxford University Press, Oxford.)

Thrombolysis for acute myocardial infarction

Thrombolysis is indicated where:
- symptoms of AMI< 12h;
- ECG criteria are met;
- no PCI availability;
- there are no contraindications (📖 see Box 8.5).

▶ Contraindications warrant immediate senior review for risk assessment and possible PCI.

Box 8.5 Contraindications to fibrinolytic therapy*

Absolute contraindications
- Haemorrhagic or stroke of unknown origin at any time
- Ischaemic stroke in preceding 6 months
- Central nervous system trauma or neoplasms
- Recent major trauma/surgery/head injury (within preceding 3 weeks)
- Gastro-intestinal bleeding within the last month
- Known bleeding disorder
- Aortic dissection
- Non-compressible punctures (e.g. liver biopsy, lumbar puncture).

Relative contraindications
- Transient ischaemic attack in preceding 6 month
- Oral anti-coagulant therapy
- Pregnancy or within 1 week post partum
- Refractory hypotension (systolic blood pressure > 100mmHg and/or diastolic blood pressure > 110mmHg
- Advanced liver disease
- Infective endocarditis
- Active peptic ulcer
- Refractory resuscitation

*Taskforce on the Management of ST-segment elevation, acute myocardial infarction of the European Society of Cardiology (2008). Management of acute myocardial infarction in patients presenting with persistent ST-segment elevation, *European Heart Journal* **29**, 9–45.

Thrombolytic agents There are two groups of thrombolytic agents: fibrin-specific, e.g. tenecteplase, and non-fibrin-specific, e.g. streptokinase (📖 see Table 8.5). Hospital policy should be reviewed as practice differs with some hospitals using only one type of agent for all patients (e.g. tenectaplase) and others using a combination of streptokinase and fibrin-specific agents depending on the location of the AMI.

Heparin for fibrin-specific agents (check local policy)
- 4000–5000 units IV bolus.
- LMWH, e.g. enoxaparin 1mg/kg bd (NB. max 100mg bd for tenecteplase in 1st 24h) or 800–1000 units/h IV adjusted to aPTT × 2 control.

Table 8.5 Thrombolytic agents

Drug	Administration	Comments
Streptokinase	Dissolve 1.5 million IU In 100mL of 0.9% saline and administer over 1h via infusion pump	High incidence of hypotension (20–25%) & anaphylaxis Slightly lower incidence of haemorrhage stroke, but less effective agent Doesn't require immediate heparin Can be given only once in patient's lifetime. Avoid if patient hypotensive. Consider a fibrin-specific agent for all anterior AMI
Tenecteplase	Weight-adjusted (increments of 10kg) single bolus agent. Given over 10sec	Requires heparin bolus pre-dose with infusion/SC doses post-administration
Reteplase	Non-weight adjusted twin bolus drug with doses given 30min apart. Given over 2min	Requires heparin bolus pre-dose with infusion/SC doses post-administration
Alteplase (rTPA)	Weight-adjusted infusion administered over 90min. Dose and rate dependent on onset of symptoms	Requires heparin bolus pre/post-administration Complex regime—has a specific role in PE

Nursing care/alerts for patients having streptokinase

Hypotension with streptokinase is common but is rarely 2° to anaphylaxis. Maintain meticulous monitoring of BP and pulse every 2–5min, initially for first 15min and then as the condition dictates. If the patient develops hypotension, do the following.

- Stop the infusion.
- Lie patient flat (if tolerated).
- Administer a fluid challenge 250–500mL 0.9% saline if required.
- Restart infusion at 50% original rate and increase once BP recovers.
- If hypotensive again call for medical assistance and review lytic agent.
- Treat true anaphylaxis with prompt IM adrenaline. Avoid steroids if possible due to increased risk of myocardial rupture post-AMI.

Indication of reperfusion

- The most sensitive/specific is 50% resolution of ST segment elevation at 90min post-thrombolysis.
- Pain-free (remember opiates given, etc).
- Arrhythmias (commonly idioventricular) also indicate reperfusion.
- Failure to demonstrate reperfusion is a medical emergency requiring immediate intervention.

Pericarditis

Pericarditis is caused by inflammation of the pericardium resulting in pain that may be associated with mild pyrexia and an audible 'pericardial rub'.

Causes

- AMI (Dressler's syndrome or large AMI involving atria).
- Bacterial or viral infection.
- TB (± HIV).
- Cancer (typically within chest cavity, e.g. lung).
- Rheumatic fever.
- Uraemia.
- Collagen disease (e.g. SLE).
- Trauma (e.g. fracture of sternum, cardiac surgery, or local radiotherapy).
- Drugs.

Signs and symptoms

- Patients complain of sharp retrosternal pain that is worse on inspiration, movement, swallowing, or lying down.
- Sitting forward/expanding the thoracic cavity may relieve pain.
- Pain may radiate or be localized.
- Tachycardia.
- A pericardial rub (like walking through snow) may be heard. Its absence does not exclude diagnosis.
- Mild pyrexia.

Investigations

- ECG, FBC, ESR, U&E, CRP, CXR, and, if in AF/flutter, thyroid function.
- Clinical history.

ECG (Fig. 8.12) classically shows concave ST elevation, which is widespread but in the early stages can be localized. T wave changes are possible (to include flattening/inversion) and PR segment depression has been noted. Careful history and ECG examination are required to avoid misdiagnosis, e.g. AMI.

Treatment is primarily pain relief with NSAID (aspirin 600mg or ibuprofen) and assessment for pathological disease. Consider echocardiogram.

Dressler's syndrome is caused by an autoimmune response to damaged cardiac tissue and consists of pericarditis, fever, and pericardial effusion. It can occur 3–14 days post-AMI/cardiac surgery and requires admission—ideally to CCU/cardiology ward.

Myocarditis is a medical emergency and can present similarly to AMI/pericarditis with ECG ST segment changes. Again the history is the key; myocarditis can be caused by bacterial or viral infection. Diagnosis can be difficult depending on severity but raised cardiac markers (CK/troponin T/I) mandate admission to CCU/cardiology ward.

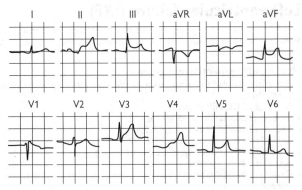

Fig. 8.12 ECG of pericarditis (Reproduced with permission from Wyatt, J., *et al.* (2005). *Oxford Handbook of Accident and Emergency Medicine*, 2nd edn, p. 77. Oxford University Press, Oxford.)

Left ventricular failure (LVF)

This is a common emergency with patients presenting with chest pain, SOB or in acute respiratory distress, anxious/agitated, and in some cases with a decreased GCS.

Nursing assessment/intervention

As for cardiovascular assessment with specific management guided by the patient's BP.
- Sit upright if GCS/BP allows.
- Give supplementary oxygen as required.
- Record 12 lead ECG, BP, pulse, RR, SpO_2.
- Gain IV access and bloods for U & E, FBC.
- Administer IV nitrates if systolic BP ≥ 100mmHg
- Administer IV furosemide.
- Opiates reduce LV pre- and after-load (ventricular stress) and decrease anxiety.

Hypertensive LVF

Patients presenting in LVF frequently have hypertension. These patients respond to aggressive management, which may include the following.
- Nitrates: initially SL GTN or 2–9mg subbuccal nitrates.
- IV nitrates are the main treatment. Record BP every 5min and titrate GTN according to systolic BP (aim for > 100mmHg).
- Administer IV furosemide.
- The hypoxic or tiring patient will benefit from CPAP (consider intubation).
- Nebulized β_2 agonist (bronchospasm is common but nebulizing β_2 agonist may increase HR).
- Treat underlying cause, e.g. AMI or fast AF.

All patients with LVF will require admission and physician review. Patients should be admitted to CCU.

Cardiogenic shock

▶▶ This is a significant medical emergency requiring immediate support from senior medical staff. Cardiogenic shock has a high mortality.

Causes are numerous with the most common being AMI with marked loss of LV function, development of a ventricular septal defect, or rupture of a papillary muscle. The most common chronic cause is decompensated heart failure 2° to a systemic illness.

Nursing assessment

These are very unwell patients who will appear clinically shocked.

Signs and symptoms

- Pale, cold clammy, and cyanosed.
- Severely hypotensive due to reduced cardiac output.
- Tachycardia to compensate initially followed by bradycardia and arrhythmias.
- Dyspnoea.

Nursing intervention

- Administer high flow O_2.
- Vital signs: temperature, BP, pulse, RR, SpO_2.
- Attach the patient to a cardiac monitor with defibrillator nearby.
- Record ECG. This may show ventricular ectopic beats.
- Assess pain and give analgesia and anti-emetic as prescribed.
- Request CXR.
- Establish IV access and collect blood for FBC, U & E (Mg priority), CK, troponin I/T, and coagulation screen.
- CVP access is desirable.
- Maintain strict fluid balance (urethral catheterization may be necessary).
- IV fluids may be needed but should be titrated to CVP and LV function.
- Ensure the administration of medication as prescribed, i.e. antibiotics, inotropic drugs.
- Offer reassurance and support to the patient and family.

Specific treatment

Depending on response to resuscitation, admission to ICU/CCU should be expedited for ongoing management.

- Treatment may include angioplasty or thrombolysis for AMI (angioplasty is preferred if available).
- Inotropic, nitrates, and vasodilatory drugs may be used to aid and support the cardiovascular system.
- Intraaortic balloon pump may be required to support the function of the left ventricle.

Shock

By definition shock is a combination of failure to perfuse and failure to oxygenate vital organs. Shock is a clinical emergency requiring prompt identification. Treatment must be aimed at the cause of shock and not generic 'blind' fluid resuscitation.

Types of shock

- Compensated shock. The body strives to meet oxygenation and perfusion and uses compensation mechanisms to achieve this: ↑ RR, vasoconstriction, and tachycardia. At this point BP is maintained with 'pulse pressure narrowing' as diastolic BP rises to meet systolic.
- Decompensated shock is the failure of the body to support perfusion. It is characterized by hypotension,
- Hypovolaemia may be due to loss of circulating fluid and not just from trauma, e.g. burns, dehydration.
- Pump failure. Typically cardiogenic 2° to AMI, although drug-induced (e.g. beta- blockers) and other causes should be considered.
- Distributive shock. Secondary movement of fluid due to vasodilatation primarily due to anaphylaxis or sepsis. It resembles hypovolaemia but fluid loss isn't visible. An early indicator of distributive shock is a widened pulse pressure as the diastolic BP decreases.
  - Neurogenic shock is another form of distributive shock and is caused by stimulation of the autonomic nervous system resulting in vasodilatation. This is often called spinal shock, although the same process occurs during 'fainting'.
- Obstructive shock is due to 'obstruction of blood flow', e.g. secondary to tension pneumothorax, PE, or cardiac tamponade.

Diagnosis

- The typical picture of tachycardia and hypotension is a late sign and indicates decompensated shock.
- Greater use of RR, capillary refill, pulse pressure, anxiety/confusion, drowsiness, and clinical suspicion is required.
- A key nursing observation is dizziness and/or drop in BP when the patient sits up.
- ABG monitoring of lactate (± base excess) can indicate degree of inadequate tissue perfusion.
- An increased early warning score can indicate shock.

Generic treatment

This is aimed at improving perfusion. Oxygenation and the treatment of underlying cause of shock are the clinical priorities.
- Administer high flow O_2.
- Fluid challenge and/or fluid resuscitation.
- Specific treatment dependant on cause of shock.
- Blood.

Fluid resuscitation

- Typically a 20mL/kg bolus of crystalloid (0.9% saline) is used to improve perfusion.
- Haemodynamic status post fluid resuscitation should be assessed.

- Fluid resuscitation has to be carefully managed: senior help is required.
- Over resuscitation with crystalloid will dilute the circulatory volume and clotting factors.
- Extreme caution is necessary in cardiogenic shock or shock related to dissection of AAA or penetrating trauma.

Recent evidence from battlefield resuscitation identifies the need for major trauma transfusion guidelines.

- Patients who are at risk of clotting problems through haemorrhage and fluid resuscitation should receive adequate FFP and supplementary platelets not just packed cells.
- Senior transfusion advice should be sought in fluid resuscitation in major trauma.

Septic shock is often missed in the early phases particularly in the elderly where hypothermia is a common symptom. If suspected, early intervention of senior medical support and ICU involvement is mandatory.

Treatment of septic shock is the same as for all types of shock but blood cultures and early administration of broad-spectrum antibacterial agents are vital .

▶▶ Do not delay antibacterial therapy if there is difficulty in obtaining blood cultures as even small delays in administration of antibiotics increase mortality.

Anaphylaxis

Anaphylaxis is caused by an adverse reaction to a foreign protein, its onset can be rapid or more gradual (min/h) (📖 see Fig. 8.13).

> The reluctance to administer adrenaline can be fatal.

Specific reactions

Respiratory Upper airway involvement is common. Systemic respiratory reactions such as lip tingling and tongue swelling are significant. Bronchospasm is common as the lung is sensitive to histamine. This can be particularly the case in those who suffer with asthma.

Skin A widespread raised red rash, itching, and angio-oedema. Widely dispersed skin symptoms indicate a systemic reaction.

GI tract Abdominal pain/cramps ± diarrhoea and vomiting are common and are due to reduced perfusion to the bowel and/or attempts to expel ingested foreign material. The risk of misdiagnosing food poisoning needs to be avoided.

Circulation Anaphylaxis results in distributive shock but BP may be maintained due to compensatory strategies. This often results in delayed administration of adrenaline.

Adrenaline

Administration of adrenaline is life-saving. It should be given immediately if the patient has any life threatening airway (stridor), breathing (bronchospasm) or circulation (shock) features. Adrenaline is administered by IM injection. IV injection is discouraged. Patients with Epi-Pens® will tend to self-administer before arrival. Additional adrenaline may be required.

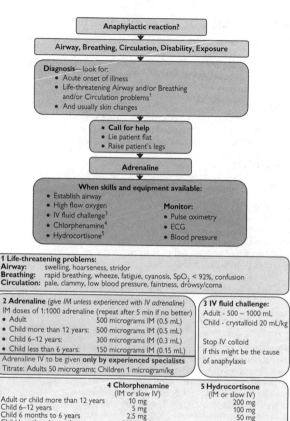

Anaphylactic reaction?

Airway, Breathing, Circulation, Disability, Exposure

Diagnosis—look for:
- Acute onset of illness
- Life-threatening Airway and/or Breathing and/or Circulation problems[1]
- And usually skin changes

- Call for help
- Lie patient flat
- Raise patient's legs

Adrenaline

When skills and equipment available:
- Establish airway
- High flow oxygen
- IV fluid challenge[3]
- Chlorphenamine[4]
- Hydrocortisone[5]

Monitor:
- Pulse oximetry
- ECG
- Blood pressure

1 Life-threatening problems:
Airway: swelling, hoarseness, stridor
Breathing: rapid breathing, wheeze, fatigue, cyanosis, SpO_2 < 92%, confusion
Circulation: pale, clammy, low blood pressure, faintness, drowsy/coma

2 Adrenaline (give IM unless experienced with IV adrenaline)
IM doses of 1:1000 adrenaline (repeat after 5 min if no better)
- Adult   500 micrograms IM (0.5 mL)
- Child more than 12 years: 500 micrograms IM (0.5 mL)
- Child 6–12 years: 300 micrograms IM (0.3 mL)
- Child less than 6 years: 150 micrograms IM (0.15 mL)
Adrenaline IV to be given **only by experienced specialists**
Titrate: Adults 50 micrograms; Children 1 microgram/kg

3 IV fluid challenge:
Adult - 500 – 1000 mL
Child - crystalloid 20 mL/kg

Stop IV colloid
if this might be the cause of anaphylaxis

	4 Chlorphenamine (IM or slow IV)	**5 Hydrocortisone** (IM or slow IV)
Adult or child more than 12 years	10 mg	200 mg
Child 6–12 years	5 mg	100 mg
Child 6 months to 6 years	2.5 mg	50 mg
Child less than 6 months	250 mcg/kg	25 mg

Fig. 8.13 Anaphylaxis algorithm (Reproduced with permission from The Resuscitation Council (2005). *Resuscitation guidelines.* Resuscitation Council, London. Available from ⏚ www.resus.org.uk)

Abdominal aortic aneurysm (AAA)

AAA is a major cause of death particularly in middle-aged/elderly males. Diagnosis is at times difficult particularly following sudden collapse. Triage nurses need to retain a high index of suspicion in middle-aged/elderly males with back or loin pain. Misdiagnosis of renal colic delays definitive treatment.

Diagnosis
- Abdominal/epigastric or back pain are classic signs and the presence of a palpable abdominal mass confirms the diagnosis if it's detectable.
- Rupture may present with epigastric pain radiating to the back.
- Abdominal ultrasound is helpful but abdominal CT provides the definitive diagnosis.
- The risks/benefits of haemodynamically unstable patients going to CT should be assessed thoroughly on a case-by-case basis.

Nursing intervention
- Administer high flow O_2.
- Assess BP, pulse, RR.
- Attach cardiac monitor.
- Obtain senior help immediately: surgeons and anaesthetists.
- Secure IV lines obtain U & E, FBC, group & save, glucose, LFT, coagulation screen.
- Order blood minimum of 10 units (follow local protocols).
- Maintain a systolic BP of 80–90mmHg using IV fluids (can be controversial due to risk of rupture).
- Assess pain and give analgesia.
- Request CXR and abdominal X-ray and obtain a 12 lead ECG.

▶▶ The priority is to move to theatre. Time in the resuscitation room should not delay transfer. Local policy may dictate that the patient is transferred to a regional hospital or that a vascular surgeon travels to the patient.

Cardiac arrest following AAA is either due to massive hypovolaemia following rupture and is rapidly fatal without surgical intervention or is due to parasympathetic activity following the tearing of the inner aortic wall, this responds promptly to atropine ± low-level fluids.

Thoracic aortic dissection

This is a tearing of the thoracic aorta and is classified as type A, involving the ascending aorta and/or aortic arch, or type B, involving the descending aorta. It is most commonly associated with hypertension and connective tissue disorders. The highest incidence occurs in individuals 50–70 years old with a male/female ratio of 2:1. In 96% of presentations pain is typically sudden, severe, and tearing in nature—radiating to the patients back. Severe hypotension on presentation is evidence of a poor prognostic outcome. Patients with types A and B can present with either hyper- or hypotension.

Investigation (to confirm diagnosis)

- CXR (this can be normal) may show pleural effusion, widened mediastinum, and/or calcified aorta.
- ECG. No specific changes associated with dissection but 30% of the time will show evidence of LV hypertrophy. A further 30% will be normal. ECG may show ischaemic changes if the coronary arteries are involved.
- Echocardiogram may enable type A to be identified.
- CTPA/MRI is necessary for a definitive diagnosis.

Nursing intervention

- Administer high flow O_2.
- Attach patient to cardiac monitor.
- Maintain frequent monitoring of all vital signs especially BP (beware a pseudohypotension due to involvement of the brachiocephalic and left subclavian arteries supplying the right and left arms, respectively).
- BP should be recorded for both left and right side. All pulses should be checked.
- Ensure the patient is given opiate analgesia and an anti-emetic.
- Secure IV access. Obtain U & E, FBC, group and save. Cross-match for at least six units and inform lab by phone of probable diagnosis.
- Assist in the insertion of an arterial line (see 📖 Chapter 20, 'Arterial line insertion and invasive blood pressure monitoring', p.578).
- Offer support to patient and keep family informed.
- Specific treatment involves BP control (e.g. IV beta-blockers) and advice from cardiologists/cardiothoracic team.
- Accompany the patient to theatre if surgery is decided on.

Deep venous thrombosis (DVT)

DVT is an increasingly common presentation in the minors area of the ED due to an increased public knowledge of the risks. It is difficult to diagnose leading to under- and overdiagnoses. The principal clinical concern is development of a PE.

Diagnosis

This is initially based on risk factors.
- Immobility (don't forget flights or chair/bedrest).
- Recent surgery (particularly lower leg/pelvis).
- Cancer.
- IV drug use.
- Smoking.
- Pregnancy/pelvic mass.
- Contraceptive pill.
- Overweight.
- Previous DVT/PE.
- Thrombophilia.

Clinical features

- Calf pain and local swelling are the classic signs of a DVT along with tenderness, warmth, and distension of superficial veins.
- Clinical signs also resemble those of cellulitis (which may coexist with a DVT), muscular injury, or ruptured Baker's cyst.

∴ clinical examination and history may be insufficient to exclude DVT. Final diagnosis is typically based on a combination of D-dimer with Doppler ultrasound/venogram and risk assessment, e.g. Wells criteria (Table 8.6). This will depend on local policy.

Treatment

Depending on risk, treatment may be started before formal diagnosis and with GP follow-up for ongoing management ± oral warfarin therapy.

Table 8.6 Wells score: a probability scoring system for DVT[*]

Clinical features	Score
Active cancer	+1
Immobile: paralysis, paresis, & plaster cast immobilization of a lower leg	+1
Recent bed rest > 3 days or post major surgery in past 4 weeks	+1
Localized tenderness along the deep vein system	+1
Entire leg swelling	+1
Calf swelling > 3cm compared to asymptomatic leg	+1
Pitting oedema—greatest in affected leg	+1
Non-varicose collateral superficial veins	+1
Possible alternative diagnosis is more likely than that of DVT, e.g. musculoskeletal injuries, chronic oedema, Baker's cyst, haematoma, superficial phlebitis, cellulitis	−2

[*] Risk stratification: high, > 3 points; intermediate, 1 or 2 points; low, < 0 points.

Musculoskeletal injuries

Introduction

Patients with musculoskeletal injuries represent approximately 25% of the ED workload.

These injuries may be simple fractures or can be life- or limb-threatening. ED nurses should be able to assess musculoskeletal injury and identify life- or limb-threatening trauma, some of which may not be immediately apparent. ENPs will be expected to assess, diagnose, treat, or refer many straightforward fractures.

This chapter differs from other chapters in that it takes into account that many patients presenting with musculoskeletal injuries and ailments may be managed solely by an ENP.

An understanding of anatomy is essential to accurate assessment of fractures and soft tissue injuries.

Anatomy

The skeletal system provides the shape and form for our bodies in addition to supporting, protecting, allowing bodily movement, producing red blood cells, and storing minerals. The human skeleton is divided into two distinct parts.

- The axial skeleton consists of bones that form the axis of the body, which supports and protects the organs of the head, neck, and trunk. These bones include: the skull, sternum, ribs, and vertebral column.
- The appendicular skeleton consists of upper limbs, lower limbs, and the pelvic girdle; the sacrum and coccyx are considered part of the vertebrae.

Internal organs are protected by the skeletal system and fracture of any bony structure may cause associated damage to soft tissue and viscera. Blood cells are produced by the marrow located in some bones. Fractures to long bones in particular can result in a significant loss of circulating volume.

Joints are the point where articulating bones meet, are encased in a capsule, and lubricated with synovial fluid. Joint movements are abduction, adduction, flexion, extension, and rotation.

Muscle Contractile tissue that attaches to tendon or bone to aid movement.

Tendon Fibrous tissue that connects muscle to bone

Ligament Fibrous connective tissue that connects bone to bone.

Fractures

A fracture is a partial or complete breach in the continuity of a bone. Fractures can be open or closed, displaced or undisplaced. They are also classified in relation to their anatomical location, e.g. proximal, distal shaft, head, or base.

Types of fractures include the following.

- Simple. Single transverse fracture of bone with only 2 main fragments.
- Transverse fracture at 90° axis of the bone.
- Oblique fracture at 45° axis of bone with only 2 main fragments.
- Spiral. Seen in long bones as a result of twisting injuries, twists around bone shaft.
- Comminuted. Complex fracture resulting in > 2 fragments.
- Crush. Loss of bone due to compression.
- Wedge. Compression to one area of bone resulting in wedge shape (e.g. vertebra).
- Burst. Comminuted compression fracture with scattering of fragments.
- Impacted. Bone ends driven into each other.
- Avulsion. Bony attachment of ligament or muscle is pulled off.
- Hairline. Barely visible lucency with no discernible displacement.
- Greenstick. Buckling or bending of immature bones; most commonly seen in children.
- Pathological. Fracture due to underlying disease (e.g. osteoporosis, Paget's disease).
- Stress. Certain bones are prone to fracture after repetitive minor injury (e.g. metatarsal).
- Fracture dislocation. Fracture adjacent to or in combination with a dislocated joint

Musculoskeletal assessment

In assessing patients with musculoskeletal injury always consider spinal injury and act to prevent further injury. ATLS guidelines should take precedence and life-threatening injuries should be dealt with immediately.

History taking should include the following.
• Recent trauma.
• Underlying orthopaedic condition.
• Relevant medical history.
• Current medications.
• Known allergy.

Ask about mechanism of injury, degree of force used, and how long the patient was exposed to the force. Inconsistencies between the history and the injury should raise suspicion of abuse especially where children or vulnerable adults are concerned.

Ask about and document pain or sensory loss—pain distal to the injury may suggest vascular involvement. Likewise any sensory loss distal to the injury may indicate neurological insult.

The five Ps

In assessing an injured extremity use the 'five Ps'.
• Pain.
• Pallor.
• Pulselessness.
• Paraesthesia.
• Paralysis.

Inspection

• Observe skin colour and note any bruising, abrasions, laceration, puncture wounds or critical skin.
• Note any deformity, swelling, or oedema around the wounded area and compare with uninjured limb.
• Observe for pain and the patient's ability to move the affected limb.

▶▶ If gross deformity, e.g. joint dislocation, get help immediately. This is an orthopaedic emergency.

Palpation Carefully palpate injured area to assess skin temperature, specific areas of pain, feel for pulses, and assess capillary refill. Absence of pulses or sensation, particularly if distal to injury, suggests neurovascular compromise. Crepitus may be felt with movement of the injured limb.

▶▶ If neurovascular compromise is identified, get help immediately.

Nursing interventions

Life-threatening features must be dealt with prior to limb-threatening features. General nursing management of musculoskeletal injuries should focus on the following.
• Pain. Immobilizing the area may give initial relief but opiate analgesia is usually indicated in bony injuries. Administer prescribed analgesia and evaluate effect.

- Vital signs. Record BP, pulse rate, respiration rate, temperature, oxygen saturation. If history of dizziness or blackout prior to injury, record ECG and capillary blood glucose.
- Establish IV access and blood tests for FBC, U & E, coagulation studies, and group and save. Commence infusion of fluids as prescribed and chart accordingly.
- Immobilization. Various splints may be used but vascular status needs to be established prior to application, and access to pulse points must be assured for ongoing monitoring. Where there is no apparent neuro-vascular injury the injured limb should be immobilized in its presenting position.
- Elevation of the injured limb aids venous return and helps to minimize swelling.
- Removal of jewellery or tight clothing. If jewellery needs to be cut off, where possible, gain written consent from patient or relative.

Additional interventions

- Where appropriate the assessing nurse should request X-rays.
- Any open wounds should be covered with sterile dressings until they can be thoroughly aseptically cleaned.
- Patients who have open fractures should be given IV antibiotics. Ensure medications are given as prescribed.
- Patient's tetanus status should be established and, where there is doubt, a booster given (🕮 see Box 9.2, p.313).
- Assist with manipulation of fracture and the application of plaster cast or traction.
- Ensure pressure area care for vulnerable patients (assess Waterlow score).
- Reassure and comfort patient and keep relatives informed.

Spinal fractures

The spinal cord is vulnerable and may be injured as a consequence of the fracture sustained or may be at risk of additional injury if not carefully handled following trauma. Nurses caring for any patient who has sustained trauma should act to immobilize the C-spine where the history, signs, or symptoms suggest possible spinal injury. It should also be borne in mind that people with degenerative conditions, such as osteoporosis, neoplasm, or other underlying conditions that affect bone, can sustain fractures with minimal trauma or even through normal activity. The commonest spinal injuries occur in the C-spine and at the thoracolumbar junction.

Most patients with a C-spine injury are young with approximately 80% of patients aged 18–25 years. Males are 4 times more likely to sustain this injury than females. These patients are most likely to be brought to the ED by ambulance but may self present.

Patients with vertebral fractures secondary to trauma should be evaluated and treated in a systematic way in line with ATLS principles. Initial priorities are twofold: attention should be focused toward the patient's airway, breathing, and circulation (ABC) while simultaneously adhering to C-spine precautions. Common findings on physical examination in C-spine injury may include the following:

- spinal shock;
- flaccidity;
- arreflexia;
- loss of anal sphincter tone;
- faecal incontinence;
- priapism;
- loss of bulbocavernosus reflex;
- neurogenic shock;
- hypotension;
- paradoxical bradycardia;
- flushed, dry, and warm peripheral skin;
- autonomic dysfunction;
- ileus;
- urinary retention;
- poikilothermia.

Specific nursing points to remember with spinal injury

- Immobilize the C-spine by placing one hand on either side of the patient's head and maintaining alignment with the rest of the body. Give the patient 100% oxygen and perform simple airway opening manoeuvres if airway is not open, whilst maintaining in line immobilization of C-spine Apply a hard collar, with head blocks and tape. Attach patient to oxygen saturation monitor.
- Observe the breathing pattern, bearing in mind that cord ischaemia/oedema can compromise breathing. Observe for diaphragmatic breathing and the use of accessory muscles of respiration.
- Insert two wide bore cannulae and commence IV fluids as prescribed and collect blood samples as needed.
- Record an ECG. Initiate ongoing monitoring of BP being mindful that hypotension may indicate hypovolaemia or neurogenic shock.

- A full neurological examination will be performed as part of the expanded primary survey or secondary survey. Assist the clinician in examining the pelvic areas, perineal areas, and extremities. Consider the need for a urinary catheter.
- A rectal examination is indicated, especially if the patient has weakness in the extremities. A full explanation should be given before this is carried out. Assist in log rolling the patient to examine the spine and rectum. Remove spinal board if it has not already been removed.
- Reassure patient constantly and ensure privacy and dignity. Keep relatives informed.
- Keep the patient warm.

Incomplete cord injury patterns

Anterior spinal cord syndrome This is usually a result of compression of the artery that runs along the front of the spinal cord. These patients usually have complete loss of strength below the level of injury. Sensory loss is incomplete. Generally, sensitivity to pain and temperature is lost while sensitivity to vibration and proprioception is preserved.

Posterior cord syndrome Injury to the posterior cord. Preservation of motor function, sense of pain and light touch, with loss of proprioception below the level of lesion.

Brown–Sequard syndrome This is incomplete spinal cord injury caused by hemisection of the cord. This results in loss of motor function, proprioception, on side of lesion and loss of sense of pain and temperature on opposite side.

Central cord syndrome This is an incomplete spinal cord injury resulting in greater neurological involvement in the upper extremities than in the lower extremities.

Fractures of the thoracic and lumbar spine

These are classified according to the pattern of injury.

- Compression fracture: the anterior aspect. The vertebra breaks and loses height. This type of fracture is usually stable and rarely associated with neurological problems.
- Axial burst fracture: often caused by a fall from height with the patient landing on his feet.
- Flexion/distraction fracture. The vertebra is literally pulled apart such as in a head-on car crash in which the upper body is thrown forward while the pelvis is stabilized by the seat belt.
- Transverse process fracture. This type of fracture results from rotation or extreme sideways bending and usually does not affect stability.
- Fracture dislocation. This is an unstable injury involving bone and/or soft tissue in which one vertebra may become displaced from the adjacent one.

Treatment is aimed at protecting nerve function and restoring alignment and stability of the spine. Compression fractures and some burst fractures are treated conservatively. Some injuries such as an unstable burst fracture, flexion-distraction injury, or fracture-dislocation may require surgical intervention. Surgery realigns the spinal column and holds it together using metal plates and screws (internal fixation) and/or spinal fusion.

Torticollis

Torticollis is an acquired condition where the neck appears to be in a twisted or bent position. It is caused by involuntary contractions of the neck muscles, leading to abnormal postures and movements of the head. If there is a history of trauma refer patient for a full clinical assessment.

If there is no trauma, exclude neurological signs and symptoms.

• Reassure patient.
• Advise on analgesia.
• Refer to physiotherapy.

Traumatic neck sprain (whiplash)

Whiplash is a common presentation in the ED. It occurs when the soft tissues in the neck are strained as a result of a sudden jerk. It most commonly occurs after RTCs but can also occur in sporting accidents.

History and examination

If there is significant mechanism of injury, e.g. fall from a height, axial loading, injury etc., or there are abnormal neurological signs, i.e. numbness or paraesthesia, or if there is cervical bony tenderness or marked pain in the midline, immobilize C-spine and refer immediately. In the absence of any of the above signs or symptoms:

- Analgesia and NSAIDs.
- Encourage the patient to resume normal routine as soon as possible.
- Refer to physiotherapy.
- Be meticulous in documenting findings as these injuries are often the subject of insurance claims.

High risk features

- Significant mechanism of injury
- Tenderness over spinous process.
- Neurological signs and symptoms.
- Severe pain.
- Holding own head.

If these features are present immobilize and refer for immediate medical assessment.

▶ Whiplash is a diagnosis after significant inury has been ruled out. Formal rules for C-spine clearance should be used to assess the need for X-ray. (📖 see p.606)

Shoulder and clavicle injuries

Clavicle fractures

Most clavicle fractures can be treated conservatively often requiring simple analgesia, broad arm sling, and orthopaedic follow-up. Occasionally, when there is severe displacement to the clavicle or tenting to the skin, orthopaedic intervention may be required.

Shoulder injuries

Dislocation of the shoulder is common in adults. This follows an injury that is compatible with shoulder displacement e.g. fall on to outstretched arm. Anterior dislocation is more common than posterior. Consider posterior dislocation if the mechanism of injury is attributed to a fit or a direct blow to the shoulder. Diagnosis can often be made clinically as the patient will have severe pain in their shoulder, holding their arm to their chest at the elbow.

On examination the contours of the shoulder appear different and less defined. Careful examination for the integrity of the axillary nerve must be made, assessing sensation to touch and pinprick over the 'regimental badge area' (the lateral aspect of the proximal humerus), and assessing the integrity of the radial nerve looking for wrist drop.

Patients with a dislocated shoulder should be given analgesia, and encouraged to relax. An X-ray should be taken to confirm diagnosis.

▶ Be aware that posterior dislocations are reasonably hard to diagnose so always seek senior support if you are uncertain.

Reduction of shoulder dislocations

- There are three common methods used to reduce shoulder dislocations: the Kocher's; Hippocratic; and using gravitational traction.
- The key to reduction is good analgesia and adequate sedation to ensure compliance.
- Post-reduction neurovascular examination must be carried out to ensure no entrapment of the axillary nerve has occurred during the reduction procedure.
- Post-reduction films should be taken.
- It is important to note that humeral head fractures can be a complication of overenthusiastic reduction procedures so proceed with caution.

Evidence suggests that immobilization of the limb in a collar and cuff for 3 weeks is beneficial. The patient should be referred to the fracture clinic for follow-up.

Acromioclavicular joint (ACJ) injury

These are reasonably common injuries associated with a fall or a heavy blow directly to the shoulder. Occasionally they result from a fall on to an outstretched hand. The patient will complain of pain and tenderness directly over the ACJ. On examination there is normally a step deformity over the ACJ with a marked loss of mobility. ACJ injuries are classified into 3 groups:

- minimal separation between the clavicle and the acromion;
- obvious subluxation of the joint;
- complete dislocation of the ACJ.

Treatment involves good analgesia and a broad arm sling. Patient advice should be given re shoulder exercise. Often physiotherapy follow-up can be helpful. For the more severe joint disruption injuries an orthopaedic opinion should be obtained.

Soft tissue shoulder injuries

Soft tissue shoulder problems are a common presentation in the ED as they can be very painful restricting daily activity. Nurses should be cautious in their assessment of shoulder problems bearing in mind that the shoulder is a complex joint and vulnerable to injury due to its wide range of movement.

The rotator cuff muscles consist of:

- supraspinatus;
- infraspinatus;
- subscapularis.
- teres minor.

These muscles strengthen the shoulder capsule and prevent dislocation. Disease/injuries to the rotator cuff apparatus can be due to degeneration (old age), trauma (impingement of supraspinatus), or acute calcification.

Minor rotator cuff strains occur commonly in athletes. They usually present with a 'twinge' felt in the shoulder area and show limitation in function.

Treatment is rest, ice, analgesia, then exercise and physiotherapy. If untreated, there is a risk of muscle thickening and scarring that may predispose the patient to rotator cuff tear. Complete and partial tears are more frequently seen in older patients caused by a process of degeneration within the tendon.

Patients complain of pain on specific ROM (range of motion) and of being unable to lie on that side.

Acute tendinitis/acute calcification Deposits of calcium hydroxyapatite appear on the tendon of supraspinatus muscle. This causes acute vascular reaction, swelling, and pain.

- History: acute pain worsening over days, then gradually resolving.
- X-ray may show calcification on the supraspinatus tendon.
- Treatment: NSAIDs or perhaps none as pain subsides over several days.

Adhesive capsulitis 'frozen shoulder' This is a spontaneous onset of pain and sensitization of the shoulder, caused by inflammation of the glenohumeral joint and its surrounding capsule. It sometimes follows an injury. There is pain and severe limitation of all movements. It also occurs after a stroke and is more common in people with diabetes.

Subacromial bursitis Inflammation of subacromial bursa. There is pain and weakness when the arm is abducted through a 60° arc and pain on deep palpation.

- If it is the tendon that is injured rather than the bursa, there is likely to be more pain when the arm is abducted against resistance.
- Treatment is rest, ice, and analgesia. NSAIDs may be helpful.

Upper limb injuries

Rupture of the long head of the biceps The tendon may rupture with activity involving the biceps muscle. Patient gives a history of sharp pain and tearing sensation. Despite obvious deformity ('Popeye sign'), which increases with contraction of biceps, the biceps strength is often maintained. Treatment is rest, ice, NSAIDs and physiotherapy. Complete tears require orthopaedic referral.

Bicipital tendinitis often occurs as a result of injury, overuse, or with ageing as the tendon loses elasticity. Bicipital tendinitis is a fairly common complaint of swimmers, rowers, throwers, golfers, and weight lifters. The patient complains of pain and tenderness along bicipital groove. The pain is worse with movement or activity and at night.

Humeral shaft fractures

❶ Any injured limb should be assessed for the presence of the 'five Ps' that might indicate neurovascular compromise:
- pain
- pallor
- pulselessness
- paraesthesia
- paralysis

Fractures to the neck and shaft of the humerus are more common in older females due to osteoporosis. The integrity of the radial nerve should be assessed.
- If any deficit or displacement is found the patient should be referred to the orthopaedic team immediately.
- If the fracture is minimally displaced and there is no neurological deficit, place in a collar and cuff and refer to fracture clinic.
- Severe angulation or displacement of the humeral head should be referred to the orthopaedic team.
- The practitioner assessing the patient should be aware that humeral fractures have been associated with elder abuse and a careful history must be taken to determine how the injury has occurred.

Elbow injuries

Elbow injuries are a common presentation in the ED. Full range of movement usually excludes serious injury. A recent study[1] suggests that, if a patient has normal extension, flexion, and supination, they do not require emergency elbow radiographs.

Supracondylar humeral fracture

This is relatively rare in adults. Such fractures often result from a fall on to an outstretched hand.

- Assess the neurovascular status of the limb. Give special consideration to the integrity of the radial and median nerve as well as the brachial artery.
- Normally, the arm is very swollen and deformed around the elbow.
- On initial assessment, give analgesia, place the patient in a comfortable position, and request an X-ray.
- Most patients will require further intervention and MUA.
- Place in an above-elbow back slab and refer to the orthopaedic team.

Dislocated elbow

Elbow dislocation, which is normally associated with significant force, will be obvious on examination, as there will be significant loss of the normal triangular contours between the olecranon and epicondyles.

- Make the patient comfortable, give IV analgesia, and request an X-ray.
- Carry out neurovascular observations throughout.
- Obtain senior support as this will need urgent reduction under controlled conditions.

Olecranon bursitis

There are many causes of olecranon bursitis, but the main causes are either direct trauma or infection.

- Most cases settle without any treatment—simple analgesia and rest normally suffice.
- If there are signs of infection, treat with appropriate antibiotics. (Follow local guidance for antibiotic use.)
- Very occasionally, if infection is severe, orthopaedic intervention is needed.

Epicondylitis Commonly know as 'tennis elbow' or 'golfer's elbow', this results from overuse/strain of the common tendinous insertions of the extrinsic extensor and flexor muscles of the lateral and medial epicondyles of the humerus. Treatment includes analgesia, rest, and supportive measures. If symptoms persist, physiotherapy and referral to a soft tissue clinic for steroid injections may be required.

Reference

1 Lennon, R.I., et al. (2007). Can a normal range of elbow movement predict a normal elbow x ray? *Emergency Medicine Journal* **24**: 86–8.

Radial head fractures

Radial head fractures are usually caused by a fall on to the outstretched hand. The patient may complain of pain on pronation and supination of the forearm. Fractures may not be obvious on X-ray but evidence of an effusion (fat pad sign) is indicative of a bony injury. Loss of full extension of the forearm is also suspicious of a fracture. Treatment is collar and cuff or broad arm sling, analgesia, and follow-up in fracture clinic. If there is significant angulation, seek orthopaedic opinion.

Radial/ulna shaft fractures

These fractures cause significant deformity or angulation to the forearm. They require immediate assessment and analgesia. Ensure no neurovascular deficit and place the arm in a broad arm sling or rest on a pillow. Refer to X-ray. Always ensure X-rays are taken of the whole forearm thus ensuring that Monteggia and Galeazzi fractures are not missed. It is important to note that in adults neurovascular injury is common. These patients will require referral to an orthopaedic surgeon.

- A Monteggia fracture is a fracture of the ulna with an associate dislocation of the radial head within the elbow joint.
- A Galeazzi fracture is a fracture of the radius with an associated injury to the distal radio-ulnar joint of the wrist.

Wrist injuries

Fractures within the wrist are often associated with falls on the out-stretched hand (FOOSH) and are often age-dependent.

- < 10 years: often present with green stick/ buckle fractures with transverse fractures through the metaphysis.
- 10–16 years: associated with fracture through the epiphysis, usually Salter–Harris II fracture (🕮 see Fig. 4.7, p.101).
- 17–40 years: more likely to be scaphoid fracture.
- Over-40s: more likely to present with a Colles' or Smith's fracture.

Colles' fractures

Usually associated with obvious clinical signs: the wrist is often deformed and swollen; the patient is unable to pronate or supinate their wrist; and is in a great deal of discomfort or pain.

- Give analgesia.
- Place the wrist in a broad arm sling.
- Carry out neurovascular observations.
- Send the patient to X-ray.
  - This fracture is associated with dorsal angulation, which produces the classical ' dinner fork deformity' on the lateral view. It is normally associated with an avulsion of the ulna styloid process.

If displaced or if there is notable impaction, manipulation under local anaesthetic with sedation and analgesia is often required.

- Manipulation under local anaesthetic is usually conducted using either a haematoma or Bier's block.
  - This procedure must be carried out in a controlled environment. An ECG and consent must be obtained before the procedure.
  - If a Bier's block is the procedure of choice two doctors must be present.
- Apply a back slab and take a post-reduction X-ray.
- If the fracture is successfully reduced, the patient may be discharged and followed up in the fracture clinic.

Undisplaced fractures can be treated conservatively with a dorsal back slab and follow-up in the fracture clinic.

Smith's fractures of the wrist are associated with a palmar or volar angulation of the distal radius. They often require surgical intervention and must be discussed with the orthopaedic team.

Barton's fracture is a fracture of the joint of the anterior margin of the distal radius with proximal displacement. Treat in a volar slab and refer to the orthopaedic team.

Hutchinson's fracture is an undisplaced fracture of the ulnar styloid commonly seen in the AP projection. Patients present with a history of a FOOSH injury and complain of pain over the ulna styloid. Treat with analgesia, dorsal back slab, broad arm sling, and facture clinic follow-up.

Wrist sprain should be treated with analgesia, wrist and hand exercises, and, if required, a wrist splint. Instruct the patient to exercise the wrist and not to keep it in the splint all the time.

Tenosynovitis is often associated with repetitive activity. Over a period of time the patient develops swelling over the wrist. The wrist becomes very painful on movement and crepitus can often be palpated. Treatment includes wrist splintage and analgesia (NSAIDs) for 7–10 days. Occasionally physiotherapy can be useful. The patient should be taught progressive exercises and given adequate advice concerning recurrence.

Scaphoid fracture

This is usually caused by a FOOSH. Signs and symptoms include:
- pain over the anatomical snuffbox and on telescoping of the thumb;
- pain directly over the scaphoid tubercle when palpated;
- pain on flexion and ulnar deviation of the wrist.

Scaphoid fractures may not always be apparent initially and requesting specialist scaphoid views may be helpful.
- 70% of scaphoid fractures involve the waist and can be associated with avascular necrosis.
- The remainder occur in the dorsal and proximal poles and are associated with fewer complications.

If there is clinical suspicion of a fracture but no fracture on the X-ray, it is usual practice to treat as a fracture and immobilize the wrist in a splint/POP. Review the patient at 10–14 days either in the ED or in fracture clinic (depending on local policy). The wrist should then be re X-rayed, by which time the fracture should be more evident due to new callus formation. Analgesia advice should be given and analgesia prescribed if required. Some departments use small limb MRI scanners to detect these fractures.

Lunate and perilunate dislocations often follow a FOOSH. Clinically the patient will present with pain and swelling over the anterior aspect of the wrist. These dislocations are rare and often difficult to detect on X-ray. The AP will appear normal; ∴ a close inspection of the lateral view is imperative. If there is any suspicion of a dislocation, give the patient adequate analgesia and seek senior advice.

Carpal bone fractures are rare and are often associated with direct trauma. Patients with a significant mechanism and associated wrist trauma need careful assessment and imaging. If there is evidence of dislocation patients must be referred to the on call orthopaedic team. Small avulsions and fractures of the hook of hamate or triquetral can be treated with a back slab or wrist support and analgesia and referred to the fracture clinic.

Hand injuries

Hand injuries are a common presentation in the ED and require meticulous assessment as injuries to nerves and tendons can be quite subtle in presentation. It is essential that the ENP examining the hand has a sound understanding of the anatomy.

- Always document the dominant hand, occupation, and social circumstances of the patient as these have bearing on treatment decisions.
- Uncomplicated lacerations and fractures will be managed by ED clinicians with specialist follow-up if needed.
- Complicated hand injuries where there is neurovascular or tendon damage or injuries with a cosmetic implication should be referred to the hand surgeon as these injuries can result in significant loss of function.

The hand is made up of multiple compartments and planes. Because of its intricate anatomical structure and wide range of function, it is essential that the examination is thorough and the ENP documents all structures examined.

- Examination should include radial, ulnar, median, and digital nerves.
- Establish and document the integrity of extensor tendons and deep/superficial flexor tendons.
- Note any vascular deficit.

Damage to any of these structures needs specialist assessment.
Initial assessment and treatment of any hand wound should include:

- analgesia;
- removal of any rings;
- temporary splinting and elevation of the injured limb.

Metacarpal fractures Fractures of the 5th metacarpal are sometimes referred to as a 'boxer's fracture' as they frequently result from punching. If the fracture is very displaced or if there is rotational deformity it needs to be referred. Treat undisplaced fractures with no rotational deformity with a high sling, neighbour strapping of the affected finger, and fracture clinic follow-up. Some metacarpal fractures may be managed more comfortably in a volar slab.

Distal phalangeal fractures Manage closed fractures to the distal phalanx with elevation and analgesia. Refer open fractures/burst fractures to the hand surgeon.

Proximal and middle phalangeal fractures Treat undisplaced fractures with analgesia, neighbour strapping, and elevation. Angulated fractures need manipulation under digital block and then neighbour strapping.

Volar plate injuries

A volar plate injury is caused by hyperextension injury to the PIPJ. It may be just a sprain to the ligaments or it may be more serious involving an avulsion fracture where the ligament has pulled off a piece of bone. Simple sprains may be treated with RICE (rest, ice, compression and elevation) and neighbour strapping. Refer more complex injuries to the hand surgeons.

Ulnar collateral ligament injury is also known as gamekeeper's thumb or skier's thumb. A partial or complete tear to the ulnar collateral ligament is most often the result of sporting injuries but can be caused by a fall. The patient will complain of pain over the base of the thumb and will have difficulty grasping objects. Partial tears may be immobilized in a cast and followed up in fracture clinic. Complete tears may require surgical intervention.

Mallet deformity Mallet finger is a closed injury to the extensor mechanism near its insertion into the distal phalanx. It is often associated with an avulsion fracture at the base of the distal phalanx. Mallet finger is a characteristic flexion deformity of the DIPJ. Apply a mallet splint or Zimmer splint and refer the patient for orthopaedic follow-up. The patient needs instruction on how to maintain full extension of the digit while changing the splint.

Avulsion/degloving injuries are often the result of high velocity RTCs and industrial accidents. Degloving injury, which can result in extensive avulsion of the skin and subcutaneous tissues, is a serious injury where an extensive area of skin is sheared from its underlying blood vessels and nerves. These patients need immediate analgesia and urgent referral to a plastic surgeon. Any delay in referral must be avoided to ensure best outcome for the patient. The injured limb should be covered in a sterile saline dressing and elevated.

Amputation of distal phalanx Refer patients presenting with partial or complete amputation of finger tips to the hand surgeon. Place the amputated portion in a saline-soaked swab surrounded by ice. Some may be suitable for re-implantation. Give the patient effective analgesia as these injuries are very distressing. Also give IV antibiotics and establish patient's tetanus status.

Paronychia is an infection to the lateral border of the nail that is usually attributable to simple trauma such as nail-biting. Artificial nails are also thought to be a cause of paronychia. A paronychia usually starts as a cellulitis, but often progresses to abscess formation, which requires incision and drainage. Infection can sometimes spread under the nail causing a subungual abscess that requires trephining.

Subungual haematoma is the result of direct trauma to the distal phalanx that causes bleeding under the nail. The presence of a subungual haematoma is suggestive of a nail bed injury and an underlying distal phalangeal fracture. It is important to identify such injuries as inappropriate management can damage nail plate regeneration. Formation of a nail bed scar may prevent plate adherence to the bed and lead to the subsequent development of onycholysis of the newly formed nail plate. Trephining the nail gives instant relief from the pain and is not contraindicated even in the presence of a fracture to the distal phalanx. However, do this under sterile conditions and consider appropriate wound care, tetanus prophylaxis, and antibiotic therapy.

Tendon sheath infections of the hand are usually the result of direct inoculation of bacteria from penetrating trauma. This is a very painful condition and needs urgent referral to a hand surgeon for irrigation, IV antibiotic, elevation and further management.

Back pain

Simple backache is a common presentation in the ED and may be managed by an ENP with appropriate training. This pain is usually attributed to heavy lifting or manual work and must be differentiated from nerve root pain or back pain that is attributed to a more serious pathology. Simple back pain is usually attributable to muscle or ligamentous 'strain'. The patient may present as follows.

- Presentation between ages 20 and 55 years.
- Pain in lumbosacral region.
- No tenderness in spinous process.
- Pain 'mechanical' in nature.
- Varies with physical activity and with time.
- Patient generally well.
- No numbness or tingling in legs.
- No bowel or bladder problems.

Simple back pain accounts for 90% of all episodes of back pain. 90% of patients make a full recovery in 4–6 weeks.

Management of simple back pain

- If the patient has no 'red flags', reassure and provide positive information on prognosis.
- Encourage early light activity.
- Educate on the nature of back pain and address psychosocial features as this has prognostic importance.
- Advise NSAIDs, muscle relaxants, and simple analgesia (as effective as opiates).
- Refer for early physiotherapy.

Nerve root pain

Nerve root pain is a more complex condition, which needs a medical assessment. The patient may present with the following.

- Unilateral leg pain worse than low back pain.
- Pain generally radiates to foot or toes.
- Numbness and paraesthesia in the same distribution.
- Nerve irritation signs.
- Reduced straight leg-raising (SLR), which reproduces back pain.
- Motor, sensory, or reflex change.
- Limited to one nerve root.

50% recover from acute attack within 6 weeks.

▶ Red flags: possible serious pathology

These patients must be seen by a doctor.

- Presentation under age 20 or onset over the age of 55.
- Violent trauma, i.e. fall from a height, RTC.
- Constant, progressive, non-mechanical pain.
- Thoracic pain.
- Past medical history of neoplasm.
- Patient is taking systemic steroids.
- Drug abuse, HIV.
- Systemically unwell.
- Weight loss.
- Persisting severe restriction of lumbar flexion.
- Widespread neurological signs and symptoms.
- Structural deformity.
- Bowel and bladder disturbance.

Pelvic fractures

Pelvic fractures are orthopaedic emergencies and, although relatively uncommon, potentially life-threatening complications of haemorrhage can occur if not immediately identified and treated. Compound fractures of the pelvis have a mortality of up to 50%. Associated bladder and urethral injury is not uncommon.

Symptoms A patient with a pelvic ring fracture will have severe pelvic pain and flank, perianal, or scrotal swelling and bruising.

Signs
- Abnormal vital signs; signs of shock.
- Differences in leg length and external rotation of a leg without an associated limb fracture.
- Look for any injury to groins, perineum, and genitalia. Swollen testicle may suggest testicular rupture requiring surgical decompression. Examine penis for blood at meatus, suggestive of urethral damage.
- Check the femoral pulses on both sides. Absent pulses may indicate vascular damage. Get help as surgery may be necessary to preserve the limb of the affected side.
- Examine vulva and inspect the vagina and urethral meatus for blood.
  - Where no evidence of urethral injury insert a urinary catheter.
  - If urethral injury is likely, suprapubic catheterization may be necessary for bladder decompression. This applies to males and females.
- A rectal examination should be performed to test sphincter tone. A reduction in tone is suggestive of a sacral fracture.
- Any blood from the rectum may be indicative of a rectal tear. This will require surgery.

Specific interventions
- Initial management focuses on fluid replacement, stabilization of fractures, and pain control.
- Give opiate analgesia as prescribed and monitor effect.
- Consider use of a pelvic splinting device.
- Fluid replacement should follow ATLS guidelines. The patient's haemodynamic condition should be continuously monitored during this period.
- Give prophylactic antibiotics as prescribed for wounds as there is a risk of infection from faecal flora.
- Patients with obvious pelvic fractures should **not** be log rolled. Enough people should be enlisted to perform a straight lift.
- Keep patient nil by mouth and prepare as appropriate for theatre.

Sacral fractures are often associated with other pelvic fractures as the result of major trauma. Transverse fractures result from directly applied forces to the sacrum. Vertical fractures occur as part of complex pelvic fractures. Stress fractures are usually vertical and near the sacroiliac joint.

MRI or bone scan are useful to detect stress fractures. Sacral fractures can be quite subtle and are easily missed.

Femoral fractures

❶ Any injured limb should be assessed for the presence of the 'five Ps' that might indicate neurovascular compromise:
- pain
- pallor
- pulselessness
- paraesthesia
- paralysis

Fractures of the femur fall into three anatomical categories: proximal; mid-shaft; and distal. Check for signs of hypovolaemia as blood loss from a shaft of femur fracture can be 1000–1500 mLs.

Management priorities

Two main management priorities exist in ED: preventing secondary damage and pain control. Preventing secondary damage includes managing blood loss by initiating IV fluid replacement. Reduction in blood loss and significant pain reduction can be achieved by correct application of an appropriate traction splint, such as a Thomas splint. These stabilize the fracture until definitive repair can take place.

In doing this, the extent of the trauma to surrounding soft tissue is minimized. Pain is reduced because bone ends are immobilized. Distal and proximal pulses, capillary refill, and sensation should be rechecked after splint application. If the fracture is open, broad-spectrum antibiotics should be given and the patient's tetanus status checked. The wound should be covered with a wet dressing. Povidine–iodine soaks are commonly used to lower the risk of infection.

Fracture of neck of femur

This is common in the elderly following relatively minor trauma. Risk ↑ because of osteoporosis, osteomalacia, and also because of ↑ rate of falls.
Many hospitals have fast-track policies for these patients.
- As these fractures can frequently be diagnosed clinically, give patients with suspected fractures effective analgesia, such as morphine sulphate, prior to X- ray.
- An in-patient bed should also be arranged at this time.
- Blood loss is significant particularly with intertrochanteric fractures so establish IV access and commence fluids as early hydration reduces mortality.
- Take blood for FBC, U & E, and cross-match.
- Monitor vital signs regularly to ensure haemodynamic stability is maintained.
- Record ECG to exclude MI or other arrhythmia.
- Undertake a Waterlow score and initiate pressure area care in the ED as these patients are very vulnerable to pressure ulcers.
- Apply skin traction early if the patient is not going to theatre (☐ see p.666).

Supracondylar fractures of the femur are assessed in the same way as shaft fractures. The mechanisms of injury are similar, with pain usually localized to the knee. These fractures do not cause the same extent of blood loss as shaft fractures and are repaired by either long leg casting or surgery.

Dislocated hip prosthesis

Hip dislocations most commonly occur in people with total hip replacements or femoral head replacements.

The patient may present in severe pain, with an internally rotated, flexed leg. Early limb relocation is indicated providing there is no associated fracture. This may be done in the ED under sedation. Once relocated, the patient should be admitted for traction. If relocation attempts are unsuccessful with sedation in the ED, then urgent transfer to theatre for closed or open reduction under general anaesthetic is indicated.

Lower limb injury: triage

History taking and examination at triage need to be brief and should focus on ensuring neurovascular function, relief of pain, and, if appropriate, referral to X-ray. A more thorough examination will be performed by the ENP or the doctor.

Knee injuries

When assessing the injury the nurse /ENP should consider a number of factors.
- Mechanism of injury; twisting injury may suggest injury to menisci.
- Valgus or varus strain may cause damage to medial or lateral collateral ligament, respectively.
- Rapid swelling to the knee post-injury is usually an acute haemarthrosis and implies significant injury.
- A more gradual swelling suggests an effusion.
- Past medical history should include pre-existing injuries to that limb, medical conditions that affect the musculoskeletal system or bone density, and factors that would influence recovery.
- Ask about current medications and any known allergies.

It is also important to establish a social history as limb injuries may adversely affect the younger person's ability to work and may limit the older person's ability to care for themselves. These factors need consideration in any treatment plan.

Examination

To examine the knee the patient needs to be partially undressed and lying on a trolley. Examine both legs for comparison.
- Look for swelling, bruising, redness, abrasions, any breaks in the skin.
- Feel skin temperature and compare with other joint. Feel for crepitus and look and feel for an effusion.
- An examination for effusion should be performed with the injured knee in extension. The suprapatellar pouch should be milked to determine whether an effusion is present.
- Assess tone and bulk of quadriceps for any sign of wasting. Compare the painful knee with the asymptomatic knee. The musculature should be symmetric bilaterally.
- Feel for joint line tenderness: may suggest injury to menisci.
- Feel for bony tenderness over the patella, the tibial plateau, and the femoral condyles.
- Assess collateral and cruciate ligaments.
- Ask patient to straight leg raise. Ability to do this against resistance generally excludes quadriceps or patella tendon rupture or transverse patellar fractures.

Medial collateral ligament The valgus stress test is performed with the patient's leg slightly abducted. Place one hand on the lateral aspect of the knee joint and the other hand at the medial aspect of the distal tibia. Then apply valgus stress at both 0° (full extension) and 30° of flexion to assess for pain or laxity in the medial collateral ligament.

Lateral collateral ligament To perform the varus stress test, place one hand at the medial aspect of the patient's knee and the other hand at the lateral aspect of the distal fibula. Apply varus stress at both 0° (full extension) and 30° of flexion to test for pain or laxity in the lateral collateral ligament.

Anterior cruciate ligament (ACL) may be injured in a twisting or hyperextension movement Use the drawer test to assess the cruciate ligaments. For the anterior drawer test, patient's knee must be flexed to 90°. Fix patient's foot in slight external rotation (by sitting on the foot) and then place thumbs at the tibial tubercle and fingers at the posterior calf. Ensure patient's hamstring muscles are relaxed; then pull anteriorly and assess anterior displacement of the tibia (anterior drawer sign).

Lachman test is another method of assessing integrity of ACL. The injured knee is flexed to 15°. Stabilize the distal femur with one hand, grasping the proximal tibia in the other hand. Then attempt to sublux the tibia anteriorly. Lack of clear endpoint indicates a positive Lachman test.

Posterior cruciate ligament (PCL) is less frequently injured than ACL. For posterior drawer test, injured knee must be flexed to 90°. Standing at side of trolley observe for posterior displacement of the tibia (posterior sag sign). Then fix patient's foot in neutral position (by sitting on it), position thumbs at tibial tubercle, and place fingers at posterior calf. Push posteriorly and assess for posterior displacement of tibia.

Ottawa knee rules An X-ray is only required for acute knee injuries with one or more of these findings.
- Age 55 or older.
- Tenderness at head of fibula.
- Isolated tenderness of patella.
- Inability to flex to 90°.
- Inability to weight bear at time of injury and in the ED.

However, consider X-raying patients > 18 years and < 55 years who are intoxicated with alcohol or have a history of degenerative bone disease.

Patellar fractures occur as a result of a fall on to the knee. Indirect twisting injury or a direct blow to the joint can also result in a fracture. The patient presents with pain, swelling, crepitus, effusion, and extension block. Inability to straight leg raise may suggest rupture of the quadriceps or patellar tendon. Do not confuse a bipartite patella with a fracture.

Treatment of patella fracture
- Immobilize in a non-weight-bearing cast and ensure patient is given written plaster instructions.
- Ensure adequate analgesia.
- Give the patient crutches and advice on how to use them.
- Arrange early follow-up in fracture clinic.

Patellar dislocation results from a direct blow to the medial aspect of the knee. The patient presents with lateral deformity, medial tenderness, and pain on attempted movement. Haemarthrosis may also be evident.

Treatment of patellar dislocation
- The patella can be relocated by extension of the knee. Analgesia and muscle relaxants should be used to relieve pain prior to procedure.
- Once relocated, a supportive bandage such as a Robert Jones or cricket splint should be applied.

Knee dislocation and tibial plateau fractures

Knee dislocation

Knee dislocations are rare. Most are due to high-energy injuries, such as RTCs or industrial accidents. They are an orthopaedic emergency as there is a high incidence of neurovascular damage associated with this injury. Multiple ligament injuries are required for knee dislocation. Usually both cruciates and one or both collateral ligaments are injured. Injury to the popliteal artery or nerve is common.

- Check and record pulses and sensation. Look also for associated bony injury of femur and lower limb.
- Reduction will require analgesia and sedation. Get specialist help.
- Post-reduction, immobilize in a full long leg back slab and continue to check and record circulation.
- Prepare patient for admission.

Tibial plateau fractures

The principal bones involved in tibial plateau fractures are the femur and tibia. Fractures of the tibial plateau commonly occur in association with other injuries resulting from a fall or an RTC. Isolated fractures of the tibia are not fatal but may be associated with injuries to neighbouring structures such as the popliteal artery, ligaments, peroneal nerve, soft tissues, and menisci.

Signs and symptoms

- Patients usually present with pain over the fracture site and inability to weight-bear.
- Swelling can vary and there is often a haemathrosis.

Treatment

- Fractures of the tibial plateau may require elevation and open reduction and internal fixation with bone grafting as the preferred management.
- Conservative treatment in POP is less preferable because of the risks of long immobilization, especially in older patients. Ensure adequate analgesia before immobilizing limb in a long leg POP back slab and refer to orthopaedic team.

Soft tissue knee injuries

Soft tissue injuries to the knee are a common presentation in the ED. Such injuries are now frequently managed by ENPs. Patients may present with an acute or chronic problem and this should be elicited in the history.

History taking

- Ask about time and date of injury.
- Mechanism of injury?
- Crack or popping sound at time of injury?
- Degree and site of pain/referral of pain?
- Ability to weight-bear?
- Instability or locking since injury?
- Swelling and speed of onset?
- Any other joint affected, i.e. hip/ankle?
- Is the condition longstanding?
- Ask about exacerbating factors such as using stairs, rising from sitting position.

Prepatellar bursitis

People who spend a lot of time on their knees often present with swelling in the front of the knee. The constant friction aggravates the bursa (lubricating sac), which is situated in front of the kneecap (patella). The bursa allows the kneecap to move smoothly under the skin. If the bursa becomes inflamed, it fills with fluid and causes swelling of the knee. This condition is called prepatellar bursitis.

Symptoms include:

- pain usually with activity
- rapid swelling on the front of kneecap
- tender and warm to the touch.

If there is any history of trauma it may be necessary to X-ray to exclude a fracture. Conservative treatment is usually effective, providing the bursa is only inflamed and not infected.

Treatment of bursitis

- Rest until the bursitis settles.
- Apply ice at regular intervals 3 or 4 times a day for 20min at a time. Do not apply ice directly on to the skin.
- Elevate the affected leg as much as possible.
- Advise anti-inflammatory medication such as aspirin or ibuprofen.

Some clinicians may decide to aspirate the bursa. Chronic bursitis may need orthopaedic referral.

Tibial and fibular shaft fractures

Tibial fractures

A direct blow to the tibia is the most common cause of fracture as the tibia has little muscle protection. Significant injury may also be caused by falls or jumps from a height and, in recent years, gunshot wounds to the lower leg. Spiral fractures to the tibia or fibula may occur during violent twisting injuries from sport.

Undisplaced stress fractures can occur, particularly in adults involved in sports, and may not always be evident on X-ray. Persistent symptoms suggestive of stress fracture should be followed up in fracture clinic.

Diagnosis of a tibial fracture is relatively easy. Inability to bear weight on the affected leg and a visible malformation of the leg are often presenting features.

Pain is usually severe but this can vary. Any wound proximal to the fracture site should be regarded as a potential open injury. A tibial fracture should be considered among the differential diagnoses after trauma, especially in a patient with an altered mental status who cannot provide a reliable history. A tibial shaft fracture will be treated according to the type of fracture and alignment of the bone.

Treatment
- POP is appropriate for tibial shaft fractures that are minimally or undisplaced and are well aligned. The cast must extend from above the knee to below the ankle (a long leg cast). These fractures tend to heal well and casting avoids the potential complications of surgery such as infection. Patients with casts must be monitored for the development of compartment syndrome and to ensure satisfactory healing of the tibia and to ensure the bony alignment is maintained.
- Open reduction and internal fixation are required when fractures are unstable. Factors that contribute to instability are type of fracture, location of fracture, and the degree of comminution—also associated fibular fractures.

▶▶ Open fractures are orthopaedic emergencies, and a specialist should be consulted immediately.
- Rarely, such fractures can be treated conservatively.
- Most patients need to be prepared for theatre for debridement and irrigation within 6h of injury. Longer intervals have been shown to increase rate of infection.
- On occasions, especially in multiple trauma, the definitive fracture treatment may be delayed. If surgery must be delayed, leg appearance and compartmental pressure must be monitored carefully.
- The risk of compartment syndrome is high. ∴ admission for 24h observation and limb elevation should be considered in very swollen proximal tibial fractures.

Fibular fractures

- These occur in combination with tibial fractures or as a result of direct trauma to the lateral aspect of the calf. Distal fibular/malleolar fractures occur with excessive rotational forces. (📖 See p.292)

- Isolated fibular fractures are not common The patient may present with pain over the fracture site. Because the fibula is not a weight-bearing bone, the patient may be walking with discomfort. Swelling is usually minimal.
- The common peroneal nerve may be damaged in proximal fibular injuries so it is important to examine specifically for weakness of ankle dorsiflexion and decreased sensation of lateral aspect of forefoot.

Depending on the degree of pain, isolated fractures are treated by either plaster cast or compression bandage.

Maisonneuve fracture is a fracture of the proximal fibula in addition to a fractured medial malleolus (or injured deltoid ligament) Patients present with proximal fibular pain in addition to medial ankle pain. This is an unstable ankle injury.

Open fractures

An open fracture (compound fracture) is a broken bone that penetrates the skin and is open to the air. Open fractures are usually caused by high-energy injuries such as RTCs falls, or sports injuries.

▶▶ Open fractures are orthopaedic emergencies requiring immediate specialist intervention because of high risk of infection and potential associated neurovascular damage. Surgical intervention is usually required to adequately assess the injury, clean the area, and stabilize the fracture. Even with prompt surgical intervention these injuries are often slow to heal and may result in some level of disability for the patient.

Nursing interventions

- Follow ATLS guidelines and ensure ABCs before dealing with the open fracture.
- Assess pain. Administer opiate analgesia and anti-emetic as prescribed.
- Immobilize wound as much as possible.
- Record baseline observations to include temperature, HR, BP, CBG. Report any abnormalities.
- Record pedal pulses half hourly on affected limb.
- Apply an iodine-based dressing to the wound to protect against further contamination. Leave fracture blisters (if any) intact as once broken they are likely to become more contaminated.
- Establish the tetanus immunization status of the patient and consider the need for tetanus immunoglobulin if the patient lacks immunity and is vulnerable because of a contaminated wound.
- Establish IV access and collect blood for FBC, U & E, group and save as patient will need surgical intervention.
- Administer IV antibiotics as prescribed.
- Record presence/absence of distal pulses before covering the wound and continue to monitor.
- Remove any obvious foreign bodies before applying a sterile soaked dressing.
- Reassure and support patient and family as these are very frightening injuries.
- Prepare patient for theatre.

Compartment syndrome

The muscles of the limbs are organized into compartments and divided by thick fascia. Compartment syndrome occurs when the pressure inside a compartment is increased above 30–40mmHg compressing the nerves and blood vessels within that space. It can occur in upper or lower limbs as the result of high energy trauma and bony injury. It can also result from tight bandages or casts. Compartment syndrome is most common in the lower leg and forearm, although it can also occur in the hand, foot, thigh, and upper arm.

The classical sign that should alert nurses to consider compartment syndrome is extreme pain in the compartment that is out of all proportion to the injury and is not relieved with analgesia and elevation. The skin overlying the compartment will be critical, swollen, and shiny. As the pressure continues to rise there may be diminished sensation, weakness, and paleness of the skin. This condition is diagnosed by inserting a needle attached to a pressure meter into the compartment. When the compartment pressure is greater than 45mmHg or when the pressure is within 30mmHg of the diastolic BP, the diagnosis is made.

Treatment for both acute and chronic compartment syndrome is usually surgery.

Nursing interventions for compartment syndrome

- Ensure adequate opiate analgesia.
- Elevate the limb.
- Remove any constricting dressings or POP.
- Prepare for, and assist medical staff in measuring compartment pressure.
- Prepare patient for surgery.
- Maintain frequent monitoring.
- Offer support and reassurance to patient.

Ankle injuries

Ankle fractures refer to fractures of the distal tibia, distal fibula, talus, and calcaneus. The true ankle joint consists of tibia (medial wall), fibula (lateral wall), and the talus, the base upon which the tibia and fibula sit. The joint allows dorsiflexion and plantar flexion movement at the ankle.

The subtalar joint consists of the talus and the calcaneus. The subtalar joint allows inversion and eversion.

- Excessive inversion stress is the most common cause of ankle injuries. This is due to the medial malleolus being shorter than the lateral malleolus, thus allowing the talus to invert more than evert. Also the deltoid ligament gives greater support to the medial malleolus than the less substantial lateral ligaments.
- The ankle is much more stable and resistant to eversion injury than inversion injury. However, when eversion injury does occur, the patient often sustains significant damage to bony and ligamentous supporting structures and joint instability.

The ankle joint may be destabilized by either a fracture to one of the bones or by injury to a ligament. Most ankle injuries occur during sports activities or when walking or running on an uneven surface. Forced rotation or angulation of the joint can result in a fracture and/or associated ligament injury. Fractures of the ankle are serious because of the implications for weight-bearing and mobility. They can be very painful and heal slowly.

The Ottawa ankle rules

Fractures account for only 15–20% of all ankle injuries so X-rays are not indicated in all cases. The Ottawa ankle rules (Fig. 9.1) are proven to be very accurate in identifying patients who may have sustained a fracture and applying the rules will assist the triage nurse in making decisions about whom to refer to X-ray.

Ottawa ankle rules are based on the assessment of ability to bear weight at the time of injury and subsequently in the ED. They also specify areas of bone tenderness that allow clinicians to determine accurately which patients are at negligible risk of fracture.

Management of ankle fractures

Management depends on clinical and radiological findings. It is important to exclude neurovascular compromise and to establish the integrity of the ankle mortise. Note any talar shift on the X-ray.

- Simple, undisplaced lateral malleolar fractures usually can be immobilized in a below knee back slab and followed up in the next fracture clinic. Large avulsion fractures of the lateral malleolus should be managed in the same way.
- Displaced fractures of the lateral or medial malleolus should be referred immediately to orthopaedics as they need open reduction and internal fixation (ORIF).
- Bimalleolar, trimalleolar, and intraarticular fractures of the distal tibia (pilon fractures) need urgent orthopaedic assessment as they require ORIF.

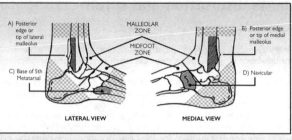

a) An ankle X-ray series is only required if there is any pain in malleolar zone and any of these findings:
1. Bone tenderness at A
OR
2. Bone tenderness at B
OR
3. Inability to bear weight both immediately and in ED

b) A foot X-ray series is only required if there is any pain in midfoot zone and any of these findings:
1. Bone tenderness at C
OR
2. Bone tenderness at D
OR
3. Inability to bear weight both immediately and in ED

Fig. 9.1 The Ottawa ankle rules. (Reproduced with permission from Stiell, I.G., *et al.* (1993). Decision rules for the use of radiography in acute ankle injuries. Refinement and prospective validation. *Journal of the American Medical Association* **269**, 1127–32.)

Ankle dislocation and sprain

Ankle dislocation

▶▶ Ankle dislocations are an orthopaedic emergency and are the result of significant trauma. Do not delay in getting specialist help.

Because of the large amount of force required and the inherent stability of the joint, dislocation of the ankle joint alone is uncommon without an associated fracture. In addition, there is also disruption of the lateral or medial ligaments or the tibiofibular syndesmosis. Examination of the joint shows obvious swelling and deformity. Tenting of the skin by the malleoli may be present. Palpation of the joint reveals tenderness along the joint line, consistent with ligamentous injury. Early reduction is imperative as delay increases risk of neurovascular compromise. In patients with vascular compromise, perform reduction prior to radiological examination.

When requesting X-rays, request anteroposterior, lateral, and mortise/oblique views.

Nursing intervention
- Establish venous access and collect blood for FBC, U & E, and FBC.
- Ensure the administration of IV opiate analgesia. Entonox® can also be administered.
- If opiate analgesia administered monitor respiratory rate and SpO2
- Assist in reducing the dislocation. Support and reassure the patient as this can be very painful.
- Apply the plaster while the alignment of the joint is maintained. When dry, a window needs to be cut in the plaster so pedal pulses can be checked.
- Record baseline observations and pedal pulses.
- Accompany patient to X-ray.
- Prepare patient for admission.

Ankle sprain

A sprain is caused by stretching of a ligament that may be torn or partially torn (Fig. 9.2). The signs of an ankle sprain are not dissimilar to those of a fracture and can include:
- pain or tenderness;
- swelling;
- bruising;
- inability to walk or bear weight on the joint;
- stiffness.

Ankle sprain is a very common injury. The severity depends on the mechanism of injury and how badly the ligaments are stretched or torn. Ankle sprains are graded as follows.
- Grade I, mild sprain. Stretch and/or minor tear of the ligament without laxity (loosening).
- Grade II, moderate. Tear of ligament plus some laxity.
- Grade III, severe. Complete tear of the affected ligament (very lax).

Treatment for ankle sprains is RICE.
- Rest the ankle, either completely or partly, depending on how serious the sprain is. Use crutches for as long as it is painful to weight bear.
- NSAIDs
- Ice. Use ice packs, ice massages, or even a bag of frozen peas to help relieve the swelling, pain, bruising, and muscle spasms. Keep using ice for up to 3 days after the injury.
  - ► Caution. never apply ice directly on to the skin: wrap in a cloth or towel before applying.
- Acute phase. There is little evidence to support the use of compression bandages/products in the acute phase.
- Rehabilitation. There may be benefit from strapping/bracing of significant sprains during rehabilitation. This should be under the supervision of the physics/orthopaedic team.
- Elevation. Raising the ankle to or above the level of the heart will help prevent the swelling from getting worse and will help reduce bruising. Try to keep the ankle elevated for about 2 to 3 hours a day if possible.

Whilst most patients make a full recovery from their injury some may experience long-term problems and recurrent sprains. Where possible, patients with moderate to severe sprains should have physiotherapy follow-up. Patient education and advice about what to expect are very important aspects of care.

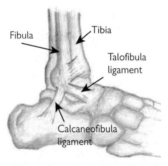

Fig. 9.2 Lateral ankle ligaments (Reproduced with permission from Bulstrode, C., et al. (2002). *Oxford Textbook of Orthopaedics and Trauma*, p. 1307. Oxford University Press, Oxford.)

Gastrocnemius muscle tears

Tears to the lateral or medial bellies of the gastrocnemius are very common. They are acutely painful commonly occurring during sport or activity. There is sudden onset of calf pain with a feeling of 'tearing'. The calf may be bruised and/or swollen. There is tenderness laterally or medially to the muscle bellies. The integrity of the Achilles tendon should be assessed and the fibula examined to identify signs of tenderness. X-rays are only necessary if there are signs of bony tenderness over the calcaenum of fibula. Treatment of a rupture is symptomatic; NSAID's, rest, +/− crutches and walking with a slightly raised heel may provide dramatic relief. Symptoms usually settle in 2 weeks.

Achilles tendon injuries

The Achilles tendon is the tendon that connects the calf muscle (gastrocnemius) to the calcaneum.
- Achilles tendinitis is an inflammation of the tendon that causes the tendon to become swollen, painful, and less flexible than usual.
- A ruptured tendon may occur when the tendon has been structurally weakened by untreated tendinitis, or due to unaccustomed activity. Patients often report hearing a pop at the back of the ankle. Symptoms include pain, swelling, and loss of function.
  - As the calf muscle is no longer attached to the calcaneum the patient finds weight bearing difficult and may be unable to stand on their toes.

Examination
- The area of the rupture may be swollen, tender, and bruised.
- A gap in the tendon may be palpable.
- X-rays, although they do not show the tendon injury, show the calcaneus. In some cases, the tendon may not tear, but may cause a small avulsion fracture of calcaneal bone.
- If the tendon has not ruptured, then the patient may have sustained only a pulling injury to the tendon causing tendinitis.
- The most reliable diagnostic test for a suspected rupture of the Achilles tendon is the Simmonds' test (also called the Thompson test or Simmonds–Thompson test). The patient lies face down with feet hanging off the edge of the bed. If the test is positive, there is no movement of the foot (plantar flexion) on squeezing the corresponding calf, indicating likely rupture of the Achilles tendon.

Treatment
Treatment options are surgical or conservative and the choice of treatment is often dependent on the clinician and local policy. Both treatments may require an initial period of equinus casting. The cast may be changed at 2–4 week intervals to slowly stretch the tendon back to its normal length. Casting may be combined with early movement (1–3 weeks) to improve overall strength and flexibility.

Equinus cast This is usually a below knee cast (occasionally extended to above knee) done with the patient's leg hanging over the end of the bed. It is designed to take the stretch off the tendon. The requirements are exactly the same as for a below-knee cast and the same method is used except for the slab, which is applied to the anterior aspect of the lower leg from the knee end first. The foot should be plantar flexed.

Plantar fasciitis

This is inflammation of the plantar fascia of the foot. It is an overuse injury causing heel pain that may radiate forward into the foot. Pain is usually worse first thing in the morning but eases as the day wears on and becomes more painful again in the evening especially after walking. Treatment is usually rest and NSAIDs. Persistent pain may need referral to orthopaedics for steroid injections.

Fracture of the lateral process of talus

This is more commonly known as 'snowboarder's ankle' and is an injury more common in snowboarders than in the general population. Most patients present with unremitting pain and swelling and what they believe is a sprained ankle. Diagnosis is usually made when the person is referred to an orthopaedic doctor and a CT scan of the ankle is performed.

- If the fracture fragments are undisplaced, treatment is conservative in a cast for 6 weeks and non-weight-bearing on crutches.
- Displaced fractures usually require surgical intervention.

Calcaneal fractures

Fractures of the hindfoot particularly the os calcis (calcaneum) are not unusual and are the result of an axial load type of injury, e.g. jumping from a height. Calcaneal fractures are serious because secondary arthritis of the subtalar joint can occur. Examine both calcanei as these fractures are often bilateral and often involve the subtalar joint. They are also often associated with burst fractures of the spine and for this reason it is important to examine the cervical spine, lumbar spine, pelvis, and hips. X-rays show a decrease in Boehler's angle to less than 20%.

Metatarsal fractures are common sporting injuries caused by direct trauma, excessive rotational forces, or overuse. Avulsion fractures of the base of the 5th metatarsal are caused by inversion injuries where the base of the 5th metatarsal is avulsed by the peroneus brevis tendon. The Ottawa ankle rules also provide guidelines for when to request foot X-rays following ankle injury (see p.292). The treatment of metatarsal fractures varies depending on the nature and location of the fracture and, in some cases, the occupation of the patient, e.g. footballers, ballet dancers. If the fracture fragments are well aligned then the treatment is an/or POP elastic support bandage backslab and restricted weight bearing for 6–8 weeks. However, avulsion fractures of the base of the 5th metatarsal are sometimes slow to heal and for this reason should be followed up in the fracture clinic.

Jones fracture is a fracture at the base of 5th metatarsal at the metaphyseal–diaphyseal junction. It must be differentiated from the more common avulsion fracture of the 5th metatarsal styloid process. Jones fractures are sometimes treated in a below knee plaster cast for 4–6 weeks but very often surgical intervention is required.

Fractured toes

As treatment of undisplaced fractures of toes is symptomatic, X-rays are only required if there is a deformity that may require reduction, or there is an overlying wound that would indicate a compound fracture.

Where there is no bony injury to toes, reassure patient and advise sensible shoes. Occasionally relief may be obtained from two toe neighbour strapping.

- Undisplaced fracture of toe.
  - Neighbour strapping and analgesia. No follow-up necessary.
  - Fractures to the great/1st toe require supportive splinting. The patient should be non-weight-bearing using crutches and be given a follow-up appointment in the fracture clinic.
- Dislocated or displaced Fracture of toes. Reduce using Entonox® or a digital nerve block and neighbour strap. Fracture clinic follow-up.

Wounds: introduction

The stages of wound healing

Assessment and management of acute wounds is an essential component of emergency nursing. It is important that nurses working in any urgent care setting have a sound understanding of the healing process.

Vascular inflammatory phase: 0–3 days Within seconds of the injury, blood vessels constrict to control bleeding at the site. Platelets unite to form clots and arrest bleeding. Neutrophils enter the wound to fight infection and to attract macrophages. Macrophages break down necrotic debris and activate the fibroblast response.

Destructive migratory phase: 2–5 days Dead tissue and bacteria are removed in this stage. Where cells die due to injury, the body acts to dissolve and eliminate necrotic matter. Macrophages migrate into the wound and play a vital role in this stage by engulfing bacteria, any foreign bodies, and necrotic tissue. With neutrophils, the macrophages attract fibroblasts and influence the growth of new blood vessels into the wound.

Proliferative phase: 3–24 days Fibroblasts proliferate in the deeper parts of the wound synthesizing small amounts of collagen, which facilitates further fibroblast proliferation. Granulation tissue also appears in the deeper layers of the wound. The proliferation phase lasts 24–72h.

Maturation phase: 24 days to 1 year During this phase, fibroblasts leave the wound, there is a decrease in vascularity, and collagen is remodelled into a more organized matrix. The wound changes from a red granulation tissue to a pink epithelialization. Finally, a white relatively avascular tissue develops, and the epidermis is restored to normal thickness.

Wound contraction, which starts during the proliferative phase and continues into this final phase of healing, is powerful and may, in certain individuals cause contracture. In some individuals the healing process can lead to the formation of excessive amounts of scar tissue resulting in a keloid scaring. While healed wounds never regain the full strength of uninjured skin, they can regain up to 70–80% of the original strength.

Wound categorization

Wounds may be categorized as acute or chronic.
- Acute wounds seen in the ED include surgical, traumatic, and thermal injuries.
- Chronic wounds include malignant wounds, pressure sores, leg ulcers, and diabetic foot ulcers. (📖 see p. 395) These wounds are attributable to systemic disease processes that require specialist intervention beyond the emergency setting and such patients must be either referred on to the appropriate speciality or primary care provider.

Pre-tibial lacerations

These are lacerations to the anterior aspect of the lower leg. They are a common presentation particularly in elderly females and are sometimes associated with long-term corticosteroid treatment. Because of this and also the anatomical position healing may be impaired and very slow. Some of these patients may need referral at some point to plastic surgery for skin grafting but skilled initial management can have successful outcomes.

- The flap often appears concertinaed backwards leaving an open wound. The flap needs to be gently smoothed over the wound after gentle cleaning with saline and removal of any haematoma.
- The skin edges of the flap should be brought together and steri-stripped, covering as much of the wound as possible. These wounds should not be sutured as this can lead to necrosis of the flap. Steri-Strips™ ensure a better outcome for the patient.
- Once steri-stripped the wound should be covered with a non-adherent well padded dressing and a support bandage. The bandage should be applied from the toes to below knee to encourage even circulation.
- The patient should be advised to mobilize as necessary but also to elevate the limb where possible to aid venous return and to prevent the development of a chronic, non-healing leg ulcer.
- Consider tetanus status and the need for antibiotic prophylaxis.
- Simple analgesia such as paracetamol is advisable to control any pain.
- Discharge into the care of the GP and practice nurse is the most appropriate option, where continuity of care is more likely than in hospital.

Health promotion in this group of patients is paramount to prevent chronic non-healing. Assessment of the patient holistically rather than considering only the wound in isolation is the gold standard and will promote successful treatment. Consider referral to occupational therapy, social services, or hospital at home in line with local policy to provide added support.

Gunshot wounds

Gunshot wounds are unfortunately an increasing presentation in the ED. In the UK the police must be notified if a patient presents with a gunshot wound. It helps to have some understanding of the nature of ballistics in caring for patients with gunshot injuries. Ballistics refers to the study of projectile motion and is divided into three categories: internal; external; and terminal ballistics. Wound ballistics is a subset of terminal ballistics and is the most important aspect of ballistics for clinicians to understand.

A bullet wound is different to a knife wound. When a projectile strikes it dissipates energy. The energy of a body is $e = mv^2$ where e is energy, m is mass, and v is velocity. Thus kinetic energy KE is proportional to mass and to the square of its velocity so injury is more dependent on velocity than mass.

Bullet injuries are most serious in friable solid organs such as the liver where damage may be caused by temporary cavitation away from the actual bullet track. Bone and subcutaneous fat are more resilient to bullet injury. Bones slow down the course of the bullet.

Assessment of gunshot wounds

As with any trauma ATLS guidelines should be observed and resuscitation of the patient is the primary objective. History may be obtained from the paramedic crew, police, or the patient if conscious or relatives /friends. In these situations it is important to ensure the safety of staff so allow only immediate next of kin into the resuscitation room. Try to establish what kind of weapon was used and check that the weapon is not still with the patient.

Nursing interventions

- Make an assessment of the general state of the patient. Remember that a young person compensates for blood loss and even tachycardia may be a fairly late feature, whilst hypotension suggests very marked blood loss.
- Give high flow O_2 and monitor saturation.
- Establish IV access as soon as possible with two wide bore cannulae for fluid replacement and collect blood for FBC, U & E.
  Cross-match for an initial 6 units.
  - In hypovolaemic shock from penetrating trauma/injuries fluid replacement should be carefully titrated to achieve a lower than normal systolic blood pressure. Boluses of 250mLs fluid can be titrated against the presence or absence of a radial pulse. There is strong evidence that reduces mortality pre-hospital. However, once in the hospital the emphasis must be on early operative intervention to control the source of haemorrhage.
- Apply pressure to any obvious bleeding points. Sucking chest wounds must be covered immediately.
- Record baseline observations and maintain frequent monitoring of vital signs; blood gases.
- Attach to ECG monitoring.
- Request CXR.
- Be prepared. Have chest drain ready and equipment for emergency thoracotomy if there is any deterioration or cardiac arrest.

- Do not consider primary closure of a wound before full exploration and debridement as bullets cause considerable tissue damage.
- Consider tetanus prophylaxis.
- Give IV antibiotics as prescribed.
- Give prescribed analgesia as needed.
- Assist in full medical examination.
- Prepare patient for theatre /ITU.

Points to consider

Chest injuries may involve the heart, lung pleura, great vessels, mediastinum, diaphragm, and abdominal contents. The most frequent injury is a haemopneumothorax from damage to lung and chest wall. This requires a chest drain. Injury to the mediastinum may cause a cardiac tamponade.

Abdominal injuries Most deep penetrating wounds of the abdomen need an exploratory laparotomy.

Limb injuries Nerves, tendons, and vessels may be damaged. Examine the limb in a good light and check for pulses, but remember that finding a pulse does not exclude vascular injury. Record sensation/skin temperature/ sweating. Apply direct pressure to bleeding points.

Blast injuries

Blast injuries are devastating and can be caused by domestic, industrial, or bomb explosion injuries. They are categorized as primary, secondary, tertiary, and quaternary.

- Primary blast injuries affect those closest to explosion and are caused by the impact of blast wave on body surface. Lungs, GI tract, middle ear, and other gas-filled structures are most vulnerable. Types of injury ensuing from a primary blast are tympanic membrane rupture, blast lung or pulmonary barotraumas, abdominal perforation and haemorrhage, eye injuries, and concussion without any apparent head injury.
- Secondary blast injuries are caused by flying debris and bomb fragments. These include penetrating or blunt injuries and shrapnel injuries. Penetrating eye injuries can be occult.
- Tertiary blast injuries are caused by people being thrown by blast. Injuries can be very severe and can include serious head injuries, amputations, and fractures.
- Quarternary blast injuries include all explosion-related injuries, illness, or disease not attributable to primary, secondary, or tertiary mechanisms. Also include exacerbation of existing conditions. e.g. angina. Injuries include partial and full thickness burns, inhalation injuries, crush injuries, and open or closed brain injuries.

Nursing interventions Management of such seriously injured patients is a team effort where ATLS guidelines apply and life-threatening injuries are prioritized. However, these patients need very intensive support and understanding and must have assigned a nurse to ensure continuity of care.

Proceed with nursing assessment as usual but give special consideration to the following points.

- Respiratory injuries. Consider blast lung in patients who are wheezing. Blast lung is the most common fatal blast injury and presents as a triad of apnoea, bradycardia, and hypotension. These symptoms may or may not be evident at initial presentation. Pulmonary contusion may evolve over a period of up to 48h so these patients need meticulous observation for the duration Be aware that wheezing may also be due to inhalation of fumes/dust/gases or pulmonary oedema.
- Renal injury. Urinalysis should be routine at initial assessment to identify any renal trauma.
- Abdominal injuries. Consider delayed perforation and intestinal mural contusions. Unexplained hypovolaemia may indicate severe intra-abdominal injury.
- Ruptured tympanic membrane. All victims of a blast should be examined by an ENT specialist.
- Ophthalmology. All victims of a blast should be assessed by a specialist.
- Head injury. Patients can suffer from concussion without having sustained an apparent head injury.

▶ Frequent recording of vital signs is paramount. It is equally essential that staff show compassion and support for these very traumatized patients.

Traumatic amputation

Traumatic amputation is the accidental severing of some or all of a body part. A complete amputation refers to the total severing of the limb. In a partial amputation some of the tissue remains attached.

Trauma is the leading cause of amputation. The majority of patients are < 30 years old and male. RTCs, especially those involving motorbikes, and the use of heavy gardening equipment and power tools are attributable causes. Industrial and agricultural workers traditionally have been more vulnerable to such trauma. More recently, traumatic amputations have been caused by terrorist explosions.

Haemorrhage is variable depending on the site and nature of injury. On arrival in the ED decisions will be made about the viability of the severed part and the potential of successful reattachment. Various limb salvage scoring systems are used to aid surgeons in making these difficult decisions. These are

- Mangled extremity severity score (MESS).
- Predictive salvage index (PSI).
- Limb salvage index (LSI).

Nursing interventions

- The injured limb should be gently cleaned with a sterile solution and covered with a moist sterile dressing.
- Loose tissue should be supported in its normal position while waiting for theatre.
- Establish tetanus status of patient and consider the need for tetanus immunoglobulin.
- An amputated body part should be wrapped in a sterile towel and sealed in a plastic bag and kept cool till definitive care.
- Analgesia.
- Elevation of the effected limb if possible.
- Offer reassurance for the patient and family.

Wound infection

Wound infection is a common presentation in the ED and ENPs increasingly manage such patients autonomously. In assessing wounds and cause of infection do the following.

- Consider that a foreign body may be present in the wound.
- Organic foreign bodies such as wood or cane will never be tolerated and will always cause infection if retained.
- X-ray for radio-opaque foreign body as appropriate. (Wood is not radio-opaque.) if unable to locate FB consider referring patient to orthopaedics for further exploration.
- Swab wound and send for culture and sensitivity.
- Record temperature and CBG bearing in mind that patients who have diabetes are more prone to infection.
- Clean wound thoroughly and apply appropriate dressing according to local protocol.

Wounds requiring antibiotic prophylaxis

- Human or animal bites.
- Lacerations involving joints.
- Compound fractures.
- Contaminated wounds.

Bites—human/animal

- Assess for extent of depth and damage to underlying tissue.
- Animal/human bites should not be sutured.
- Refer bites to face or gaping wounds with deep structural involvement to the faciomaxillary surgeon as appropriate.
- Give antibiotics as prescribed.
- Human bites will require hepatitis B vaccination with an accelerated course if the patient does not already have immunity.

Superficial bites

- Clean well.
- Apply antiseptic dressing.
- Elevate/rest according to affected area.
- Check tetanus status and consider tetanus immunoglobulin in unimmunized patients.
- Educate patient regarding signs and symptoms of further infection and emphasize the importance of review of the wound.
- Review all bites following day.
- Consider the need for IV antibiotics and medical review if systemically unwell and if there are signs of cellulitis, lymphangitis.

Abscesses

An abscess is a collection of pus that has formed in the tissues. Abscesses can form in almost every part of the body and may be caused by infectious organisms, parasites, and foreign bodies such as splinters. Abscesses in the skin are easily identifiable as they are red, raised, and painful. Abscesses in other areas of the body may not be obvious, but they may cause significant pain and organ damage.

Incision and drainage of abscess
- Where there is clearly a collection of pus, incision and drainage is indicated.
- Small abscesses may be incised and drained in the ED but some abscesses require specialist referral.
- The following are not suitable for treatment by the ENP and should be referred to the appropriate specialist.
  - Breast.
  - Perianal.
  - Facial.
  - Neck.
  - Labial.
  - Pulp and palmar.
- Always check for diabetes mellitus.

Good anaesthesia is essential to effectively incise an abscess. It can be achieved by lidocaine injected circumferentially around the abscess and/or Entonox® breathed for 2min prior to the incision.
- Make an incision.
- Express all the pus and curette gently.
- Irrigate the cavity with saline and pack with a hydrogel compound.
- Redress next day and refer back to GP as necessary.

Infected sebaceous cysts Treat as for abscesses.

Skin infections

Cellulitis is an inflammation of the connective tissue under the skin. It is usually caused by a bacterial infection. It can be caused by normal skin flora or by other bacteria where the skin integrity has been broken by cuts or insect bites, or at sites of IV cannula insertion. The most common location for cellulitis is the lower limb but it can occur in any part of the body. Cellulitis may be superficial but it can spread to the lymph nodes and bloodstream and the patient can be systemically unwell.

Early symptoms may be redness, swelling, and pain in the affected part but as the infection spreads other symptoms can include pyrexia, nausea, and headaches. In advanced cases of cellulitis, red streaks (tracking) may be noted travelling up the affected area. The swelling can spread rapidly. Treatment is with the appropriate antibiotics but many patients may need admission for elevation and IV antibiotics.

Bites and stings

Patients frequently present to the ED having been bitten or stung by an insect. They are often worried that the sting /bite is poisonous There are many insects whose bites or stings can cause problems but also others that cause only itching and erythema (📖 see Box 9.1).

> **Box 9.1 Bites and stings**
>
> *Venomous*
> - Wasps
> - Hornets
> - Bees
> - Ants
>
> *Non-venomous*
> - Lice
> - Sand fly
> - Chiggers
> - Fleas
> - Ticks
> - Mosquitoes
> - Bugs

The difference between a bite and a sting is based on the nature of the bite or sting.
- Venomous insects such as wasps attack as a defence mechanism, injecting poisonous venom through their stings that can be extremely painful and can, in rare cases, cause an anaphylactic reaction.
- Non-venomous insects such as the mosquito bite in order to feed on the blood. Whilst mosquitoes are not venomous they are dangerous as they transmit such diseases as yellow fever, malaria, and filariasis dengue.

Local irritation and allergic reactions can result from non-venomous bites. Severe reactions such as anaphylactic shock only result from venomous stings.

Bees leave the sting and venom sac attached after stinging the victim. Venom continues to be released until the sting is removed. Bees die after they sting. Wasps and hornets, however, don't leave their stings behind and can sting repeatedly.

Treatment of bites

- Pruritis is usually the most common symptom. Topical antihistamines provide some relief as do anti-inflammatory gels.
- Systemic reaction with symptoms such as facial/tongue swelling, wheezing, or shortness of breath will need urgent treatment and should be nursed in an appropriate high observation area (📖 see p.248).

Treatment of stings Remove the sting and treat with analgesia and antihistamines Pain, swelling, and itching are the main complaints.

Removal of ticks

Ticks are notoriously difficult to remove intact. One method that works well to place a small forceps along the skin with the ends either side of the tick's head. Press down into the skin, and firmly grip the head of the tick. Apply even traction perpendicular to the skin until the tick is finally removed. The aim is to remove the tick intact and not leave any part behind. If this is not successful it may be necessary to infiltrate the area with local anaesthetic and excise the tick.

Needlestick injuries

Needlestick injuries are an occupational hazard that exposes health care workers to a number of blood borne pathogens that can result in serious or fatal infections. It is estimated that 600 000–800 000 needlestick injuries occur each year, half of which are not reported. Many infections can be transmitted via a needlestick injury but the infections that pose the greatest risk are:

- hepatitis B virus (HBV);
- hepatitis C virus (HCV);
- human immunodeficiency virus (HIV)—the virus that causes AIDS.

HBV vaccination is recommended for all health care workers (unless they are immune because of previous exposure). HBV vaccine has proved highly effective in preventing infection in workers exposed to HBV. However, no vaccine exists to prevent HCV or HIV infection. Taking precautions to prevent needlestick injuries is the best protection. Health care workers should avoid:

- recapping needles;
- transferring a body fluid between containers;
- failing to dispose of used needles properly in puncture-resistant sharps containers.

Health care workers should:

- avoid the use of needles where safe and effective alternatives are available;
- use devices with safety features provided by your employer;
- plan for safe handling and disposal of needles before using them;
- promptly dispose of used needles in appropriate sharps disposal containers;
- report all needlestick and sharps-related injuries promptly to ensure that you receive appropriate follow-up care;
- tell your line manager about any needlestick hazards you observe;
- participate in training related to infection prevention;
- get an HBV vaccination.

Management of needlestick injuries

- Follow local guidelines and report injury to occupational health.
- Wash the wound thoroughly with soap and water, allowing it to bleed under the water. Do not suck the wound or apply a pressure to cause bleeding. Wash mucous membranes with copious amounts of water.
- Take baseline blood for serology. If the source is possibly HIV positive, take blood for FBC, U & E, LFTs, and amylase.
- If the source patient is known and also considered to be high risk, discuss post-exposure treatment with the infectious diseases specialist on call. Prophylaxis is most effective if started 1h post-exposure but can be considered after that for up to 2 weeks.
- If the source is high risk and prophylaxis is commenced advise the patient to use barrier contraception and not to donate blood until seroconversion is excluded.
- Organize counselling for the patient.
- Ensure HBV accelerated vaccination.

Tetanus prophylaxis

Tetanus is an acute and often fatal disease, which is now rare in developed countries because of immunization. The disease is caused by tetanus toxin, which is released following infection by the bacterium, *Clostridium tetani*, which is found in soil and animal manure. Typically tetanus spores may be introduced into the body through a puncture wound, a burn, or a laceration. The wound may seem innocuous and not serious and the infection mild but the bacteria attacks the nervous system and the condition is characterized by general rigidity and muscle spasm, which can involve the jaw and neck.

While most patients born in Western countries are immunized, tetanus has not been eradicated and never will be as the spores live in the soil. Anyone can contract tetanus but farmers and those working with soil are at increased risk. It must also be borne in mind that people from the developing world may not have adequate immunity. Certainly, children and young adult refugees from war zones may be particularly at risk because of interrupted vaccination programmes.

High risk tetanus-prone wounds include:
- puncture-type wounds, especially where there has been contact with the soil or manure;
- wounds or burns that show a degree of devitalized tissue;
- wounds containing foreign bodies;
- compound fractures;
- wounds /burns in patients who are systemically septic;
- wounds/burns in patients that require surgical intervention that is delayed > 6h.

Box 9.2 lists indications for tetanus immunization.

Box 9.2 Indications for tetanus immunization

Patient fully immunized (5 doses at appropriate intervals)
- Clean or tetanus-prone wound: vaccine not required
- High risk tetanus-prone wound: give human tetanus immunoglobin

Primary immunization complete; boosters incomplete but up to date
- Clean or tetanus-prone wound: vaccine not required (unless next dose due and convenient to give now)
- High risk tetanus-prone wound: give human tetanus immunoglobin

Primary immunization incomplete or boosters not up to date
- For clean and tetanus-prone wounds give a reinforcing dose of vaccine and further doses as required to complete the recommended schedule to ensure immunity
- In addition, for tetanus-prone wounds, give one dose of human tetanus immunoglobin in a different site

Patient not immunized or immunization status unknown or uncertain
- Clean or tetanus-prone wound: an immediate dose of vaccine, followed, if records confirm the need, by completion of a full 5 dose course to ensure future immunity
- In addition, for tetanus-prone wounds, give one dose of human tetanus immunoglobin in a different site

For further information see www.dh.gov.uk Green Book, Chapter 30

Gastrointestinal emergencies

Overview

Gastrointestinal (GI) problems are frequently encountered in emergency care areas and patients can present with wide-ranging symptoms. Symptoms that suggest an underlying GI problem can include: abdominal pain; nausea; vomiting; diarrhoea; melaena; haematemesis; constipation; jaundice; and abdominal distension. Abdominal pain is a common ED presentation and can be the cause of a wide variety of GI problems. Pain is usually present when there is a disorder within the GI tract but its severity is not a reliable indicator of the seriousness of the condition. However, the site and characteristics of the pain can often indicate the cause. Pain usually arises from an organ within the abdominal cavity that is either inflamed, distended, perforated, or ischaemic. Abdominal wall pain arises from irritation of the peritoneum and/or abdominal musculature from inflamed organs, free blood, or leaked gastric contents. Pain can also be referred from an organ outside the abdominal cavity, e.g. an inferior MI can present as epigastric pain.

The acute abdomen

The acute abdomen is a term given to sudden severe pain in the abdomen. This requires swift diagnosis and treatment usually involves emergency surgery. Causes of acute abdomen may include: appendicitis; pancreatitis; PUD; gall bladder pathology; intestinal ischaemia; DKA; diverticulitis; ruptured ectopic pregnancy.

The gastrointestinal system

The abdomen (Fig. 10.1) contains the structures bordered by the diaphragm superiorly, pelvis inferiorly, vertebral column posteriorly, and abdominal muscles anteriorly. The abdomen can be divided into three cavities: peritoneum; pelvis; and retroperitoneum.

- The peritoneum contains liver, spleen, stomach, gallbladder, small intestine, transverse colon, and sigmoid colon.
- The pelvis contains rectum, bladder, uterus, ovaries, and iliac vessels.
- The retroperitoneum contains part of the duodenum, ascending and descending colon, kidneys, pancreas, ureters, abdominal aorta, and inferior vena cava.

For purposes of examination the abdomen is divided into 4 quadrants: right upper quadrant (RUQ); left upper quadrant (LUQ); right lower quadrant (RLQ); and left lower quadrant (LLQ).

- The **oesophagus** travels through the posterior of the mediastinum and passes through the diaphragm to join the stomach at the level of the T10 vertebrae.
- The **diaphragm** is a dome-shaped structure with 3 foramina (holes) at T8 for the vena cava, T10 for the oesophagus, and T12 for the aorta. The phrenic nerve passes through the thorax along both sides of the pericardium and divides into the anterior and posterior branches. Each phrenic nerve is the sole motor nerve to its own half of the diaphragm.
- The **stomach** is located in the LUQ and is divided into four parts: the cardia; fundus; body; and pylorus.
- The **liver** is the largest intra-abdominal organ and is extremely vascular. The liver tissue is very friable and is surrounded by a fibrous capsule. The liver lies at the level of the 6th–10th ribs on the right, 7th–8th on the left. Circulation is via the hepatic artery and portal vein, Blood flow is ~ 30% of cardiac output. The liver has 5 main functions: detoxification; carbohydrate and fat metabolism; protein synthesis; and bile secretion.
- The **gallbladder** lies under the liver and stores 50mL of bile. Bile drains from the liver via the common hepatic then cystic duct into the gallbladder. Bile drains from the gallbladder via the common bile duct, meeting the pancreatic duct to drain into the duodenum.
- The **biliary system** (Fig. 10.2) is a collective term for the common hepatic duct, cystic duct, common bile duct, gallbladder, and pancreatic duct.
- The **spleen** is located in the LUQ and is in close proximity to the 7th–10th ribs. The splenic pulp is friable and vascular supply is via the splenic artery. The splenic capsule is 1–2mm thick
- The **pancreas** lies at the level of L1 against the posterior abdominal wall. Pancreatic juice is rich in digestive enzymes. The pancreas also produces insulin and several other hormones.
- The **kidneys** lie at the level of T12 to L3. The right kidney is slightly lower due to the liver.
- The **small intestine** is 7m long. It is divided into three sections: duodenum; jejunum; and ileum. Some of the duodenum is retroperitoneal. The small intestine is located in all four quadrants.

- The **appendix** is a 10cm, blind-ended tube connected to the caecum. It is a remnant of embryological development and is not known to have a function.
- The **large intestine** is 1.5m long and consists of the caecum; ascending, transverse, and descending colon; rectum; and anal canal.
- The **peritoneum** is a serous membrane that lines the abdominal cavity and covers the abdominal organs.
- The **bladder** when empty lies in the pelvic cavity; when full it extends into the abdomen.

❶ The last six ribs overlie abdominal structures. ∴ injuries to this area can cause significant intraabdominal pathology.

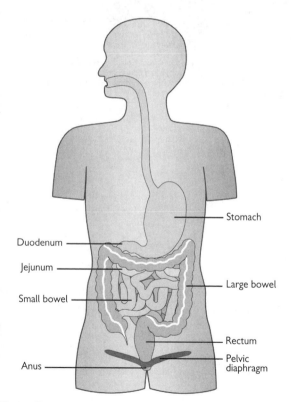

Fig. 10.1 The gastrointestinal tract. (Reproduced from Collins, S., et al. (eds.) (2008). *Oxford Handbook of Obstetrics and Gynaecology*, 2nd edn. Oxford University Press, Oxford with permission from the Burdett Institute of Gastrointestinal Nursing, King's College, London.)

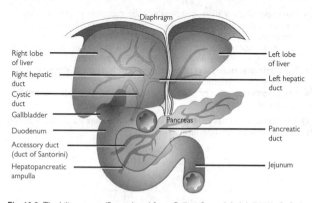

Fig. 10.2 The biliary tract. (Reproduced from Collins, S., et al. (eds.) (2008). *Oxford Handbook of Obstetrics and Gynaecology*, 2nd edn, Oxford University Press, Oxford with permission from the Burdett Institute of Gastrointestinal Nursing, King's College, London.)

Nursing assessment: history

▶▶ Some patients with a GI problem will require immediate resuscitative interventions. ∴ a brief ABC assessment should always be undertaken (⬚ see Chapter 3, 'Management of the patient with multiple injuries, p.40). The most common life-threatening consequence of a GI problem is hypovolaemic shock. Severe pain also requires immediate intervention, usually with opiate analgesia.

It can sometimes be difficult to identify whether a patient's symptoms are GI in origin. The nurse should always be alert to the possibility that the symptoms may originate outside the GI system.

History

The presence of any of the following features is relevant and can help to direct further assessment and investigations.
- Abdominal pain (⬚ see 'Abdominal pain' below).
- Nausea (the feeling of wanting to vomit).
- Vomiting; projectile suggests gastric outflow obstruction. Large volumes or faeculent fluid suggest intestinal obstruction. NB. Nausea and vomiting without abdominal pain may not be of GI origin.
- Diarrhoea: duration; frequency; presence of blood; consistency.
- Constipation. When were bowels last opened?
- Melaena.
- Haematemesis.
- Coffee-ground vomit.
- Fever, shivers.
- Indigestion.
- Weight loss.
- Loss of appetite.
- Dysphagia.
- LMP.
- Dysuria.
- Medications, particularly NSAIDs.
- Alcohol intake.
- Travel.

The PQRST mnemonic is a useful tool in the assessment of pain.
- **P**rovocation.
- **Q**uality.
- **R**adiation/relief.
- **S**ite/severity/other symptoms.
- **T**ime.

Abdominal pain Comprehensive assessment of abdominal pain can help indicate source of pain, guides investigation, and enables prescription of effective analgesia.
- Organ pain caused by stretching or inflammation. Often described as dull, not aggravated by movement, and tends to occur around midline.
- Abdominal wall pain. Cause: activation of pain-sensitive fibres in peritoneum. Well localized pain aggravated by movement or stretching. Pain described as sharp and stabbing. Palpation is extremely painful and exacerbated when palpating hand is removed (rebound tenderness).

Assessment of abdominal pain

- Where is the pain (site)?
  - Helps to localize an area/quadrant.
- What is the pain like (quality)?
  - Colicky pain comes and goes,
  - Spasmodic pain can be 'squeezing' in nature and suggests obstruction of a hollow structure.
  - Sharp pain is localized and suggests peritoneal irritation.
  - Dull pain is less localized and suggests organ disorder.
- When did the pain start (time)?
  - Sudden onset suggests acute perforation or rupture.
- How long does the pain last (time)?
  - Is it intermittent or persistent.
- Where does the pain go (radiation)? 📖 See Table 10.1.
- What makes the pain better or worse (relief and provocation)?
  - Eating can relieve pain in PUD or make pain from pancreatitis or small bowel obstruction worse.
  - Breathing can aggravate pain if the disordered organ lies next to the diaphragm.
  - Movement that makes pain worse suggests peritonitis.
  - Position. Flexing the legs may relieve pain from peritonitis. Lying flat can increase pain from pancreatitis.
- What else is going on (other symptoms)?
  - Nausea, vomiting, fever, diarrhoea, GU symptoms, LMP.

Table 10.1 Referred pain

Site of pain	Structure
RUQ, epigastric area, → shoulder tip pain, pain between shoulder blades	Gallbladder
LUQ, (left) shoulder tip pain (Kehr's sign)	Ruptured spleen
Lower anterior chest/epigastric region; mimics angina	Upper GI structures (oesophagus, duodenum, gallbladder, pancreas, biliary tree)
Epigastric radiating through to back	Pancreatitis; peptic ulcer
Throughout upper chest to back	Aortic aneurysm
Flank pain	Kidney
Loin to groin pain	Ureters (renal colic)
Periumbilical & shift to RLQ	Appendicitis
Testicles	Duodenal injury

Physical assessment, investigations, and nursing interventions

Physical assessment
Inspection
- Observe for abdominal distension, which can be caused by fat, flatus, faeces, fetus, or fluid.
- Ascites.
- Scars from previous surgery.
- Surface trauma to the abdomen or lower ribs: wounds; bruising; abrasions; impaled objects.
- Evisceration.
- Jaundice. Cholestatic jaundice is either directly related to a problem within the liver, e.g. cirrhosis, or due to extrahepatic causes, e.g. bile duct stone, pancreatitis, or carcinoma.

Palpation
Although not a skill routinely practised by ED nurses, palpation of the abdomen by the assessing clinician can identify the specific site of pain, pain patterns on examination, and the presence of any masses. In health abdominal organs are not usually palpable except in the very thin.

Pain patterns
- Tenderness. Pain may be localized to an abdominal organ or a quadrant on palpation.
- Guarding is the normal tendency to contract the abdominal muscles on examination. Guarding (increased abdominal muscle tome) despite relaxing/reassuring the patient accompanies intraabdominal disease.
- Rebound tenderness reveals deep-seated inflammation and is elicited on abrupt withdrawal of the palpating hand.
- Rigidity. Generalized 'board-like' rigidity implies peritonitis; the abdomen does not move on respiration.

Auscultation All four quadrants should be auscultated for bowel sounds. Absent bowel sounds are highly suggestive of intraabdominal pathology. Tinkling bowel sounds suggest obstruction.

Percussion
- Dullness indicates fluid or an enlarged organ; hyperresonance suggests air in the abdominal cavity.
- Percussion can be extremely painful, especially in the acute abdomen.

Investigations
Assessment of the patient with abdominal pain can be complex. Even those apparently well and triaged into a low priority category *should* have a full set of vital signs. Even slight abnormalities, e.g. tachycardia, should not be dismissed. The elderly, critically ill, and immuno compromised may not develop a fever even in the presence of overwhelming infection.
- Pulse.
- Temperature.

- Respiratory rate.
- Blood pressure.
- Pain assessment and score.
- Urinalysis.
- ECG if pain is epigastric.

Not all patients will require all of the following investigations. Assessment and examination by the assessing clinician may be required to indentify what, if any, investigations are indicated.

- FBC, U & E, β-HCG, amylase/lipase.
- Lactic acid is useful in helping diagnose bowel ischaemia especially in the elderly.
- Capillary blood glucose (DKA can present as an acute abdomen).
- AXR; erect CXR
- ABG if the patient is shocked.

⚠ Every year women still die of ruptured ectopic pregnancy, some having attended an ED with symptoms that were not fully explored. All females of child-bearing age who present with abdominal pain should have an ectopic pregnancy actively ruled out as a cause of their pain. A pregnancy test should be done in the ED. ***Beware***. Ectopic pregnancies can present atypically as genitourinary or gastrointestinal upset, e.g. diarrhoea and vomiting, dysuria.

General nursing interventions

- Analgesia. Opiate analgesia should be given IV, titrated to response. An anti-spasmodic can be useful in colicky pain.
- Anti-emetics.
- IV antibiotics. May be indicated in perforation, infection.
- IV fluids, fluid resuscitation if indicated. Patients who are dehydrated, NBM, vomiting, or shocked will require IV fluids.
- Oxygen therapy if the patient is shocked.
- Psychological support. Patients will need support and explanation about procedures and treatment. During examination the presence of the ED nurse is vital in maintaining the patient's privacy and dignity.
- Insertion of urinary catheter. In shock this is essential; hourly urine measurements are required.
- Monitoring of fluid balance. An 'input/output' chart should be commenced.
- NG tube placement is indicated in bowel obstruction, perforation. (📖 see p.638.)

Epigastric pain

Epigastric pain is a very common presentation both in primary care and the ED. A wide variety of problems can present with epigastric pain, some relatively benign, e.g. indigestion, others much more serious, e.g. pancreatitis, inferior MI, PUD.

Nursing assessment

Nursing evaluation should take into account the need to assess for a range of problems and may need to include some or all of the following.
- Vital signs.
- ECG.
- Pain assessment and score.
- CXR/AXR.
- Capillary blood glucose.
- FBC, U & E, amylase/lipase, LFTs.

Nursing interventions

- Analgesia.
- Antacid.
- Anti-emetic.
- IV fluids.

Gastrointestinal bleeding

Bleeding can occur from any part of the GI system. Acute upper GI bleeding can present as haematemesis ± melaena. It is commonly caused by PUD (50%), oesophageal varices (10–20%), gastric erosions (15–20%), and Mallory–Weiss syndrome (5–10%). Chronic GI bleeding usually presents as anaemia. Iron deficiency anaemia in men and post-menopausal women is usually of GI origin and investigations of the upper and lower GI tract may be necessary to identify the cause if it is not apparent from history and examination.

Massive acute lower GI bleeding is rare and is most commonly seen in the elderly. A small amount of bleeding from haemorrhoids is much more common and is a frequent cause of anxiety that prompts an ED attendance. Massive lower GI bleeding is usually due to either diverticular disease or ischaemic colitis. Patients require the same rapid assessment and resuscitation as those with upper GI bleeding.

▶ Patients who present with GI bleeding require an initial rapid assessment to identify those who are shocked and require resuscitation (📖 see p.246 for assessment of shock).

Haematemesis Vomiting fresh blood or darker blood (sometimes called 'coffee grounds') occurs after bleeding in the oesophagus, stomach, or duodenum. Darker/coffee ground vomit occurs as blood is altered in the stomach over time by gastric acid.

Melaena is abnormally black, tarry stools with a distinctive offensive odour. The stools contain digested blood that has usually originated from an upper GI bleed that may be acute or chronic.

Mallory–Weiss syndrome is bleeding from a tear in the mucosa at the gastro-oesophageal junction. It is usually caused by protracted vomiting/retching and is often associated with the prolonged vomiting that results from excessive alcohol intake! Blood loss may be large but in most patients it stops spontaneously. Diagnosis is by endoscopy, which then allows early discharge from hospital.

Massive GI bleeding

▶▶ Bleeding from PUD or oesophageal varices accounts for up to 70% of upper GI haemorrhage. Urgent resuscitation is required prior to any in-depth assessment as to the cause.

Bleeding from ruptured varices can be phenomenal—like a hose pipe! Loss of > 40% of blood volume is immediately life-threatening and blood loss is often underestimated. Early involvement and advice from a haematologist can guide blood replacement and help manage derangements in clotting that are often a consequence of massive transfusion (📖 see p.586).

- Airway protection. In patients with massive haemorrhage and a reduced level of consciousness urgent intubation may be required to protect the airway (📖 see p.570).
- Oxygen administration may be difficult if there is continued vomiting. Nasal prongs may be a useful way of administering low flow oxygen.

- IV access. × 2 large bore cannulae (green or grey) into large veins will allow the rapid infusion of warmed fluids, blood, and FFP. Immediate central access may be indicated if the bleeding is significant.
- Bloods sent for FBC, U & E, LFTs, cross-match, clotting.
  - ❶ *Ensure* samples are labelled correctly as mislabelling is the most common transfusion risk. If resuscitation is prolonged with multiple interventions these bloods will need to be repeated regularly.
- ABGs.
- IV fluids. Give warmed crystalloid or colloid followed by blood. Blood transfusion is indicated when 30% of circulating volume is lost. O-negative blood can be given almost immediately, followed by type-specific, then fully cross-matched blood.
- Replacement platelets/clotting factors. Platelets, FFP, and cryoprecipitate may need to be given in massive blood loss (usually when > 100% blood volume has been lost) These replace essential clotting factors and can help prevent the development of DIC.
- CVP monitoring.
- Arterial line to enable continuous invasive monitoring.
- Urinary catheter. Aim for a urine output > 30mL/h.
- Nasogastric tube.
- Keep the patient warm. Hypothermia increases the risk of serious complications, e.g. DIC.
- Further cardiovascular support may be needed with inotropes and vasopressors.

Monitoring of patients with massive blood loss
- Pulse.
- Respiratory rate.
- SpO_2.
- Blood pressure (usually invasive).
- Skin colour.
- CVP.
- Urinary output, monitored hourly.
- GCS.
- Continuous cardiac monitoring.
- 12-lead ECG.
- CXR.
- Repeated bloods.
- Repeated ABGs.
- Record fluid balance meticulously.

Peptic ulcer disease (PUD)

Peptic ulcer disease (PUD) is a collective term given to ulcers in the stomach (gastric ulcers) or the duodenum (duodenal ulcers; DU). The most common cause of upper GI bleeding is peptic ulcers, accounting for about 50% of cases.

In health a balance exists between peptic acid secretion and gastro-duodenal mucosal defence. Inflammation and ulceration occur when the balance is disrupted. Factors such as NSAIDs, *Helicobacter pylori* infection, and alcohol can alter the mucosal defence by allowing acid to diffuse back and cause epithelial cell injury.

- Gastritis is superficial inflammation of the mucosa.
- In ulceration there is a complete break in the mucosa down to the muscular layer.

Inflammation tends to respond well to antacids.

Signs and symptoms

- Epigastric pain—the patient may point directly to the epigastrium. Pain can be relived by eating. Severe sudden pain may indicate perforation.
- Nocturnal pain—classically occurs with a DU.
- Nausea.
- Heartburn.
- Anorexia and weight loss.
- Melaena.
- Haematemesis.
- Shock in perforation.
- Fever in peritonitis.
- Rebound tenderness, rigidity in peritonitis.

For the management of massive GI bleeding ☐ see Gastrointestinal bleeding, p.328.

⚠ Some patients may have been asymptomatic and present acutely with a perforation; this is more likely in the elderly or those on regular NSAIDs.

Peritonitis

Peritonitis is a common consequence of perforation of the GI tract and can be caused, for example, by a perforated ulcer, appendix, or diverticulum.

Signs and symptoms of peritonitis

- Severe abdominal pain.
  - ⚠ In the elderly or those with underlying inflammatory bowel disease it may be more insidious.
- Rigid 'board-like' abdomen.
- Rebound tenderness.
- Absent bowel sounds.
- Hypovolaemic shock.
- Septic shock as time progresses.
- Fever.
- Vomiting.

- Tachycardia.
- Tachypnoea.

Nursing assessment

Patients with simple gastritis may require little more than antacids and GP follow-up. However, nursing assessment should be aimed at ensuring that all serious underlying problems are ruled out prior to discharge.

- Vital signs.
- Evaluate for signs of hypovolaemic or septic shock.
- Pain assessment and score.
- Bloods: FBU; U & E; amylase/lipase.
- ABG.
- Erect CXR. In 75% of patients with an acute perforation free gas can be seen under the diaphragm.
- AXR.

Nursing intervention for patients with perforation

Patients with an acute perforation exhibit signs of peritonitis due to the leakage of gastric contents that irritate/infect and inflame the peritoneum.

- IV analgesia.
- Antiemetic.
- IV access.
- Oxygen therapy.
- Ensure bloods sent and group and save.
- IV antibiotics.
- Fluid resuscitation.
- NG tube.
- Urinary catheter.
- Prepare for theatre.

Oesophageal varices

Acute bleeding from oesophageal varices is a fairly common ED presentation and accounts for 10–20% of acute upper GI bleeding. There is usually a history of alcohol abuse and cirrhosis. 90% of patients with alcoholic cirrhosis develop varices over a 10-year period, during which they develop and enlarge. ∴ patients with severe cirrhosis and large varices are most likely to bleed. Interestingly, the majority of patients with alcoholic cirrhosis who stop drinking have a reduction in the size of their varices—sometimes they disappear completely.

Varices develop as necrosis of liver cells damages the structure and function of the liver. In patients with cirrhosis all the functions of the liver are disrupted, e.g. clotting is deranged as protein synthesis is affected. Because the structure of the liver is grossly abnormal, blood flow is affected. Portal hypertension develops as blood can no longer drain freely from the GI tract via the portal vein into the liver. As the blood 'backflows' and portal pressure increases, the venous system dilates and a collateral circulation develops. The most common site of this collateral circulation is at the gastro-oesophageal junction. Because these gastro-oesophageal veins are superficial they tend to rupture. 50% of patients with portal hypertension will bleed from their varices.

- Mortality is extremely high: 50% of patients die following the first episode of bleeding.
- Primary prophylaxis tends to be with propranolol or surgery.
- Patients who present to the ED with massive upper GI bleeding, whatever the cause, require immediate airway protection and fluid resuscitation. For the management of massive GI bleeding 📖 see p.328.

Nursing interventions

⚠ Specific nursing interventions for oesophageal variceal haemorrhage depend on the availability of urgent endoscopy.

Urgent endoscopy available If endoscopy is urgently available then the varices will be either ligated or subject to sclerotherapy (chemical injected into the vein to cause it to narrow/clot).

Urgent endoscopy not available
Several pharmacological interventions are available to control acute bleeding.
- Vasopressin ± GTN infusion.
- Somatostatin, octreotide.

Insertion of a 3 lumen Sengstaken tube can be used if endoscopy is not available and drug treatment is contraindicated or has failed. A Sengstaken tube is usually refrigerated as it is stiffer and easier to insert when cold. The procedure is very unpleasant for the patient but can be life-saving in the presence of severe haemorrhage. It stops bleeding in 90% of cases although re-bleeding occurs in 50% of patients on deflation of the tube (📖 see p.664).

Prophylactic antibiotics reduce mortality and morbidity.

Ruptured oesophagus

Although rare, this complication of vomiting or, even more rarely, blunt or penetrating trauma has significant morbidity and mortality.

Signs and symptoms
- Severe chest pain.
- Surgical emphysema in the neck.
- Normal ECG, which rules out cardiac causes of chest pain.
- Abnormal CXR: pneumomediastinum, pneumothorax.
- There may be history of vomiting.
- Signs of shock.

Nursing interventions
- Oxygen.
- IV analgesia.
- IV fluids.
- IV antibiotics.
- Cardiothoracic opinion.

Appendicitis

Appendicitis is a common ED presentation in children (📖 see Chapter 4, 'Surgical emergencies', 'Appendicitis', p.110) and young adults. It is less common in patients over 40 years.

- Appendicitis is the most common surgical emergency and should be considered as a cause of an acute abdomen in all patients if it has not been removed.
- The presentation can range from mild/moderate right iliac fossa (RIF) pain to generalized peritonitis with associated shock.
- Presentations are often atypical, symptoms vary, and up to 45% of appendices that are removed are normal. In sexually active women acute salpingitis associated with sexually transmitted infections is a common cause of RIF pain. Pain can be bilateral and there is an associated vaginal discharge.

❶ The diagnosis of appendicitis is a clinical one unless a CT scan has been performed and excludes it. ∴ Do not allow the surgeon to delay assessment by insisting on waiting until blood results are available.

Signs and symptoms
- Nausea.
- Vomiting.
- Abdominal pain. Classically pain begins vaguely centrally/periumbilical and then localizes to the RIF.
- Fever.
- Diarrhoea occasionally occurs.

Nursing assessment

Accurate nursing assessment should enable differentiation between patients with localized pain in the RIF and those with more serious pathology, e.g. generalized peritonitis and shock. Assessment should also include investigations that may point to another cause.
- Vital signs.
- Pain assessment and score.
- Urinalysis.
- LMP; risk of pregnancy.
- FBC. The WCC may be raised but it isn't always.
- U & E.
- $_\beta$HCG

Nursing interventions
- IV access.
- Analgesia.
- IV fluids if NBM or dehydrated.
- IV antibiotics reduce the risk of postoperative complications associated with infection.
- Prepare for admission.
- Preoperative preparation may be required if theatre is arranged imminently.

Biliary colic and acute cholecystitis

Gallstones are very common and are present in many people, often remaining asymptomatic throughout life.

- However, in some people they move out of the gallbladder and cause severe pain when they become lodged in the gallbladder neck, common bile duct, or cystic duct. This is often termed biliary colic and is usually a temporary obstruction. The term 'colic' can be confusing when used in this context as it usually does not 'come and go' but is constant, severe, and increases in severity.
- Acute cholecystitis is the term given to inflammation of the gallbladder that results from a stone preventing the gallbladder emptying. When the cystic duct is blocked the gallbladder distends, becomes inflamed, and then may become infected and even distended by pus.

Signs and symptoms of biliary colic

Patients tend to be systemically well and can even be discharged home for GP follow-up and further investigation if their pain subsides, examination is normal, and blood results are not significantly abnormal.

- Pain is usually epigastric but can be localized to the RUQ. Pain may radiate to the right shoulder/through to the back.
- Pain may be related to eating food with a high fat content.
- Nausea and vomiting in more severe cases.

Signs and symptoms of cholecystitis

Initially the signs and symptoms are similar to those of biliary colic. However, as time passes severe pain localizes to the RUQ. There is overlying peritonitis due to inflammatory changes in the gallbladder. Patients tend to be systemically unwell and require admission. Occasionally there can be septic shock, which requires resuscitation (☐ see p.246).

- Severe RUQ pain.
- RUQ guarding and rigidity.
- Fever.
- Mass in the RUQ. Occasionally there is a palpable mass.

Nursing assessment

- Vital signs.
- Pain assessment and score.
- LMP. Ruptured ectopic can present with shoulder tip pain.
- ECG to rule out MI.
- FBC, U & E, LFTs, amylase/lipase.
- AXR. Stones may be visible.
- USS is the most useful investigation as it can confirm cholecystitis.

Nursing intervention

- IV access.
- Analgesia, usually opiate.
- IV fluids if NBM, dehydrated.
- Fluid resuscitation of shocked.
- IV antibiotics if infection suspected.

Pancreatitis

Pancreatitis can be acute or chronic and episodes can be recurrent. In the ED the differentiation between an acute episode or one that develops on a background of chronic disease is difficult and probably unnecessary. Patients who have had previous episodes of pancreatitis are quick to recognize their symptoms and may present regularly to the ED, particularly those with chronic alcohol problems.

- The most common causes of acute pancreatitis in the developed world are alcohol, gallstones, and trauma.
- Gallstones that obstruct the pancreatic duct can cause pancreatitis.
- Increased alcohol intake is frequently associated with chronic pancreatitis.
- The severity of pancreatitis is wide ranging: inflammation may be mild and self-limiting but in its severest form it has a mortality of 40–50%.
- Consider a diagnosis of pancreatitis in all patients with epigastric pain.

Signs and symptoms

Mild disease may present with minimal signs and symptoms. 25% of all patients with pancreatitis will have severe disease; they will be critically ill requiring resuscitation and intensive care. The earlier severe disease is identified, the sooner aggressive treatment can begin. However, in those with only mild symptoms it is difficult to predict who will develop severe complications. The ED nurse needs to be vigilant in the ongoing assessment of the patient's physiological status. Predictive tools can be used to assess the severity of pancreatitis but most are of limited value on presentation.

- Pain. Classically it is epigastric and radiates through to the back.
- Nausea and vomiting.
- Tachycardia.
- Hypotensive
- Septic.
- Oliguric.
- Widespread abdominal tenderness, guarding, rigidity.
- Absent bowel sounds.
- Jaundice if there is obstruction within the biliary tract or associated cirrhosis.

Nursing assessment

- Vital signs.
- Pain assessment and score.
- Urine output.
- FBC, U & E, LFT, glucose, clotting, lactic acid, calcium.
- Amylase.
- Lipase is sensitive and specific to pancreatitis and can be more accurate in diagnosis than amylase, especially in chronic disease.
- ABG.
- Erect CXR. Excludes perforation, which can also cause a rise in amylase.
- ECG.

Nursing interventions
- Oxygen.
- IV access.
- IV fluids.
- IV antibiotics.
- Fluid resuscitation if shocked.
- Analgesia.
- Anti-emetic.
- NBM.
- NG tube.
- Urinary catheter.
- CVP monitoring in the critically ill, which can guide fluid resuscitation.
- Prepare for possible HDU/ICU transfer.

Alcoholic liver disease (ALD)

The harmful effects of alcohol are wide ranging and the impact is social, psychological, and physical. Women are much more prone that men to the harmful physical effects of alcohol. Not everyone who has an increased alcohol intake develops ALD. Approximately 30% of 'alcoholics' develop cirrhosis. Men drinking in excess of 8 units (4 pints) per day for 10 years have a high risk of developing cirrhosis; for women this is only 4 units.

Alcoholic liver disease (ALD) is a collective term given to a spectrum of diseases that result from excess alcohol intake.

- Fatty liver occurs with minimal amounts of alcohol. Fat is present in the liver but there is no damage to the liver cells. The fat disappears when alcohol intake is stopped. There are often no symptoms.
- Alcoholic hepatitis is next in the continuum of ALD. As well as fatty change there is liver cell death. Symptoms may be mild; there may be general ill health, signs of chronic liver disease, and some jaundice. Abstinence from alcohol can reverse all the effects.
- If the patient continues to drink then cirrhosis is likely. Alcoholic cirrhosis is the irreversible, end stage of ALD. The liver is grossly abnormal, there are problems with blood flow (portal hypertension), and liver function is deranged. General signs of chronic liver disease include fever and jaundice.
  - In compensated chronic liver disease there is a range of signs that are present in the skin, abdomen, and endocrine systems. People with compensated cirrhosis should lead a normal life.
  - When chronic liver disease becomes decompensated, ascites develops and neurological function is markedly impaired.
  - Long-term survival from cirrhosis depends on complete alcohol abstinence. 5-year survival is 70% in those who abstain.

Signs and symptoms of chronic liver disease

- RUQ pain.
- Anorexia, weight loss.
- Ascites.
- Ankle oedema.
- Jaundice.
- GI bleeding (haematemesis, melaena, varices).
- Spider naevi.
- Palmar erythema.
- Dupuytren's contracture.
- Splenomegaly.
- Portal hypertension.
- Gynaecomastia.
- Disorientation, drowsy progressing to coma (Wernicke's encephalopathy). (📖 see p.534–535.)

Nursing assessment

- Vital signs.
- AVPU/GCS.
- FBC, U & E, glucose, LFTs, clotting, ammonia level.

Nursing intervention
- IV access.
- IV fluids.
- IV thiamine (can cause anaphylaxis).
- Lactulose. Reduces the production of ammonia in the GI tract which is the main cause of encephalopathy.

Intestinal obstruction

Intestinal obstruction is a common cause of acute abdomen and has different causes in the small and large bowel.

- Small bowel obstruction is very commonly caused by adhesions. Less common causes are strangulated hernias and intussusception.
- Obstruction of the colon is commonly caused by tumour, sigmoid volvulus, or diverticular disease.

The bowel becomes distended above the obstruction, inflamed, infiltrated by bacteria, and, in strangulation, ischaemic and gangrenous.

Signs and symptoms

Signs and symptoms are dependent to some extent on the site of the obstruction. If there has been previous abdominal surgery adhesions are usually the cause. Obtaining hospital notes can be helpful.

- Abdominal pain. Severe pain suggests strangulation.
- Abdominal distension.
- Vomiting, especially in small bowel obstruction.
- Constipation.
- Signs of shock.
- Signs of peritonitis.
- Fever.
- Bowel sounds may be 'tinkling' or absent.

Nursing assessment

- Vital signs.
- Pain assessment and score.
- LMP.
- FBC, U & E, LFTs, amylase/lipase, group and save.
- ECG.
- CXR.
- AXR may reveal distended loops of bowel above the obstruction. Fluid levels may be seen.
- ABG.

Nursing intervention

- IV access.
- Oxygen.
- Analgesia.
- Anti-emetic
- IV fluids.
- Fluid resuscitation if shocked.
- IV antibiotics.
- NG tube.
- Urinary catheter.

Diverticulitis

Diverticulitis is a common GI disease, thought to be a result of increased pressure in the lumen of the colon associated with lack of dietary fibre. Increased luminal pressure contributes to the development of 'pouches' or diverticula on the outside of the colon. When these diverticula get blocked with food particles or faeces they become infected. The severity of the symptoms depends on the extent of the infection and development of any complications, e.g. peritonitis from perforation. Diverticulitis is more common in the middle-aged and elderly. Older patients and the immunosuppressed may not mount a pyrexia or have obvious signs of peritonitis.

Signs and symptoms

- LLQ pain (usually the diverticula are in the sigmoid colon).
- Fever.
- Nausea.
- Constipation or diarrhoea.
- Peritonitis if the diverticula perforate.
- A tender palpable mass in the LLQ may indicate abscess formation.

Nursing assessment

- Vital signs.
- Pain assessment and score.
- LMP.
- FBC, U & E, group and save, blood cultures.
- Erect CXR may help to identify free gas in a perforation.
- AXR may help to identify perforation or obstruction.
- ABG.

Nursing intervention

- IV access.
- NBM.
- Analgesia.
- Anti-emetic.
- IV fluids.
- Fluid resuscitation if shocked.
- IV antibiotics.
- NGT.
- Urinary catheter.

Complications

- Perforation.
- Intestinal obstruction.
- Massive PR bleeding.
- Fistula (small bowel, vaginal, bladder).

Inflammatory bowel disease

Inflammatory bowel disease (IBD) covers two main diseases, ulcerative colitis and Crohn's disease. Ulcerative colitis affects the colon only and Crohn's disease can affect any part of the GI tract from the mouth to the rectum. Patients with established IBD may present to the ED with a severe exacerbation of their disease. However, most patients remain relatively well and live a normal life when in remission. Patients may also present with their first episode and may require referral ± admission for assessment and diagnosis of their symptoms.

Signs and symptoms
- Diarrhoea: when the colon is affected this is usually bloody. In ulcerative colitis there is usually mucus.
- Abdominal pain.
- Weight loss.
- Malaise.
- Lethargy.
- Nausea.
- Vomiting.
- Fever.
- Signs of intestinal obstruction.
- Signs of shock.
- Anaemia.
- Tachycardia.

Nursing assessment
- Vital signs.
- Pain assessment and score.
- FBC, U & E, LFTs, amylase/lipase, CRP, ESR.
- AXR.

Nursing intervention
- IV access.
- IV fluids.
- Analgesia.
- Anti-emetic.
- IV antibiotics.
- NG tube.
- Urinary catheter if shocked.

Gastroenteritis

Gastroenteritis is a very common presentation in primary care and the ED. Acute infection of the GI tract (gastroenteritis) may present with diarrhoea ± vomiting. The most common cause in adults is bacterial infection although viruses are increasingly common. Norwalk (Norovirus) virus is particularly virulent and is responsible for causing outbreaks of diarrhoea and vomiting on cruise ships, schools, hospitals and nursing homes. Patients may have fever and abdominal pain. Children and the elderly are most vulnerable to the affects of gastroenteritis. The elderly can also present with diarrhoea when they have a UTI, constipation, or a chest infection.

Patients who present to the ED with diarrhoea ± vomiting where the cause is thought to be infectious should be asked to wash their hands if they are ambulatory and are remaining in the waiting room. Patients who require further nursing/medical assessment should be nursed in a cubicle with strict infection control measures (Ⅲ see p.34).

Signs and symptoms

A careful history may reveal the cause of the gastroenteritis, duration of symptoms, drugs, travel, contacts, or contaminated food.

- Diarrhoea: frequency, consistency, watery, bloody, mucus.
- Vomiting.
- Abdominal pain.
- Fever.
- Dehydration (Ⅲ see Box 10.1).
- Shock.

Box 10.1 Dehydration

Identifying the presence and extent of dehydration is important as it guides the approach to rehydration and the need for hospital admission. In children it is more common to classify dehydration as mild (< 5%), moderate (5–10%), or severe (> 10%). However, the following classification can also be used in adults:

- Mild. Thirst, dry lips/mouth, reduced urine output
- Moderate. Lethargic, tachycardia, tachypnoea, postural hypotension
- Severe. Hypotension, drowsy, anuria.

Nursing assessment

- Vital signs.
- Pain assessment and score.
- Assess degree of dehydration (Ⅲ see Box 10.1).
- FBC, U & E if dehydrated.
- Stool for culture (not usually necessary) only if recent foreign travel, from residential/institutional care, severe illness.

Nursing intervention

- Strict infection control precautions.
- IV access.
- Oral rehydration if possible.
- IV fluids.
- Fluid resuscitation if shocked.

Admission Patients with mild dehydration unable to tolerate oral fluids or those with moderate to severe dehydration require admission for IV fluids and monitoring of electrolyte balance.

Discharge Patients with mild dehydration who are able to tolerate oral fluids can be discharged with advice about oral hydration and when to seek further medical assessment.

Rectal bleeding

The most common cause of bleeding and/or melaena from the rectum is the passage of blood from acute upper GI bleeding. Only 20% of GI bleeding is from the lower GI tract. The passage of bright red blood from the rectum usually indicates lower GI tract bleeding. Diverticulitis, carcinoma, and IBD are the most common causes. Patients with signs of hypovolaemic shock require urgent fluid resuscitation (□ see p.246).

Haemorroids

Haemorrhoids are the most common cause of painless rectal bleeding that may prompt an ED attendance. Increased pressure in anal veins causes them to bulge, protrude, and bleed. Blood from haemorrhoids is bright red and usually reported on toilet paper or on the outside of faeces; it is not mixed in the stool. Pregnancy, Crohn's disease, and ulcerative colitis are often associated with haemorrhoids.

Signs and symptoms
• PR bleeding, bright red.
• Pain.

Haemorrhoids can bleed, prolapse, or thrombose. Simple bleeding usually requires conservative management. Prolapsed or thrombosed haemorrhoids may require surgical referral to assess the need for surgery.

Nursing assessment involves identifying if the cause is likely to be haemorrhoids, i.e. painless, bright red blood not mixed with stools, or if the bleeding is likely to be from higher in the GI tract and requires further assessment/investigation.

Nursing interventions
• Analgesia.
• Advice about stool softeners.
• Surgical referral in some cases.

Pilonidal abscess

Patients can either present to the ED or GP with pain and swelling at the coccyx. It more commonly affects males in late teens to early twenties and can cause acute embarrassment. Systemic illness as a consequence of the infection is rare.

Signs and symptoms
- Pain and tenderness.
- Swelling.
- Area of fluctuant pus.
- Discharge.
- Surrounding cellulitis.

Nursing assessment and interventions
- Pain assessment, score and analgesia.
- Preparation for admission.

Abdominal trauma

Abdominal injury is the third leading cause of death in trauma. Blunt trauma to the abdomen from either compressive (punch to stomach) or deceleration forces (high speed RTC) are the most common mechanisms injuring abdominal organs. The kidneys are relatively mobile structures and are prone to injury from deceleration forces, which can cause tears in the renal arteries. The increasing use of guns and knives has resulted in a rise in number of patients who present with penetrating injuries to the abdomen. All multiply injured patients should have their abdomen evaluated to assess for organ injuries as part of a trauma assessment (📖 see p.40).

Patients can present with an isolated abdominal injury where the mechanism is clear, e.g. elbow to the abdomen during rugby tackle. More complex and difficult to diagnose are patients with multiple injuries who may or may not have a significant intra-abdominal problem.

- Life-threatening injuries can occur without any signs of trauma to the abdomen.
- Where bleeding is confined to the retroperitoneal space examination of the anterior abdomen may be entirely normal.
- Abdominal injuries should be suspected and assessed for in any patient with trauma between the 4th rib and hips. This will ensure that patients with lower chest injuries have their abdomen appropriately assessed as the liver and spleen could be injured.
- Assessment of flanks is also crucial to detect any retroperitoneal injury.
- Penetrating injuries to the chest have the potential to damage both thoracic and abdominal organs.

Vascular abdominal organs The liver and spleen are solid, extremely vascular organs enclosed in a fibrous capsule. Injuries range from haematomas, to lacerations, to burst type injuries. Blood loss can be significant.

Fluid/gas-filled abdominal organs The stomach and the small and large bowel are vulnerable to perforation from penetrating injuries. Rupture of the stomach or intestines can also occur from blunt forces. A transient rise in intraluminal pressure causes perforation. Leakage of abdominal contents into the peritoneal cavity causes peritonitis, which develops over a number of hours.

Signs and symptoms of intra-abdominal injury

Signs and symptoms highly suggestive of intra-abdominal pathology are pain, blood loss, and absent or diminished bowel sounds. However, signs of injury are often subtle and can even be absent initially. The abdomen can sequester large amounts of blood without any obvious distension and all symptoms can be absent if there is a retroperitoneal haematoma, competing pain from another injury, drugs/alcohol, reduced level of consciousness, or spinal cord injury. Physical findings are not always accurate. ~ 20% of patients with a significant abdominal injury only have trivial signs.

These are common signs and symptoms of intra-abdominal injury.

- Surface trauma to the lower chest, abdomen, or flanks, e.g. bruising, seatbelt markings, wounds, impaled objects.

- Absent bowel sounds. Direct bowel injury or blood or digestive secretions in the peritoneal cavity can decrease peristalsis.
- Pain and the pattern: guarding, rebound tenderness, rigidity.
- Referred pain (📖 see Table 10.1, p.323).
- Hypovolaemic shock.
- Dullness on percussion may indicate fluid within the abdomen.
- Hyperresonance on percussion may indicate air within the peritoneum.
- Haematuria can indicate renal, urethral, or bladder injuries.
- Scrotal bruising can indicate urethral trauma.

Nursing assessment

- Vital signs.
- Pain assessment and score.
- Urinalysis.
- FBC, U & E, amylase/lipase, LFTs group and save, cross-match, ABG.
- Erect CXR may detect air under the diaphragm.

Nursing interventions

- Oxygen.
- IV access.
- Fluid resuscitation

⚠ Aggressive fluid resuscitation in an unstable patient with a penetrating injury can worsen their prognosis. A systolic BP of 90mmHg in a conscious patient is acceptable prior to transfer to theatre.

- Analgesia.
- NG tube.
- Urinary catheter.
- IV antibiotics.
- Secure impaled objects. These should only be removed in theatre.
- Cover wounds.
- Prepare for USS, DPL, or CT.
- Prepare urgently for theatre patients with signs of peritonitis and/or hypovolaemic shock.

Further investigations

- USS is increasingly performed at the bedside in the resuscitation room. It is non-invasive and repeatable. It is operator-dependent and may miss some bowel and pancreatic injuries
- DPL although invasive allows early bedside diagnosis of intraabdominal bleeding and is 98% accurate. It may miss retroperitoneal injuries. (📖 see p.610.)
- CT scan with contrast is often used and has a high accuracy. However, it usually takes time to organize and perform. Therefore the patient has to be relatively stable.

Genitourinary emergencies

Overview

Patients with a genitourinary problem may present with relatively minor complaints or more significant problems. Management priorities include:

• analgesia and symptom control;
• information regarding investigations;
• health promotion pre-discharge or preparation for admission.

Few patients need resuscitation unless they are shocked, e.g. sepsis, toxic shock and, rarely, pyelonephritis.

However, although not usually life-threatening, it is important to recognize that sexual health issues may cause extreme embarrassment to the patient and it is important that nurses respond sensitively to minimize any distress.

The field of genitourinary medicine (GUM) also offers the emergency nurse the challenge of recognizing and acting on subtle clues. Some patients may fall within the 'see and treat' category and be sent to another facility but consideration needs to be given to the vulnerable patient.

Those with child protection issues, mental health issues, or post sexual assault may see the ED as a place of safety or the first part of contact to access information, reassurance, or other services, particularly as most GUM services are closed at the weekend or out-of-hours.

If registration takes place before nurse triage, the real reason for presentation may not be revealed due to embarrassment, shame, and/or lack of privacy at reception. Sensitivity needs to be employed when obtaining a relevant patient history along with recognition that, while people are becoming sexually active at a younger age, elderly people have sex too and can become unwell. Cultural issues may also prevent patients being frank about their presenting complaint and language barriers may present additional challenges.

▶ Be vigilant and mindful. The patient labelled as an 'inappropriate attender' may need your professional awareness, understanding, and compassion.

Assessment

History taking

Discussing what are usually intimate and private details with a stranger (albeit a health professional) risks patient dignity and requires privacy and sensitivity. Social norms have changed positively in recent years, information and reassurance can reduce perceived shame and embarrassment in relation to genital injury, sexual assault, and STIs.

- Family/friend input into history taking can be useful, particularly if a patient is in pain.
- Caution needs to be employed with maintaining patient confidentiality in the ED.
- Patients who present with symptoms that necessitate sexual history taking or sexual health promotion advice require a professional and non-familial interpreting service.
- Allowing a minor to interpret for a parent should also be avoided and, again, professional interpreting advice should be sought.

Physical examination

Rarely is a bimanual examination required for the ED genitourinary assessment unless there are signs or symptoms to suggest lower abdominal or pelvic pathology (□ see Figs. 11.1 and 11.2). The nurse should be familiar with the indications for this and they should sign their name in the notes if acting as a chaperone. The examination should preferably take place in a private room with a door, or screens if in the resuscitation room. Give the patient privacy to undress and use blanket/drapes to maintain the patient's dignity. Do not assist the patient to undress unless consent is obtained and it is clear the patient needs assistance.

Further reading

Vaginal and pelvic examinations: guidance for nursing staff ⏚ www.rcn.org.uk.

General Medical Council (2001). *GMC guidelines on intimate examinations*. GMC, London.

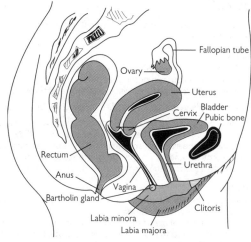

Fig. 11.1 Assessment of the genitourinary tract. Female genital anatomy. (Reproduced with permission from Pattman, R., et al. (2005). *Oxford Handbook of Genitourinary Medicine, HIV, and AIDS*, p. 51. Oxford University Press, Oxford.)

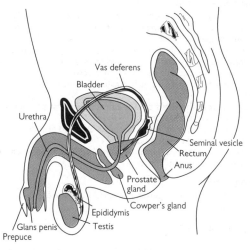

Fig. 11.2 Assessment of the genitourinary tract. Male genital anatomy (Reproduced with permission from Pattman, R., et al. (2005). *Oxford Handbook of Genitourinary Medicine, HIV, and AIDS*, p.53. Oxford University Press, Oxford.)

Renal colic

⚠ New onset flank pain in the elderly (≥ 60 years) may represent a leaking aortic aneurysm.

Prevalence
- In men 3:20 and in women 1:20.
- Peak age 20–40 years but can occur at any time.
- Half of those who develop stones will experience a recurrence.

Risk factors include dehydration, gout, UTI, previous or familial episodes.

Cause Renal colic is caused by calculi or blood clots, which may occur at any point in the renal tract. The pain is most often caused by ureteric spasm secondary to the irritation and inflammation caused by obstruction. Symptoms are not dependent on the size of the stone, which may range from a particle to a stone in the bladder.

Presentation
- Patient usually presents with unilateral and rarely bilateral loin pain from obstruction and/or haematuria.
- The location and type of pain depend on the location of the stone.
- Pain has been likened to that of childbirth and is acute. It is intense, constant, and dull associated with excruciating colicky pain that can radiate to the abdomen or refer to the respective iliac fossa, testis, and tip of the penis or the labia.

Nursing assessment
- Family history or a past medical history of renal disease or GI problems.
- Patients are often unable to sit still, are restless with pain, and may be standing upright and pacing.
- The patient may be pale, sweaty, or experience intense nausea and/or vomiting as a result of acute renal capsule or ureteric distension and spasm with a sympathetic nervous system response.
- Frank haematuria. Microscopic haematuria is present in only 80% on dipstix.
- Dysuria and/or other signs of UTI with acute, intense pain and strangury suggest a urethral stone.
  - Symptoms usually resolve if the stone is passed or if the stone has caused complete obstruction.
  - The urinary flow is interrupted with a urethral stone and, if large, acute urinary retention may occur.

Investigations
- Bilateral BP and femoral pulses. Examination for lower limb mottling may indicate AAA.
- TPR.
- IV access U & E, FBC.

Nursing intervention

▶▶ Ensure symptom control as soon as is possible.

- Diclofenac, usually PR/IM, is the analgesia of choice. It is effective with few side-effects but, as with all analgesia, its effect must be assessed. Sterile abscess incidence is 0.001% as a result of IM administration.
- An anti-emetic if nausea/vomiting are present.
- Start an IVI if persistent vomiting and check postural BP and pulse.
- IV opioid analgesia.
- Antispasmodics and anticholinergics are of no benefit.
- Fever if present indicates a complicated renal colic. An antipyretic can also promote patient comfort.

Investigations (continued)

- Urinalysis for red blood cells indicates renal tract trauma. A negative test does not exclude calculi.
- Sieving urine for passed stones and sending them for laboratory analysis is no longer practised in most areas. Check: urinalysis pH < 5 suggests uric acid stones and a pH > 7.5 indicates co-infection.
- CT of the abdomen is the diagnostic gold standard but usually a kidneys, urine, and bladder (KUB) X-ray film is done. This will identify 90–95% of renal calculi: 75% are calcium and are radio-opaque.
- This is followed by an IVU. Two X-rays are taken at 20min and 1h post contrast injection to examine the renal tract for the site and size/ degree of the obstruction.
- Doppler/USS can be used in pregnant patients or those with renal disease.

Discharge

- Discharge with renal outpatient follow-up, those who are symptom-free and whose IVU shows no obstruction.
  - Advise a fluid intake of 2–3L daily if no medical contraindications.
  - Nutritional advice for prevention is best provided by GP referral to a dietician.
- Prepare patients with infection, sepsis, renal impairment, or persistent pain for admission.

Urinary tract infection/cystitis (community-acquired)

Urinary tract infection/cystitis in women

- 25–35% of women aged 20–40 years have a history of UTI.
- This is not a sexually transmitted infection but coitus > 4 times a month increases risk of infection.
- 90% of UTIs are related to bacterial infection, particularly *Escherichia coli*, usually through self-transmission.
- 1:25 women will develop UTI in pregnancy.
- The use of spermicides with diaphragms can change vaginal pH, increasing susceptibility to *E. coli* infection.

Symptoms

- Symptoms of acute uncomplicated cystitis include dysuria, urinary frequency and urgency, lower back or suprapubic pain, cloudy or offensive urine, haematuria.
- If loin pain, renal angle tenderness, fever, rigor, malaise, and vomiting are present, ascending infection/pyelonephritis is indicated with the need for analgesia, antipyretics, IV antibiotics, and admission.

Investigations

- Urine dipstick: likely to be positive for nitrates and/or white cells and/or blood. Leucocytes/proteinuria is not indicative of infection.
- MSU should be taken and sent for laboratory analysis prior to starting antibiotics.

Health education

- Fluid intake may be reduced for duration of oral antibiotic treatment to promote comfort but thereafter increased to 2–3L daily if no medical contraindications.
- Advice that may reduce risk of recurrence:
  - postcoital voiding (twice);
  - personal hygiene: wiping/washing genitals from front to back; no vaginal douching; wearing cotton pants changing tampons more frequently.
- In those already experiencing recurrences the above advice does not apply.
- There is no good clinical evidence that oral cranberry juice prevents UTIs. Anecdotally, patients are often advised to try cranberry juice to prevent UTI.
- The use of oral probiotics is controversial.

Dysuria alone is suggestive of urethritis. Consider sexual history and need for STI screening— 📖 see p.370.

Urinary tract infection/cystitis in men

Uncommon in males under 50. Thereafter it may increase 2° to incomplete bladder emptying and prostatitis.

Factors suggesting UTI

- Sexual history: longstanding stable sexual relationship/not sexually active.
- Age > 50 years (prostatism with UTI more common).
- Symptoms: increased frequency, loin pain, pyrexia, malaise.

Factors suggesting sexually acquired cause

- Presentation. Increased likelihood if new sexual risk/suspicion about a partner. Urethritis arising within 4 weeks (usually).
- Age. Most commonly found in men from late teens to early 50s.
- Symptoms. Usually prominent dysuria and/or urethral discharge (may just be found on examination). Increased urinary frequency and systemic symptoms unusual.

Investigations

- Urine dipstick: likely to be positive for nitrates and/or white cells and/or blood. Leucocytes/proteinuria is not indicative of infection.
- MSUs should be taken and sent for laboratory analysis prior to starting antibiotics.
- Fever indicates ascending infection.

Pyelonephritis—upper tract infection

- **Cause**. Ascending renal tract infection/UTI.
- **Symptoms**. Loin pain, high fever, rigors, malaise, vomiting, and/or haematuria.
- **Management**
  - Baseline vital signs, symptom control, and fluid balance monitoring.
  - Keep the patient comfortable when shivering with sheet/blankets and remove them when rigoring has stopped.
- **Treatment**. Prepare for admission for IV antibiotics, symptom control, and observation.

Patient support and information

UK National Kidney Federation. Tel: 0845 601 02 09. www.kidney.org.uk.

Acute retention of urine

In men, complaints are of suprapubic pain and a reduced or incomplete ability to pass urine. This may be secondary to tumour, urethral stricture, or as a post-operative complication. Other causes seen in men and women are post-trauma, burns/scalds, uterine fibroids, infection, e.g. painful herpetic lesions, and blockage of long-term catheters.

Nursing assessment

History

- Last micturition, amounts of urine passed. Previous history.
- Consider a deliberate foreign body (📖 see p.367) or a blocked indwelling catheter (IDC).
- Again provide privacy and a room with a door.
- Bladder decompression with an IDC is required if no contraindications, e.g. trauma or strictures.

Observation/inspection

- Obvious discomfort/distress. Exceptions are patients with chronic retention; this may be painless.
- Use bladder scan to assess size of bladder.
- Abdominal percussion may reveal a distended bladder.
- Cloudy urine or pus with infection.
- Frank haematuria.
- Genital trauma, urethral bleeding in the unconscious patient.
- Palpation. Tender enlarged bladder.
- Percussion:
  - suprapubic and above may be dull;
  - reduced or absent bowel sounds with constipation.
- Pyrexia indicates infection. Tachycardia due to this, pain, or haemorrhage 2° to infection, tumour, accidental or deliberate trauma.

Management (📖 see p.596)

- An IDC will provide pain relief. Insert using an aseptic technique. Observe urinary output for amount and frank haematuria.
- Document catheter gauge and residual urine amount.
- Clamp after 1L has drained. Blood vessels previously compressed may now vasodilate with rebound hypotension.
- Remove clamp after 30min.
- Confirm/exclude infection on urinary dipstix and send MSU specimen to the laboratory.

Bladder/urethral/genital injury

- Be mindful of the mechanism of injury and consider sexual assault in adults and NAI/abuse in children with genital injury.
- Cultural practices such as female circumcision are illegal in the UK but may still be seen in diverse communities. It is important that nurses respond in a culturally competent way.[1]

Nursing assessment

Inspect

- Signs of foreign body, bleeding/trauma, and/or discharge.
- Inflammatory response secondary to scalds/burns. ▶▶ Immediate referral to a specialist burns unit. Meanwhile consider IDC if appropriate, analgesia and fluid replacement.
- IDC contraindicated post blunt trauma resulting in anterior pelvic fracture with concomitant bladder/urethral trauma—blood visualized at urethral meatus.

Reference

1 Female genital mutilation: an educational resource for nurse and midwives. ⊕ www.rcn.org.uk

Priapism

Persistent painful erection not related to sexual desire.

Cause

In the ED this may be:
- iatrogenic;
- related to spinal or perineal trauma;
- drugs, e.g. cocaine, cannabis, or phenothiazines;
- disease such as sickle cell, leukaemia, pelvic tumour, myeloma, renal dialysis.

Nursing assessment and intervention

- Apply ice-packs and give analgesia.
- If related to sickle cell give oxygen; this may resolve the priapism.

Management

- If the nursing interventions are unsuccessful or the patient presents > 6h post-onset this is an emergency.
- The nursing interventions just listed are not appropriate with priapism due to parasympathetic nervous system stimulation in spinal shock. Refer to the urology team as aspiration of corpora is needed. Rarely, surgery may be required.

Testicular torsion

- Testicular torsion is more common in men < 20 years of age but can occur at any age.
- This is a paediatric/adolescent emergency.
- Presentation. Acute onset of severe testicular pain ± vomiting. Pain from the testicles may be referred to the abdomen. Ask about (or examine a child for) red, tender, swollen testis.

Testicular torsion is seen mainly in neonates, children, and young men around puberty. In older males it may be related to an undescended testicle.

- If not treated early the testicle may need to be surgically removed, reducing future fertility and/or affecting body image.

Management

- Reassure the child or young person, give analgesia and/or anti-emetics, and give information to the patient or carer.
- ▶▶ An immediate surgical referral is required.

Epididymo-orchitis

- In men < 35 years of age epididymo-orchitis is usually related to bacterial STIs.
- In men > 35 years of age it is most often related to bacteria that cause UTIs or viral mumps orchitis.
- Sexual health history in all cases is important.
- Non-infective causes can be seen in men with Behçet's disease or in relation to recent catheterization, other trauma or high dose amiodarone treatment.

Symptoms

- Unilateral scrotal pain and swelling (usually less severe and acute than torsion).
- If it is STI-related, symptoms of urethritis or a urethral discharge may be present but usually are not.
- Mumps orchitis: fever, myalgia, and malaise.
  - Parotiditis usually precedes the onset of orchitis by 3–5 days.
  - Incidence has reduced since introduction of MMR vaccination.

Investigations

- MSU for M, C, & S.
- Doppler USS to exclude torsion of the spermatic cord.
- Referral to outpatient GUM clinic for STI screening, treatment, and partner notification if appropriate.

Management and advice

- Bedrest, scrotal elevation, and ice packs to promote comfort.
- Nonsteroidal anti-inflammatories (NSAIDs) to provide analgesia and antipyretic benefits.
- Advise to avoid unprotected sexual intercourse until patient and their partner have completed treatment and follow-up.
- Patient should return for reassessment if no improvement after 3/7 antibiotic treatment.
- Reassure patient that full recovery is usual, that complications are uncommon, and that sterility is uncommon after acute epididymitis.

Bartholin's cyst/abscess

The Bartholin's glands lie at 4 and 8 o'clock within the vaginal vestibule. Damage or infection to the ostium of the gland ducts causes blockage and a cyst occurs that may become infected. Found commonly in women aged 20–29, abscesses occur three times as often as cysts.

The onset is rapid over days or hours. Unilateral labial oedema precedes swelling and superficial dyspareunia, and painful swelling develops. The patient may have a wide-legged gait.

Staff should be cautious in attributing infective causes to *Neisseria gonorrhoeae/Chlamydia trachomatis*.
- STI screening can be arranged if sexual health history indicates.
- Nursing intervention should focus on prompt recognition and pain control.
- If STI screening is deemed necessary reassure patient that these infections are treatable with a short course of antibiotics.

Management

This depends on the size of the cyst.
- If small and no signs of infection, no action is taken; these cysts may rupture spontaneously.
- Marsupialization is considered as the best technique in preventing recurrence.
- More recently the *Word* catheter technique is gaining in popularity in cyst management.
- In women over 40, excision and histology to exclude malignancy is performed.

Foreign bodies

Genital foreign bodies in adults can result from retained menstrual tampons, sexual practices, self-harm, or smuggling. These can include the following.
* Vaginal: tampons, contraceptive devices, and supportive pessaries.
* Vaginal/anal: condoms (after sex or containing drugs), sex toys.
* Urethra: self-harm, e.g. pens, paper clips.

Patients who are not compromised

The nurse's role with the well patient is to act as a chaperone and advocate, giving information and providing reassurance throughout the foreign body removal.
* Ask patient to empty their bladder for removal of vaginal objects or to check for urethral obstruction.
* Check for haematuria if bladder injury is suspected.
* Consider Entonox® and/or other analgesia to promote a pain-free and speedy removal. Gather equipment needed for this.
* Ensure privacy in a room with a lockable door.
* Reassure patient that you will not be interrupted.
* Provide good lighting behind the practitioner removing the object.

Patients who are compromised

* The patient may be confused or unconscious, demonstrating signs of *toxic shock*.
* The effects of hidden, stored drugs would not be seen if they had not been orally ingested and passed through the GI system.
* Consider toxic shock syndrome if the patient is distressed, disorientated, confused, pyrexial, hypotensive (signs of shock) with a blanching generalized rash.
* Ask about LMP and retained tampons and act as chaperone and assist with a PV examination, which may find PV discharge, forgotten pessary, or, rarely, a tumour.

Known drug users and/or attempting to avoid police arrest
* These patients may present with decreased GCS, respiration with pinned pupils (with no evidence of head injury).
* IV access, naloxone.
* The patient may return or be returned to police custody once medically cleared.

Self-harm and haemorrhage
* Measure baseline vital signs and monitor level of consciousness and for signs of shock if bleeding is evident.
* Consider patient's mental health needs if self-harming and gain consent for mental health assessment.

Genital candidiasis

Thrush/moniliasis/candidosis is a fungal infection caused by a yeast, usually *Candida albicans* (80–90%). Candida commonly lives in small numbers around the genitals, especially the vagina, and is asymptomatic until it multiplies and penetrates the skin surface (🕮 see Box 11.1).

Epidemiology 75% of women have at least one episode of genital candidiasis with 40–50% having one or more recurrences. Men present with symptoms much less frequently.

Clinical features—women

- Symptoms.
  - Vulval pruritus and burning, with external dysuria and dyspareunia. These usually start/worsen from mid-cycle and improve with menstruation (oestrogen level related).
  - 20% have vaginal erythema, with a thick, white, curdy, adherent discharge in 20%, increasing to 70% if pregnant. Discharge may be purulent or watery.
- Signs. Most commonly vulval erythema and oedema with fissuring that can extend to labial majora and/or perineum.
- In recurrent candidiasis (> 4 times annually), vulval pruritis with burning is common. Signs are less common.

Clinical features—men

- In colonized men the most common symptom is postcoital itching/burning.
- It presents clinically as direct infection of the glans (balanitis) and/or prepuce (posthitis).
- More common in the uncircumcised presenting as a glazed erythematous rash, sometimes with white papules/discharge, and, if severe, fissuring, oedema, and 2° phimosis.

Box 11.1 Transmission and predisposing factors—answering frequently asked questions

- Thrush is not usually sexually transmitted, particularly in women, although it is associated with recent cunnilingus
- Partners do not need treatment unless they have signs and symptoms themselves
- Low (usual) level oestrogen combined contraceptive pill does not increase rate of thrush
- Studies have shown that a yeast-free diet will not decrease rate
- The effectiveness of oral/topical yoghurt is controversial; PV use on a tampon may just soothe irritation
- There is a small association with broad-spectrum antibiotics

Vulvovaginitis

Vulvovaginitis in *children* arises in certain rare circumstances:
- insertion of foreign bodies by the child herself;
- threadworm infestation;
- sexual interference.

▶ The possibility of non-accidental injury needs to be considered in any infection in children.

Sexually transmitted infections

Triage

- While screening is not provided by the ED, post-exposure prophylaxis (PEP) for HIV/hepatitis B infection should be given priority at triage.
- Remain mindful and vigilant of *child protection issues in those underage* and remember that female and male patients may present for STI screening *post sexual assault/rape*. These patients are a triage priority. The patient may be distressed or aggressive and de-escalation techniques may need to be employed.

Triage nurses need to be aware that, due to lack of privacy at reception, the patient may not have given their true reason for attending the ED.
- Taking a full sexual history is not appropriate at triage.
- The patient often realizes that they may need to attend elsewhere but needs reassurance that this is the case. ED staff awareness and input can demystify the GUM process for patients, reducing fear and misunderstandings so that they access specialist services protecting their health and future fertility.

GUM clinic or ED?

STI prevalence in the young is increasing. Many infections are symptomless with chlamydia and gonorrhoea being predominant.
- Most GUM clinics now have a same day, one-stop service with dedicated young person, male, and female clinics.
- Over the counter chlamydia urine screening is now available for 16–24 year olds at some chemists offering 70% sensitivity.
- Other patients may see the ED as an anonymous, safe place.
- Optimum screening time post-exposure/infection is usually within 10–14 days.
- Reassure patients regarding confidentiality in GUM practice, explaining that being known as only a number ensures privacy.

▶ Patients complaining of abdominal pain need to see a doctor.

Risk factors for STIs

- Age < 25 years. The highest rates of gonococcal and chlamydial infections occur in females aged 16–19 years and in males aged 20–24 years.
- Being single, separated, divorced, or not in a stable relationship (compared with marital, stable relationship, or widowed status) is associated with higher rates of STI.
- ≥ 2 partners in preceding 6 months.
- Use of non-barrier contraception.
- Residence in inner city.
- Symptoms in partner.
- History of previous STI.
- Ethnicity or migration. Prevalence of several infections, notably syphilis, gonorrhoea, and HIV infection, is higher in certain ethnic minority groups and immigrants.
- Sexual orientation. For example, syphilis, gonorrhoea, HIV, and hepatitis B virus infections are more prevalent among homosexual men.

Genital herpes

- Patients may present with genital lesions and/or pain, itching ± vaginal or anal discharge.
- A vesicular swab must be taken but treatment can be commenced on clinical grounds in the ED.
- GUM follow-up can be arranged for full STI screening, an internal examination, and long-term support.
- Codeine phosphate analgesia (with advice on its constipating effect), saline lavage, and micturition (if painful) in a warm bath can be advised to promote comfort.

Inspect/measure

- Pyrexia, tachycardia, hypotension. Consider sepsis secondary to pelvic inflammatory disease.
- In other patients a sexual health history may be important and information about sexual practices may be a priority in order to prevent/minimize offence. For example, if there is exudating, pustular sore throat or painful, hot, swollen, non-traumatic joint in a sexually active person, consider gonorrhoea.

If treatment is started, patient details need to be taken so that GUM referral can be made facilitating patient follow-up regarding co-infection screening, treatment, surveillance, and partner notification.

Fraser guidelines

For under 16 year olds follow the Fraser guidelines (previously known as Gillick competence) in offering treatment/contraception.

Staff must respect their duty of confidentiality to a person under 16; this is as great as that owed to any other person. The guidelines exist to protect the practitioner and patient, ensuring best practice. If treatment is to be given to a person under 16 without the consent/knowledge of their parents, these guidelines must be followed.

- Maturity. The young person demonstrates understanding of the practitioner's advice.
- The practitioner has discussed the possibility of obtaining parental consent with the patient.
- The patient has begun or is likely to begin/continue having sexual intercourse.
- Unless the patient receives treatment/contraception their physical/mental health is likely to suffer.
- Treatment/contraception is in the best interests of the patient.

Useful websites

Staff information—British Association for Sexual Health and HIV, ⊕ www.bassh.org

National Sexual Health Strategy DOH (2001). ⊕ www.dh.gov.uk

Emergency contraception

Emergency contraception is used in coital exposure whether from unprotected sex, condom breakages, omission or delay in taking/receiving contraception pills or depot injections, complete or partial expulsion of IUCD, and post-sexual assault/rape.

Oral progesterone-only emergency contraception

Oral progesterone-only emergency contraception (POEC) has replaced the combined emergency contraceptive. POEC is 99.6% effective and has reduced the rates of associated nausea and vomiting. Legally, POEC is a contraceptive and not an abortifacient as it prevents ovulation and/or implantation of a fertilized egg.

- The term 'morning after pill' is discouraged as POEC can be used up to < 72h post unprotected sexual intercourse (UPSI).
  - The earlier it is taken the greater its effectiveness.
  - The risk of pregnancy increases by 50% for every 12h delay with POEC.
- POEC is available over the counter but, if women present to ED, consider age, vulnerability, socioeconomic factors, and availability of participating pharmacies before sending patient from ED to the local pharmacy.
- Some patients who present saying pregnancy is their 'problem' are in fact asking for emergency contraception.
- POEC needs to be prescribed or given under PGD in the ED.
- Give POEC < 72h after unprotected sexual intercourse (UPSI) but first ask and consider the following.
  - Was the sexual intercourse consensual?
  - When was the last menstrual period (LMP)? If within the last 4 weeks a urine HCG is not required.
  - Ensure no previous UPSI or POEC in last cycle. POEC may be used if clinically indicated.
  - Past medical history. A double dose is needed for patients taking enzyme-inducing drugs or antibiotics, e.g. St John's wort, anticonvulsant therapy, antiretrovirals, and some TB medication.
  - Warfarin users should have their INR checked within 3–4 days as it may alter significantly or they may have an IUD instead of POEC.
  - Also consider alcohol and drug issues and the need for referral to community drug or alcohol services.
  - < 16 year olds (📖 see p.370) Consider child protection issues.
- Give 1.5mg levonorgestrel (now 1 tablet) as soon as possible. A PV examination is not required. A few discreet questions can establish whether the patient is in a safe, consensual sexual relationship.
- On discharge tell the women to:
  - return for a repeat prescription if she vomits within 3h;
  - return if abdominal pain develops consider risk of ectopic pregnancy if patient returns. If the next period is light or late, a pregnancy test should be taken.
- Before discharging, discuss safer sex and raise awareness of local family planning services.

> 72 hours post-UPSI

Refer to a local family planning centre for a copper intrauterine device (IUD) within 5 days (120h) of:
- the first sexual exposure within a menstrual cycle or
- the earliest calculated ovulation date. (Take the earliest next menstrual start date, subtract 14 days, and add 5 (useful in cycles of 21–30 days)).

Skin emergencies

Overview

Skin problems are a frequent adult and paediatric presentation in urgent care settings either due to the severity and acuteness of the condition, e.g. deep dermal burn, or its disruptive nature, e.g. itchy rash. A huge array of skin problems can present over the course of a shift. Some of these need urgent treatment and are covered in this chapter. Other less urgent but common presentations are also covered. However, many of the latter require follow-up by the GP for ongoing management or dermatology referral.

The skin

The skin is composed of two layers: the epidermis lies superficial and the dermis lies deep. Underneath these layers lies the subcutaneous tissue, composed of adipose and connective tissue and blood vessels.

Epidermis does not contain blood vessels, but receives its nutrients from the dermis. It is made up of 5 layers of cells. New cells are formed in the deepest (basal) layer and migrate upwards until they are shed from the skin surface (horny layer). The entire epidermis is replaced every 3 weeks.

Dermis is composed of connective tissue, capillary loops, lymph vessels, nerve endings, temperature and touch receptors, sebaceous glands, sweat glands, and hair follicles. Fibroblasts produce collagen; a network of collagen and elastic fibres give skin its strength and elasticity. Fibroblasts and macrophages move around within the dermal layers and are essential to wound healing.

Nursing assessment

❶ Occasionally patients may present with a skin condition that is associated with a life-threatening problem that requires immediate ABC assessment and resuscitative intervention.

- A patient with a burn must be assessed for the presence or risk of a pulmonary injury as this can develop rapidly, causing partial or complete airway obstruction.
- Upper airway swelling and laryngospasm associated with anaphylaxis may present initially as an urticarial rash.
- Purpuric or petechial rashes in an 'unwell' patient should be treated as a potential presentation of septic shock until proven otherwise.

History

The assessment and management of burns are dealt with separately in this chapter, 📖 see Burns, p.380, Major burns, p.386, and Minor burns, p.388. For other skin problems the following features from the history help guide further assessment and management.

- Onset. This will indicate the acuteness of the condition. Rapid development can point to a more serious problem.
- Trauma—whether an injury preceded the problem.
- Main complaints: itching, weeping, oozing, crusting, burning, blistering, skin peeling, lesions, pain, swelling, bruising, petechiae, purpura.
- Site of skin problem; grouping, distribution, and extent of the spread.
- Relieving factors. Has any treatment improved the symptoms?
- Aggravating factors. Has anything made the symptoms worse?
- Systemic upset. Are there any systemic symptoms, e.g. fever?
- Contacts. Is there a possibility that the skin problem is infectious?

Physical assessment

Inspection

Depending on the site and extent of the spread the patient may need to be fully undressed to ensure that all affected areas are inspected. Careful inspection can identify the type of lesion/s present (📖 see Box 12.1).

The exact site and shape/grouping of the lesion/s should also be noted. Drawing the site of the lesion/s can aid accurate description.

Palpation Examining the lesion/rash can identify whether it is solid, fluid-filled, painful, blanching, or oedematous.

Assessment/investigations

- A full set of vital signs should be obtained if infection is present or patient is systemically unwell.
- Pain assessment and score.
- Wound swab of any exudate.

Nursing interventions

- Analgesia given according to pain score.
- Wound dressing if appropriate.
- Antibiotics if infection is present.
- Antihistamine can help relieve the itch/swelling associated with urticaria.

Box 12.1 Types of lesions

- Macule. Purely a colour change. Flat, < 1cm, e.g. freckle, petechiae
- Patch. Macule > 1cm, e.g. Mongolian blue spot
- Papule. A solid elevated swelling < 1cm, e.g. mole, wart
- Plaque. Papules that merge to form a surface elevation, e.g. psoriasis
- Nodule. Solid, elevated hard or soft lump > 1cm
- Tumour. > 2cm; soft or firm; deeper into dermis. Benign or malignant, e.g. lipoma
- Wheal. Superficial, raised, transient, and erythematous. Irregular in shape due to oedema, e.g. allergic reaction
- Hives. Wheals that merge to form an extensive reaction. Intensely itchy
- Vesicle. Fluid-filled elevated cavity < 1cm containing clear fluid, e.g. early chickenpox (varicella)
- Bulla/blister. Fluid-filled elevated cavity > 1cm. Superficial in the epidermis. Thin-walled; ruptures easily, e.g. burn blister
- Pustule. A small pus-filled elevated cavity, e.g. acne
- Abscess. A larger cavity containing pus
- Cyst. Encapsulated fluid-filled cavity tensely elevating the skin, e.g. sebaceous cyst
- Ulcer. Crater-like skin lesion. Healing is often delayed, e.g. pressure ulcer, leg ulcer
- Crust. Hard, dry exudate from vesicles or pustules that have burst, e.g. impetigo
- Scale. Compact, dry flakes of skin, e.g. psoriasis.

Burns

Burns are an extremely common presentation in urgent care settings and range from the minor to life-threatening. Then can be acutely painful, painless, or limb-threatening. Some require no further assessment or management. Others, however, require intensive resuscitation in the ED and transfer to a tertiary regional burns centre many miles away.

Flame burns and scalds cause the majority of burns. Chemical and electrical burns account for only ~ 5%. Children < 5 years often attend with contact burns or scalds sustained at home. In the summer months patients can attend with burns from the sun or barbecues. In November, Bonfire night can cause a rise in the number of patients attending with burns from fireworks or fires.

❶ As with any injury, consider NAI. Children and the elderly are most vulnerable. 10% of children with an NAI also have a wound or burn.

Nursing assessment of a patient with a burn

Rapid ABCDE assessment following ATLS guidelines is required to identify those with any life- or limb-threatening problem. Subsequent assessment involves identifying the site, extent, and depth of the burn and deciding how and where the burn should be managed until it's healed.

There are several life-threatening consequences of an acute burn injury that need to be anticipated in all but most minor of burns. The ED team has to identify which, if any, are present or, more challengingly, which may develop over minutes or hours following the burn. The main pathophysiological effects are airway obstruction, pulmonary injury, and hypovolaemic shock.

Airway obstruction Any patient who may have inhaled superheated air or smoke /toxic fumes is at high risk of upper airway burns and possible upper airway obstruction. Early intubation is the key to successful management as the oedema that accompanies airway burns develops rapidly and can make passage of the ETT impossible if left too late.

Pulmonary injury Damage to lung tissue from the inhalation of the chemical byproducts of combustion causes significant damage to the lower airways resulting in atelectasis, reduced ciliary clearance, and loss of surfactant. This predisposes the patient to infection and sepsis. Carbon monoxide poisoning can result from inhalation injury leading to severe hypoxia and brain injury. Pulmonary injury is associated with significant morbidity and mortality and can be present without any burns to the skin. Intensive care treatment is required and is mainly supportive aimed at preventing hypoxia, infection, and atelectasis.

Hypovolaemic shock Major burns cause hypovolaemic shock some hours after injury due to damaged capillaries leaking plasma and protein. Protein leakage causes more fluid to shift from the intravascular spaces to the interstitial spaces and oedema develops. The rate of fluid loss is dependent on the size of the burn and the time since burn injury. The prevention of hypovolaemic shock begins in the ED with a fluid resuscitation regimen and continues for 24–48h.

History

- Time of burn. Has there been a delay in presentation?
- Type of burn: chemical, electrical, radiation, flame, scald, contact.
- Where did the burn happen? Was it in an enclosed space? Is there a risk of inhalation of smoke, fumes, heat?
- Other complaints. Has the patient any other injuries/problems?
- Site. Are the face, mouth, or airways involved?
- 1st aid measures. Immediate cold water can reduce the depth and extent of the burn.
- Non-accidental injury. Are there any features of the history that suggest the cause may be non-accidental?

Electrical burns

- Where did the electrical injury occur: domestic or industrial?
- What was the path of the current?
- Are there entrance/exit wounds?

Electrical burns are almost always full thickness, the extent of the tissue damage is rarely visible in the ED. Significant electrical burns can cause cardiac conduction abnormalities and myoglobinuria due to extensive tissue and muscle damage, which can cause renal failure. Significant/high voltage electrical burns require aggressive fluid resuscitation. Most require referral to a regional burns centre and advice will be given about a suitable fluid resuscitation regimen.

Chemical burns

- What chemical was involved? Alkali substances usually cause deeper burns.
- 1st aid. How long was the burn irrigated prior to attending?

Chemical burns should be treated with copious irrigation for at least 20min. The regional poisons centre or www.toxbase.co.uk can be contacted for specific advice regarding the chemical involved.

Cement burns are common and not initially noticed as cement falls inside a work boot and slowly erodes the skin surface. They can be full thickness if not treated quickly with irrigation. Due to the nature of a chemical injury and the difficulty in completely removing the burn agent, the depth of a chemical burn can continue to progress over several days. Patients should be warned of this and early involvement of a regional burns centre is advised.

Pulmonary injury

A pulmonary/inhalation injury should be suspected if any of the following are present

- History of being in an enclosed space where hot, toxic fumes could have been inhaled.
- Burns to the face, nose, lips, palate.
- Singed nasal hairs, eyebrows, eyelashes.
- Burns/erthyema to the mouth/nose.
- Hoarse voice.
- Stridor.

Burn assessment

Extent of the burn

This is described as a % of the total body surface area (TBSA) burnt. In adults the simple Wallace 'rule of nines' can be used to quickly estimate the % of the body burnt. Each area of the body is awarded a multiple of nine (📖 see Fig. 12.1(a)).

Alternatively, the palmar surface of the patient's hand with the thumb adducted represents approximately 1% of their TBSA; this can be used in adults and children as an initial estimate of TBSA burnt.

Ideally a burn assessment tool should be used to shade the areas of the body burnt and allow for an estimate of the TBSA burnt. The Lund and Browder chart offers an alternative tool and provides a more accurate assessment as it makes allowances for the variation in body shape with age. % TBSA burnt using this method can be done in ED and will be done in the regional burns centre (📖 see Fig. 12.1(b)).

> ❶ Major burns require immediate referral to a regional burns centre from the ED.
> • A major burn in an adult is one ≥ 15% TBSA
> • A major burn in a child is one ≥ 10% TBSA

Inspection

Depth of the burn

The depth of a burn is dependent on the degree of heat applied and the duration of contact. Burns are commonly describes as superficial, superficial partial thickness (SPT), deep dermal, or full thickness (📖 see Table 12.1). Burns are usually of mixed depth.

Accurate identification of the depth of the burn can be difficult even for the experienced ED clinician. Due to continued damage to the microcirculation over the first 48h burns can be deeper than first estimated. For this reason all but the most superficial of burns should be reviewed at 48–72h.

Site of burn

Identifying the exact site of the burn is important in all but superficial burns as 'special areas' of the body may require management by a burns specialist regardless of the size and depth. The following burn sites should be discussed with the regional burn centre.
• Face.
• Hands.
• Feet.
• Perineum.
• Nipples.
• Any flexure, especially the neck or axilla.
• Circumferential burns.

Circumferential burns

Extremity burns that are circumferential can cause compartment syndrome. Patients with deep dermal or full thickness burns are at greatest risk of a compartment syndrome that compromises perfusion to the limb. A significant compartment syndrome will require an urgent escharotomy.

This may have to be done in ED but more commonly the procedure is performed in theatre. Circumferential burns to the chest can significantly compromise ventilation and may also need urgent escharotomy, in some cases palliative.

Palpation of the burn (with sterile gloves) identifies: texture; blanching; degree of pain; and ability to discriminate between blunt touch and pin-prick.

Auscultation Wheezing, stridor, and tachypnoea can point to an inhalation injury.

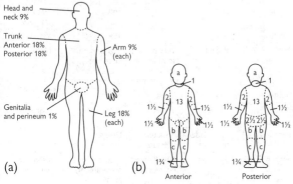

Relative percentage of body surface area (% BSA) affected by growth

Body Part	Age				
	0 yr	1 yr	5 yr	10 yr	15 yr
a = ½ of head	9½	8½	6½	5½	4½
b = ½ of 1 thigh	2¾	3¼	4	4¼	2½
c = ½ of 1 lower leg	2½	2½	2¾	3	3¼

Fig. 12.1 (a) The Wallace 'rule of nines'. (b) The Lund and Browder chart.

Table 12.1 Estimating the depth of burns

Characteristic	Superficial (e.g. sunburn)	Superficial partial thickness	Deep dermal	Full thickness
Skin layer	Epidermis	Epidermis & superficial dermis	Epidermis & dermis	Epidermis, dermis, & deep structures
Colour	Red	Red	White, creamy, mottled	White, grey, black, brown
Texture	Soft	Soft	Soft	Hard, leathery
Skin loss	None	Yes	Yes	Yes
Pain	Painful	Very painful; sensitive to air & temperature	Slight; some insensate areas. Poor discrimination	None
Moisture	Dry	Moist	Moist	Dry
Blisters	None	Immediately	Large, easily liftable	None
Blanching	Brisk under pressure	Brisk under pressure	Delayed	None
Healing time	3–7 days	10–21 days if no infection	> 30 days; may be preferable to skin graft	Won't heal without graft

Major burns

Following physical assessment of the patient a decision has to be made regarding subsequent management. This is based on whether the patient needs referral to a burns unit (Box 12.2) or can continue to be managed by the ED. If an opinion about referral is sought from the regional burns centre further assessment and investigations are usually decided by them. The following assessment/investigations can act as a guide even if a regional burns centre is involved.

> **Box 12.2 Criteria for referral to a regional burn centre**
> - A burn in an adult is one ≥ 15% (not including superficial burns)
> - Dermal or full thickness burn > 10% in an adult
> - A burn in a child is one ≥ 10% (not including superficial burns)
> - Dermal or full thickness burn > 5% in a child
> - Deep dermal or full thickness burns of the face, hand, feet, perineum, nipple/s, any flexure, especially the neck or axilla; circumferential burns of the limb, torso, or neck
> - Chemical injury > 5%
> - High tension electrical injury

Assessment/investigations

Assessment of ABCDE following ATLS guidelines is crucial to identify those with potential or actual airway obstruction, pulmonary injury, and hypovolaemic shock. Assess patients who have been burned during an explosion or who have jumped from a burning building for other injuries using the the the standard ABCD approach (📖 see p.40). Carry out following assessments and investigations on patients with suspected major burn.
- Pulse, temperature, respiratory rate, BP.
- Pulse oximetry.
- Glasgow coma scale—may indicate developing cerebral hypoxia.
- Cardiac monitoring.
- Pain assessment and score.
- FBC, U & E, clotting, cross-match.
- Capillary blood glucose.
- CXR—will act as a baseline.
- ABG if the patient is shocked or inhalation is suspected.
- ECG if an electrical injury has occurred.
- Tetanus status.

Nursing interventions

- Airway management. Suction may be required if the patient unable to clear their own airway.
- Airway protection. Rapid endotracheal intubation will be required in patients with actual or potential airway or pulmonary burns. An ETT of (📖 see p.676) a small circumference is often needed if the airway is already oedematous. The ETT should not be cut as a longer length is required as the airway and face swell over time.
- Administer oxygen in patients with suspected inhalation injury.

- Ventilation is required for patients with airway burns, pulmonary injury, or hypoxia.
- IV access. To allow administration of analgesia and IV fluids, patients with major burns will require × 2 large bore cannulae. Cannulaes can be inserted into burned tissue as a last resort.
- Fluid replacement. Patients with a major burn require fluid resuscitation to prevent the development of hypovolaemic shock (📖 see Box 12.3). Hartmann's solution is most commonly used.

Box 12.3 Fluid resuscitation in major burns

The most common fluid resuscitation formula is the Parkland (Baxter) formula.

4mL/kg/%TBSA is given during the first 24h. Half is given in the first 8h after the burn injury occurs. The remaining half is given over the next 16h.

❶ It is important to remember that the fluid calculation is from the time of injury. If the patient arrives in the ED 1h after injury, for example, half of the fluid needs to be give over the next 7h

Sample burn calculation
A 70kg man has a 35% TBSA burn, which he sustained in a house fire at 11 pm. He arrives in the ED at 12 midnight. His fluid requirement is as follows

$4 \times 70 \times 35 = 9800mL$ over the first 24h

4900mL is needed in the first 8h. 2h have now lapsed since the burn so that 4900mL is required over 6h which equals 817mL/h

---

- Analgesia. Opiate analgesia should be given IV, titrated to response.
- Large doses of morphine > 30mg may be required.
- Wound care. Initial cleansing can remove soot and debris to enable clearer assessment of extent and depth. Burn should be covered as soon as possible. Large burns requiring transfer to regional burns centre can be covered in cling film. Smaller burns need non-adherent dressing in contact with burn surface and secondary dressing that is absorbent enough for the burn exudate over the first 48h.
- Tetanus immunization. Burns are classified as tetanus-prone due to the degree of devitalized tissue. Patients who have not got adequate immunity require tetanus vaccination and immunoglobulin (📖 see p.313).
- Maintain body temperature. Patients with major burns lose their ability to maintain temperature. This is compounded by the initial and sometimes prolonged cooling of the skin, infusion of cool IV fluids, and skin exposure in the ED. Infusion of warmed fluids, a warm environment, and keeping patient covered can help prevent hypothermia.

Minor burns

The most common burn encountered in ED practice is the minor burn, one that does not fulfil the criteria for urgent referral to a burns centre (📖 see Box 12.2, p.386). However, all but the most superficial of burns require careful management to ensure optimal healing.

General management of the minor burn

- Analgesia given according to pain score.
- Cleansing to remove any debris, soot, or topical first aid treatments.
- Debridement if appropriate.
- Dressing (📖 see Box 12.4).
- Tetanus immunization if appropriate (📖 see p.313).
- Discharge advice.
- Follow-up arrangement.

> ### Box 12.4 The ideal burn dressing
>
> There is no one dressing ideal for all sites and types of burn and the stage of healing. Compromises will need to be made and products changed as the burn heals. Ideally a burn dressing should achieve as many of the following characteristics as possible
> - Non-adherent
> - Provide thermal insulation
> - Provide a moist environment but not create maceration
> - Impermeable to bacteria
> - Comfortable, conformable, and acceptable to the patient
> - Hypo-allergenic
> - Absorbent (exudate is most prolific in the first 48–72h) but not dry the burn
> - Cost-effective and available in the right size
> - Does not require frequent dressing changes

Debridement of burn blisters

There remains great controversy over the management of burn blisters. Research highlights beneficial effects of leaving blisters intact and, in contradiction to this, there are reports of the beneficial effects of removing them. Equally there are studies that suggest that leaving a blister intact is deleterious to wound healing and other studies that suggest that deroofing blisters is equally harmful. How to manage burn blisters is not an easy question to answer. However applying the following principles can aid in decision-making.

- Dead/devitalized tissue can act as a focus for infection and therefore should be removed.
- Total blister debridement can be painful.
- The depth of a burn is not easily assessed if there are intact blisters—they may need removing.
- Small blisters that do not restrict function can be left intact.
- Large blisters that restrict function may need to be removed.
- Burns that are allowed to dehydrate can become deeper. Therefore, if a blister is removed, an appropriate dressing is required.

Discharge advice

Patients/parents should be advised to:
- keep the burn clean and dry;
- attend a treatment room dressing service for a dressing change if it leaks;
- elevate the burn if it is on a limb;
- attend any follow-up arrangement;
- return immediately if they become 'unwell'.

A rare but life-threatening consequence of a minor burn, or wound or sometimes associated with tampon use is toxic shock syndrome (TSS). There are 15–20 recorded cases per year for all causes in the UK. Some of these will be from minor burns and result in the death of the patient. TSS is seen more commonly in children as they have not built up immunity to the TSS toxins. Without alarming parents or patients clear written and verbal advice needs to be given about the signs and symptoms of TSS and when to return to the ED.

▶▶ You should return immediately to the ED if any of the following symptoms develop.
- High temperature.
- Rash.
- Loss of appetite.
- Nausea or vomiting.
- Abdominal pain or diarrhoea.
- Sore throat.
- Tiredness.
- Aches or pain.

Follow-up for minor burns All but the most minor burns require follow-up at 48–72h to confirm the depth and size of the burn. Dressings usually need changing at this stage as they can be saturated with exudate.

Infected burns

Occasionally burns can become infected and require investigation (wound swab) and treatment with antibiotics. Signs of a burn wound infection include:
- increased pain;
- cellulitis;
- erythematous wound margin;
- ↑ exudate;
- discoloration of the burn, e.g. dark brown or black;
- delayed healing;
- conversion of a partial thickness burn to a full-thickness burn.

Treatment of an infected burn requires a course of flucloxacillin (or erthromycin if penicillin-allergic). Review at 48–72h and give clear written and verbal advice about the need to return sooner if the patient becomes systemically unwell.

Skin infections

Skin infections and abscess are commonly seen in urgent care settings and most are easily diagnosed and treated. Local skin infections such as paronychia, cellulitis, abscesses, wound infections, and bites and stings are covered on 📖 see p.308 and p.310.

Erysipelas is a less common skin infection, worthy of mention due to its rapid onset and site of presentation. Necrotizing fasciitis is a rare but life-threatening tissue infection that requires rapid diagnosis and treatment.

Erysipelas is a streptococcal bacterial infection of the dermis that can spread rapidly causing swelling, redness, and pain. Erythematous lesions enlarge rapidly and have raised well demarcated edges (this is what distinguishes it from cellulitis) often described as having the texture of orange peel. There is usually rapid spread through the lymphatic vessels. Facial areas around the eyes, ears, and cheeks are susceptible and facial swelling can be very dramatic. Treatment is with antibiotics usually for a prolonged period as recurrence can occur in one-third of patients.

Necrotizing fasciitis A very rare, rapidly advancing soft tissue infection that causes widespread necrosis of the fascia and septicaemia. At first the skin is acutely painful becoming swollen, blistered, red, and then purple. Patients are acutely unwell, with fever and signs of septic shock. Mortality can be as high as 70%. Treatment involves early antibiotics, surgical debridement and/or amputation of an affected limb, and intensive care.

Impetigo

Impetigo is a common skin infection, more often seen in children than adults. It sometimes follows a recent upper respiratory infection. It is a superficial, infection involving the top layers of the skin with streptococcus, staphylococcus, or both. Impetigo is contagious. The infection is carried in the fluid that oozes from the blisters.

Symptoms
- Skin lesion on the face or lips, or on the arms or legs, spreading to other parts of the body.
- It begins as a cluster of tiny blisters that burst, followed by oozing and the formation of a thick honey- or brown-coloured crust that is very tenacious.

Treatment is with oral flucloxacillin (or erythromycin if allergic) and topical fusidic acid.

Rashes

A rash is any change to the appearance, colour, or texture of the skin. Adults and children with skin rashes frequently attend the ED and urgent care facilities due to concerns that the rash is a sign of a serious problem, e.g. meningococcal septicaemia, or because the rash is causing significant irritation/discomfort.

In patients who present with a rash it can be quite difficult to make an accurate diagnosis in an ED setting. ED assessment involves identifying any sign or symptom that needs immediate treatment, e.g. a purpuric rash or a skin infection that requires antibiotics. ED management involves the treatment of immediate symptoms, in-patient referral for continued management or further investigation, or out-patient treatment, usually with antihistamines, and referral back to primary care.

Skin infestations

There are several common skin/hair infestations that can present to emergency care areas. Most require only simple advice and over the counter treatment from a pharmacy.

Scabies

Scabies is a common mite infestation that produces tiny reddish papules and severe itching as young mites hatch just under the skin. Scabies spreads easily from person to person via physical contact or shared objects. The mites are destroyed by normal laundering.

Signs and symptoms

- The most common symptom of scabies is intense itching, which is usually worse at night.
- Thin lines with a lump at the end can sometimes be seen on the skin. These are the burrows of the young mites.
- Common sites are the webs between the fingers and toes, the wrists, ankles, buttocks, and, in males, the genitals.
- Intense itching can lead to a bacterial skin infection'

Treatment

- Scabies can be cured by applying a topical cream containing an insecticide, which is left for 12–24h (depending on the preparation) and then washed off. One treatment is usually enough although a second application 1 week later may be required.
- An antihistamine can help with itching, which can persist for several weeks.
- Any person with close physical contact should be treated as well.
- Clothing and bedding used during the preceding few days should be washed in hot water and dried in a hot dryer.

Head lice

Head lice can reach epidemic proportions in schools and are extremely common. Lice are commonly detected by parents or a letter can be sent from school informing parents of a recent outbreak.

Signs and symptoms Severe itching is the most common symptom especially at night when the louse are feeding. Lice can be visible in the hair and eggs are attached to the hair shaft close to the scalp.

Treatment is with topical solution and/or a metal 'nit' comb. The whole family will need treatment.

Threadworms

Threadworms are the most common worm infestation in humans. They are 5–10mm long and resemble tiny pieces of white cotton. They most commonly infect children and spread from person to person or via an object, e.g. toilet seat, towels. They are not caught from animals. The threadworm eggs are swallowed and hatch in the intestine; the female threadworm migrates to the anus where thousands of eggs are laid.

Signs and symptoms The main symptom is intense itching around the anus, especially at night. Itching can disturb sleep and may cause bed wetting in children. The threadworms may be visible on faeces; they look like moving pieces of white cotton.

Treatment

- Over the counter treatments are available. Advice should be sought from a pharmacist as to which is the most suitable, e.g. for young children or pregnant women.
- General hygiene measures are vital to stop the spread or any re-infection, e.g. separate towels, regular change of bedding washed on a hot cycle, strict hand hygiene.

Urticaria

The rapid appearance of erythematous, itchy swellings/wheals that are blotchy and vary in size and shape is an urticarial rash. An urticarial rash is usually transient and can disappear within hours. Drugs, foods, infection, or emotional stress can be a cause. Occasionally angio-oedema to the lips and mouth can be present. If the tongue and upper airways are affected this can be a life-threatening feature.

Urticarial rashes usually respond well to antihistamines. Patients who do not respond to antihistamines may benefit from a short course of systemic steriod. Treatment with adrenaline is indicated if angio-oedema threatens the airway.

Leg ulcers

A leg ulcer is defined as any break in the skin above the malleoli and below the patella that does not heal within 4 weeks. Leg ulcers are extremely common and affect 1% of the adult population and 3.6% of people > 65 years. They are debilitating and painful and can significantly reduce quality of life. The cost to the NHS is estimated as £400million per year. 90% of ulcers are caused by venous, arterial, or neuropathic disease.

Patients may attend the ED with a concern about an already established ulcer, e.g. infection. Patients may simply attend requesting a dressing change or the ED nurse may coincidently discover an untreated ulcer in a patient presenting with another problem. Another important consideration for the ED nurse is the identification of patients with an acute wound to the lower limb that is likely to have delayed healing and develop into an ulcer. In these situations its important to give appropriate discharge advice and signpost the patient to a community leg ulcer treatment facility.

Patients with an acute lower leg wound who are predisposed to the development of a leg ulcer

- Previous leg ulcer.
- Previous DVT.
- IV drug user.
- Varicose veins.
- Varicose eczema.
- Venous flare.
- Lower limb skin staining (haemosiderin pigmentation).
- Lower limb pale areas (atrophie blanche).
- Fibrotic areas to the lower limb (lipodermatosclerosis).

Management

- Leg ulcers of venous origin (the most common aetiology) heal more rapidly with compression bandaging as this aids venous return.
- Compression bandaging should only be started after a comprehensive assessment of the lower limb and exclusion of an arterial disease as the cause.
- Ulcer assessment and management is usually done by specially trained community/tissue viability nurses and should not be attempted in the ED by the non-specialist.

ED management of a leg ulcer involves treating any infection, applying a temporary absorbent dressing, and referring to the nearest leg ulcer service.

Ophthalmological emergencies

Introduction

Eye problems are common presentations in emergency care areas. Adults and children frequently attend with minor injuries to the eye, visual problems, and other painful/red eye conditions. Assessment of patients with eye problems requires the clinician to have some basic eye assessment skills, e.g. lid eversion (📖 see p.618), and access to a slit lamp to enable a complete assessment of the eye/s to be made. If a slit lamp is not available or the clinician is not familiar with how to use it the patient will need referral to a centre with comprehensive eye assessment facilities.

Fig. 13.1 shows the anatomy of the eye.

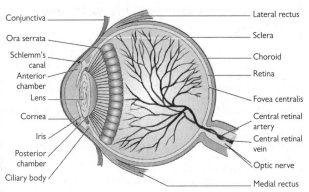

Fig. 13.1 The globe, looking down on the right eye, showing major anatomical structures. (Reproduced with permission from O'Connor, I.F. and Urdang, M. (2008). *Handbook of Surgical Cross-Cover*, p. 271. Oxford University Press, Oxford.)

Assessment of the patient with eye problems

▶ Assessment of visual acuity (VA) is *mandatory* and should be undertaken at the point of triage for any patient presenting with an eye problem. A VA should be established before any other investigations or treatment (except irrigation or instillation of local anaesthetic) are carried out. An accurate triage category cannot be assigned without an accurate VA and an assessment of whether this is normal for the patient

History taking

An accurate history is important. Questions should include the following.
- How long have the symptoms been present?
- Are they getting better/worse/stable?
- How did the problem begin and over what period of time?
- The degree, type, and location of any pain?
- Whether vision is reduced and to what degree?
- Is there any discharge or watering?
- Is the patient photophobic?
- Has the patient had this, or a similar problem before?
- Are there any concurrent systemic problems?

Examining the eye

It is very easy to assume a diagnosis from the history and miss less obvious problems. Eye examination, therefore, must be systematic starting at the outside (eye position and surrounding structures) and working inwards to consider the globe itself. The clinician should consider the following points.

Eyes
- Position normal for the patient?
- Enophthalmos (may indicate orbital fractures) or exophthalmos (may indicate orbital bleeds in trauma, thyroid eye disease)?
- Restriction of movement or double vision in any of the 8 gaze positions?

Lids
- Integrity. Lacerations of lid and lid margin?
- Position. Entropion/ectropion?
- Lash line. Intact? Ingrowing lashes/infestation/crusting?
- Swelling. Whole or part of the lid/one or both lids?
- Puncta visible and correctly sited?

Conjunctiva
- Integrity.
- Structure. Smooth? Follicles or papillae?
- Other features. Conjunctival cysts, pingueculae, pterygia?
- Inflammation. Generalized or local?
- Subconjunctival haemorrhage?
- Discharge. Type, frequency?
- Fornices. Both lower and subtarsal area. Concretions or foreign bodies may be visible.

Cornea
- Integrity. Lacerations, abrasions, ulcers?
- Clarity?
- Foreign bodies?

Anterior chamber
- Depth. The distance between the curved cornea and the iris. Generally equal in both eyes.
- Contents, e.g. white or red blood cells; any cells are abnormal.

Iris and pupil
- Colour. Similar to other eye?
- Position. Should be round and regular but may be slightly off centre (check both eyes).
- Integrity. Normal for patient? Previous surgery may change its appearance.
- Size and shape. Smaller or larger than the other eye; round or oval?
- Reaction to light and to near.

Always compare both eyes. What appears to be an abnormality may be bilateral and normal for the patient.

The injured eye

By far the most common ophthalmic problem to present to EDs and minor injury units is the injured eye. Adults and children frequently sustain minor injuries to the surface of their eye from foreign bodies or 'poking' type mechanisms. A carefully elicited history should enable the assessing clinician to determine if the injury is likely to be 'minor' and assessment can proceed without specialist intervention. Many minor eye injuries are successfully managed by ENPs. Obtaining a clear minor, mechanism is key to ensuring that a potentially more serious injury is not missed.

History

It is crucial to identify and document the following.
- What happened, e.g. poke in the eye or felt FB go in the eye.
- Where did it happen: was the injury at work, home?
- Was any eye protection used?
- Was any first aid administered at the time?
- When did the injury occur? Generally the longer an FB has been in situ, the harder it is to remove and the more likely an eye infection.
- How was the injury sustained; is there a risk of a penetrating eye injury?
- Past ophthalmic history. Has the patient any previous or current eye problems?

Blunt injuries to the eye, e.g. a punch to the face, can cause significant facial fractures as well as eye injuries. The orbit tends to protect the eye from the force of larger objects. However, small balls, e.g. squash balls or golf balls, can cause significant globe trauma. Is there a history of a high velocity injury? Hammer and chisel use typically causes small fragments to travel at high speed. Glass, knives, darts, and pencils are other causes of penetrating eye trauma and will require urgent ophthalmic referral.

- Common mechanisms for minor eye injuries include being poked in the eye with finger, hairbrush, plants, bushes, twigs
- Grinding injuries can cause metallic or brick foreign bodies (FBs)
- Other common FBs are dust, grit, flakes of metal/paint

Symptoms

The following are the most common symptoms of corneal injury or corneal FB.
- Pain. Injury to the cornea is acutely painful.
  - Large superficial abrasions are intensely painful (Fig. 13.2).
  - Deep lacerations with little epithelial loss are only mildly painful (Fig. 13.3).
- Visual disturbance.
- FB sensation.

Other symptoms include redness, watering, blurred vision, discharge.

Examination
- VA.
- Examine the eye systematically (📖 see Assessment of the patient with eye problems, p.400)

- Slit lamp examination to identify the depth of the injury and presence of any FB.
- Lid eversion to identify any subtarsal FBs.
- Fluorescein staining to reveal the extent of corneal injury.

Treatment of corneal injuries is based on the management of three areas: pain; prevention of infection; and optimization of healing.

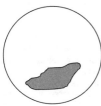 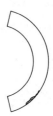

Fig. 13.2 Large superficial abrasions.

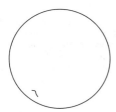

Fig. 13.3 Deep laceration.

Management of a corneal injury

Prevention of infection

Any corneal damage requires treatment with topical prophylactic antibiotic (chloramphenicol or fusidic acid). Fusidic acid is useful for children as it only requires a twice daily application.

If perforation is suspected or confirmed, a single drop of unpreserved, single dose chloramphenicol may be instilled before transfer to the ophthalmic unit. Both preservatives and ointment are toxic to ocular tissues and should not be used.

Pain

- Topical anaesthesia is for for examination purposes only and to obtain an accurate VA assessment. Repeated instillation will result in dose-related toxicity and delay in epithelial healing.
- Cyclopentolate 1% will relieve ciliary spasm and associated pain.
- Topical NSAIDs qds also provide a significant degree of effective pain relief.

Padding

- Is for comfort only.
- There is no evidence that it aids healing.
- Pad those patients who have significant pain advising that, if the pad makes the pain worse, they should remove it.

Double eye pad A double eye pad should always be used, one pad folded over the closed lids and the other open on top of it. The whole is taped firmly to the face so that the patient cannot open the eye underneath the pad. If comfortable, the pad should be left intact for 24h and then removed and instillation of medication commenced. There is no need to pad the eye just because a topical anaesthetic has been instilled.

Optimization of healing

Reviewing simple corneal abrasions depends very much on the individual clinician. Large abrasions can be reviewed to ensure that healing is taking place and that there is no loose epithelium that needs debriding. Small abrasions heal very quickly.

At review, if there is any loose epithelium visible or any sign of infection, increase in pain, or reduction in VA, it is safer to refer the patient for an ophthalmic opinion.

Recurrent abrasion syndrome is common in those patients who have an animal or vegetation-based cause for their abrasion (e.g. plants or fingernail). This can be prevented by using ointment at night before sleeping to keep the eye lubricated. 'Simple' ointment, or 'Lubri tears®' or 'Lacrilube®' (ointment base without drugs) should be used for a period of up to 3 months.

Referral of corneal injuries Each emergency care area will have guidelines about which types of corneal injuries should be referred for ophthalmic assessment and follow-up.

Foreign bodies

Conjunctival foreign body

These are usually superficial.
- Instil topical anaesthetic.
- Remove from conjunctiva by wiping with a dampened cotton bud (any swab/cotton bud used on the eye should be pre-moistened with a saline minim or the residue of an anaesthetic minim—otherwise, epithelial tissue sticks to the swab rather than the eye and significant injury can result).
- Stain after the FB has been removed to identify extent of damage.
  - If there is minimal stain, a single application of chloramphenicol ointment may be instilled.
  - If there is significant stain, chloramphenicol ointment should be prescribed qds until the eye feels back to normal.

Deeper FBs on the conjunctiva may be removed using a 21G hypodermic needle, often mounted on the end of a cotton bud to form a longer and more easily manipulated tool.

Corneal foreign body

- Assess depth using slit lamp. The depth of the cornea may be seen within the slit lamp beam.
- If the FB is anything other than superficial, it should be refereed to the local eye unit for further assessment and removal.

⚠ The cornea is only 1mm thick at its thickest. Accidental perforation does occur and can be devastating.

Foreign body removal should always take place at a slit lamp to provide magnification and stability for the patient's head. If this is not possible, consideration should be given to referral to a more appropriate setting.
- Instil topical anaesthetic.
- Use a 21G needle, bore upwards, to gently lift off the FB from the cornea.
- Metallic foreign bodies may need slightly more forceful removal.
- Rust must be removed at some point. This can be facilitated by giving the patient chloramphenicol ointment or drops to use for 2 or 3 days and then reviewing in the ED or in the eye unit. Rust is much easier to remove at this stage. Again, antibiotic or ointment should be prescribed until the eye feels back to normal.

Once a FB is removed treatment is the same as for a corneal abrasion and should be focused on preventing infection, relieving pain, and optimizing healing.

Superglue injuries

History Superglue may be instilled into the eye as its containers often resemble eye drop containers.

Signs and symptoms
- Pain.
- Eyelids stuck together.

As the eye is permanently wetted by the tear film, the glue does not generally stick to the tissues of the eye but hardens, forming a plaque inside the lids and abrading the cornea as the eye and lids move. The glue usually glues the eyelashes together and therefore holds the lids together.

Management
- Instil topical anaesthetic to the lids allowing it to drain between them to act on the cornea. This relieves pain and allows examination and treatment.
- Trim the eyelashes very close to the lid margin.
- Pick off the remaining glue to allow the lids to open. This must be done very carefully and may take some time. A very fine pair of scissors is required and a laceration of the lid margin must be avoided. This may be a lengthy procedure necessitating repeated topical anaesthetic and much patience.
- When the lids are open remove the plaque of glue and all particles of glue.
- VAs.
- Treat resulting abrasions as corneal abrasions.

Children may be much less cooperative than adults and may need a general anaesthetic for this procedure. Referral to an ophthalmic unit should be considered.

⚠ Superglued eyelids will take a considerable time to open on their own and practitioners should not be tempted to 'let nature take its course'. The abrasions are likely to be extremely painful, the glue plaque will abrade as long as it is in the eye, and the loss of corneal epithelium provides an entry point to the eye for pathogens.

Ultraviolet radiation injury (welding flash/arc eye)

History
- Exposure to welding arcs.
- Exposure to UV 'sunlamps'.

The UV radiation is absorbed by the corneal epithelial cells, some of which are damaged or destroyed. There is a latent period before symptoms are experienced, which depends on the amount of exposure and explains the typical late-night presentation of these patients.

Signs and symptoms
- Gritty sensation to one or both eyes.
- Intensely painful eye(s).
- Photophobia.
- Watering and blurred vision.
- Lid swelling.
- Redness.

Examination
- Instil topical anaesthetic.
- VA and examine the eye systematically (☐ see p.400).
- Instil fluorescein.
  - Fluorescein reveals punctate staining on the surface of the cornea where some cells have been destroyed.

Management
- Treatment is as for a corneal abrasion.
- A mydriatic drop will provide comfort.
- Antibiotic ointment as prophylaxis and for comfort.
- Padding may help, but both eyes should not be padded simultaneously.
- Advise complete recovery is usually within 24–36h.

Chemical injury

History
It is almost irrelevant what chemical is splashed into the eye and no time should be wasted in the ED trying to find out. Chemical splashes in the eye can result in devastating injury and the time to irrigation is the most important factor in minimizing ocular problems.

Irrigation The initial treatment of ocular chemical injuries involves irrigation to dilute the chemical and remove any solid debris (📖 see p.616).

Examination
- Visual acuity.
- Examine the eye systematically (📖 see p.400).

Management Superficial injury may be treated with chloramphenicol ointment qds until the eye feels back to normal.

- All but the most trivial chemical injuries should be referred to an ophthalmologist.
- Solvent injuries are generally much less damaging than those due to acid and alkaline chemicals.

Blunt trauma

Blunt trauma may result in disruption to any or all of the ocular tissues. Any patient presenting with blunt trauma to the eye or surrounding tissues with any reduction in vision should be referred to an ophthalmologist for specialist assessment.

Traumatic hyphaema

Signs and symptoms
- Blood in the anterior chamber, detected by slit lamp or visible with the naked eye, to the extent of filling the whole of the anterior chamber.
- Reduced VA.
- A raise in intraocular pressure as red blood cells block the trabecular network.
- Severe pain.
- Irregular or sluggish pupil.

Management
- Urgent referral to an ophthalmologist is required.
- Sit the patient upright in order to allow the blood cells to settle and absorb away from the visual axis. This will reduce any staining of the corneal endothelium with haem pigment, which may affect vision.

Regular review is undertaken to monitor intraocular pressure and treat any rise in pressure.

Traumatic uveitis is a common effect of blunt trauma and may be the only sign of trauma. Treatment is as for any uveitis, with pupil dilatation and topical steroids.

Iris and pupil abnormalities Traumatic mydriasis or miosis may occur as a consequence of blunt trauma and the pupil may be irregular when compared with the fellow eye due to partial or complete rupture of the iris sphincter.

Lens abnormalities

The impact of the iris on the lens as the eye distorts and then moves back into shape may leave a circle of iris pigment, which can be seen after dilatation (Vossius ring).

Traumatic rupture of the zonules holding the lens in place may occur and luxation or subluxation of the lens may take place. Raised intraocular pressure may occur if the lens blocks the pupil. Iridodonesis (iris tremble) may be visible.

▶ Urgent referral to an ophthalmic unit is required for any iris, pupil, or lens abnormalities.

Major trauma

Orbital injury
Both facial and skull trauma can result in orbital injury.

Medial orbital fractures The lacrimal secretory system (especially the nasolacrimal duct) may be damaged and the medial rectus muscle may be trapped within the fracture.

Orbital floor fractures Often referred to as blowout fractures because they are produced by transmission of forces through the bones and soft tissues of the orbit by a non-penetrating object such as a fist or a ball. These fractures may be complicated by the entrapment of muscles and orbital fat which limits ocular motility (📖 see p.471).

Signs and symptoms
These include:
• diplopia;
• enophthalmos;
• infraorbital anaesthesia.

A classic presentation involves an injured patient, who perhaps would not have presented to the ED otherwise, blowing their nose and then attending because their eyelids have swollen alarmingly as air from the sinus has been driven into the tissues of the lid.

The patient should be given advice about the avoidance of the Valsalva manoeuvre, such as blowing the nose or straining at stool.

> Any patient with an orbital fracture and any degree of double vision should be referred to an ophthalmic unit.

Orbital apex trauma
All clinicians in the ED must be alerted to the possibility of ocular involvement from indirect trauma such as base of skull fractures, as well as from more direct trauma where the eyes themselves do not appear to be involved.

Fractures of the orbital apex may result from direct, non-penetrating blunt trauma or from penetrating trauma, e.g. with large orbital FBs. Orbital apex fractures present differently depending on the degree of injury to the vascular and neural structures within the orbital apex and a number of different presentations are possible.
• Optic nerve injury may occur, commonly due to traumatic optic neuropathy from indirect trauma (such as fractures of the base of the skull). Haematoma may compress the nerve or it may be damaged by FB or from a fracture, which can result in a spectrum of injury from minor trauma to the nerve to complete transection.
• Injury to the cranial nerves present in the orbit, (III, IV, and VI) may present as extraocular muscle palsy with double vision.
• Injury to the trigeminal nerve (V) presents as sensory disturbance to areas it supplies.

Collaboration of ophthalmic units with the ED is important in order to ensure that patients with this type of injury do not lose vision unnecessarily.

⚠ Patient complaints of loss of or reduction in vision must be taken very seriously. In order to quantify this, VA must be checked on arrival, as a baseline and then hourly. Ophthalmology opinion must be obtained immediately if vision is involved.

Retrobulbar haemorrhage

This may occur from direct or indirect trauma to the orbit and can progress rapidly.

Signs and symptoms
- Pain.
- Proptosis of the globe.
- Congested conjunctival vessels.
- Lid and conjunctival swelling.
- Subconjunctival haemorrhage may be dense and may extend beyond the visible conjunctiva.

Management
- Regular observation of the appearance of the eye patient with direct or indirect trauma to that orbit is required to minimize complications of the injury.
- VA should be measured as a baseline and the patient should be encouraged to report new symptoms and any reduction in vision.
- ▶▶ If the globe begins to proptose after trauma, an ophthalmologist should be involved immediately. CT or MRI scan may be required urgently and the patient's VA should be checked very frequently (every 10min).

If VA reduces, emergency decompression by lateral canthotomy (a horizontal incision at the lateral canthus, through skin and conjunctiva and then through the lateral canthal tendon, under local anaesthetic) will be required to relieve pressure on the optic nerve. Equipment for this procedure will not be needed very often but should be readily available in the ED so that avoidable loss of vision may be prevented.

Open trauma

An open eye requires immediate assessment. No attempt should be made to remove any retained materials protruding from the globe.

Management

- Stabilize any protruding material as far as possible, perhaps by taping it to the cheek or by covering the whole area with a plastic shield or small receiver.
- No pressure should be put on to the eye and an eyepad should only be used if absolutely no other method of covering the eye exists. The pad must be loose and taped well away from the globe—any pressure on the globe may result in further injury and/or loss of ocular contents.
- Manage pain and nausea. Vomiting with an open eye is likely to lead to loss of the ocular contents.
- Lie the patient flat or propped up at around a 30° angle. This can minimize any rise in intraocular pressure.
- Do not cover both eyes unless they are both extensively damaged. A patient with one damaged eye is unlikely to be relaxed, comforted, or reassured by being unable to see anything or anyone around them.

▶▶ Immediate referral to an ophthalmologist is required.

Small penetrating injuries

Penetrating injuries and intraocular FBs may cause damage to globe by:
- tissue disruption at the time of injury;
- formation of scar tissue causing long-term damage—retinal scars may contract and cause retinal detachment; corneal scars will distort or disrupt vision;
- introduction of foreign material to which the eye reacts;
- allowing pathways for infection to enter the globe.

Large penetrating eye injuries are very obvious, but small perforations may be easily missed as the eye may look completely intact. The wound may have self-sealed or may be obscured by the upper lid.

Examination must always include all aspects of the anterior part of the globe by asking the patient to look in each different direction so that all segments may be examined. As the patient looks down, the upper lid should be retracted so that the upper portion of the globe may be seen. All penetrations of the lid should lead to a high index of suspicion about the state of the globe.
- Corneal perforations always leave full thickness scar, even if very small.
- Scleral perforations may be masked by overlying subconjunctival haemorrhage.
- A small hole in the iris may mark the passage of a FB.

▶ Analgesia and anti-emetics should be considered as vomiting may lead to expulsion of the contents of a perforated globe.

▶▶ Patients with penetrating trauma should be referred urgently to an ophthalmologist.

The red eye

Another common eye problem that presents frequently to emergency care areas is the 'red eye'. Patients cannot identify any specific injury and can complain of varying symptoms, e.g. redness, pain, itch, watering, discharge swelling, headache, and visual disturbance.

Allergies

Allergic conjunctivitis presents in several ways.

- Red eyes with itching and watering and an appearance of large bumps(papillae) on the subtarsal conjunctiva are particularly common during the 'hay fever season' and may therefore be associated with a runny nose , sneezing, and other allergic symptoms. Treatment is with systemic antihistamines and/or topical treatment such as emadine or opatanol.
- A more severe chronic atopic reaction, most often seen in children, is the appearance of 'cobblestone papillae'. The appearance of the subtarsal conjunctiva is of massive papillae arranged in a cobblestone fashion. This is intensely irritating and often requires complex management. Patients presenting in this way should be referred to an ophthalmologist urgently.
- An acute atopic reaction involves massive chemosis or swelling of the conjunctiva which the patient or parent often describes as 'jelly' on the eye. This is due to an allergen transferring directly to the eye on fingers or by blowing in. This is completely self-limiting. It resolves quickly (over a period of hours) and reassurance and information is all that is required.

Conjunctivitis

Inflammation of the conjunctiva is by far the most common cause of red eyes. Common organisms involved in infective conjunctivitis include viruses, bacteria, and chlamydia (📕 see Table 13.1). Almost all conjunctivitis in adults is caused by a virus, often a type of adenovirus, and unless there are large amounts of green/yellow discharge present all day, the infection should be presumed not to be bacterial. Conjunctivitis in children is more likely to be bacterial.

△ Eye pads should never be suggested for patients with conjunctivitis. The warm, damp atmosphere underneath an eye pad will allow further organism growth and exacerbate the condition.

Viral conjunctivitis

Signs and symptoms

- Gritty sensation to the eye/s.
- Profuse watering.
- Dry feeling to the eye/s.
- Stickiness often only in the morning when the watery discharge has dried and the lids are stuck together.
- Some types of adenovirus also cause URTI and general malaise.

Examination

- On lid eversion the conjunctiva covering the lids will appear very bumpy rather than smooth. This roughness of the conjunctiva is what makes the eye feel gritty and irritable.
- There may be punctate erosions (small staining areas) on the cornea when stained with fluorescein.

Management

- Symptom relief with artificial tears and advice about very frequent use (hourly or even more frequently).
- Advice about the self-limiting nature of the condition. The patient should be aware that viral conjunctivitis may persist for 3–6 weeks and that the symptoms of dryness may last much longer. There is no point in prescribing antibiotic eye drops.

△ Adenovirus is highly infectious and infection control is of paramount importance, both for the patient and the emergency care setting. Handwashing is vital to stop the spread of viral conjunctivitis Major epidemics of viral conjunctivitis associated with ophthalmic units have been linked with poor handwashing. All equipment should also be cleaned between each patient. It is not necessary to take eye swabs for culture and the patient should not be followed up.

Bacterial conjunctivitis

Signs and symptoms

- Redness.
- Irritable gritty eye.
- Profuse, purulent discharge; the lashes may be coated with discharge.

Management A broad spectrum antibiotic such as chloramphenicol or fusidic acid, applied topically in the form of drops. The condition is self-limiting and no investigations are required.

Chlamydial conjunctivitis

Signs and symptoms

- Unilateral.
- Chronic (the patient may have had a red and irritable eye for some time which has reached a irritating stage but not progressed to a severe viral infection).
- Large pearly follicles are present on lid eversion.

If chlamydia is suspected from the clinical picture (📖 see Table 13.1), a chlamydial swab should be obtained from the eye. The patient's details should be checked to ensure that they are contactable should the result be positive. Patients should be referred to GUM for treatment.

Table 13.1 Types of conjunctivitis

	Viral	Bacterial	Chlamydial
	Bilateral & acute	Rare, bilateral	Unilateral & chronic
Lids	May be swollen Follicles	May be swollen	Unlikely to be swollen
Conjunctiva	Injected	Injected	Injected
Cornea	May have keratitis (punctate staining of cornea)	No involvement	No involvement
Discharge	Watery, sticky in morning	Green/yellow discharge all day	Watery, stuck together in mornings
Vision	May be affected by corneal involvement	Unlikely to be affected	Unlikely to be affected
Pain	Gritty, dry; may be intensely irritating	Gritty & very sticky	Mild irritation
Investigation	None: clinical diagnosis only. Identification of organism does not change management	None: clinical diagnosis only. Identification of organism does not change management	If clinical appearance suggestive of chlamydia, swab for chlamydia
Treatment	Artificial tear regime Information Reassurance	Antibiotic drops	Artificial tear regime On positive identification appointment with GUM

Subconjunctival haemorrhage

Patients may present with a spontaneous subconjunctival haemorrhage with a deep red patch of blood under the conjunctiva, which may be quite small and circumscribed or may be severe enough for the conjunctiva to appear like a 'bag of blood'. Providing that there is no history of trauma, no treatment is needed unless the haemorrhage is severe or the eye irritable in which case artificial tears are useful to provide comfort and lubrication.

Subconjunctival haemorrhage may occasionally be associated with hypertension so it might be useful to check the patient's BP. Patients with clotting disorders or those on anticoagulants may be prone to repeat episodes. Subconjunctival haemorrhages may take some weeks to resolve and, because the conjunctiva is an elastic membrane, the blood may spread under it and the haemorrhage appear worse, before it begins to resolve.

Anterior uveitis (also known as uveitis, iridocyclitis, iritis)

Uveitis is an inflammatory condition, which may be associated with systemic disease or as response to trauma but is often idiopathic. It is unusual to encounter uveitis (especially as a primary attack) in an elderly patient.

Signs and symptoms (☐ see Box 13.1)

- Photophobia.
- Pain (due to ciliary spasm).
- Conjunctival redness (injection), which may be more marked around the limbus.
- Decreased vision due to protein and white blood cells in the anterior chamber.
- Small pupil that reacts sluggishly because of spasm and inflammation.

Examination When the cornea is illuminated with a torch, the reflection will be bright and there will be no staining with fluorescein.

Treatment The patient must be referred on to an ophthalmic unit for investigation and treatment.

Box 13.1 Characteristics of uveitis

- Lids normal
- Conjunctiva injected
- Cornea normal
- Anterior chamber deep
- Iris may look 'muddy'
- Pupil: slight miosis (compared with fellow); sluggish
- Pain: deep pain in eye
- Discharge: may water
- Photophobia
- Systemically well

Corneal ulcers

There are three main types of corneal ulcer that are likely to be seen in the emergency care settings. All should be referred to an ophthalmologist urgently. Differentiation between the different types of corneal ulcer is sometimes difficult and the treatment is completely different.

A careful history will usually identify symptoms of a 'red eye': pain; redness; visual disturbance; and no history of injury. Ulcers are seen in contact lens wearers and the clinician should always be alert to the possibility of a corneal ulcer if there has been a history of lens wearing. On staining a defect is seen on the cornea, which may have a characteristic shape.

▶ Any corneal defect that cannot be explained by a history of injury should be discussed with an ophthalmologist.

Bacterial ulcers

On staining, bacterial ulcers occur as 'fluffy' white demarcated areas. They are caused by a number of organisms, e.g. *Pseudomonas,* which is very difficult to treat, and are most commonly, but by no means exclusively, seen in contact lens wearers. The patient should be urged to leave their contact lens out of their eye while waiting to be seen in the ophthalmic unit but should keep it with them as it is likely to be sent for culture.

▶▶ Delay in treatment of infected corneal ulcers can result in devastating intraocular infection.

Viral ulcers (dendritic ulcers)

These are caused by the Herpes simplex virus. They are known as 'dendritic' ulcers because of their branching, tree-like shape when stained with fluorescein. They are treated with aciclovir eye ointment, and should be referred to an ophthalmologist for treatment and follow-up.

Marginal ulcers appear as ulcerated areas that stain with fluorescein and are usually close to the limbus. They are part of a hypersensitivity response by the eye to staphylococcal exotoxins and are treated with steroidal or nonsteroidal anti-inflammatory eye drops by an ophthalmologist.

Glaucoma

Glaucoma describes a rise in the pressure inside the eye, causing damage to the neural tissue that makes up the retina and resulting in permanent reduction in the field of vision.

There are two main types of glaucoma.

- Chronic, open angle glaucoma where the rise in pressure is small, damage is done to the retina over a large period of time, and visual field loss is insidious.
- Acute, closed angle glaucoma, which is an ophthalmic emergency.

Chronic open angle glaucoma

This type of glaucoma is only likely to be encountered in the ED if the patient has run out of eye drops or as an incidental part of history taking.

Although it cannot be recommended that patients manage without the appropriate medication for their condition, it cannot be considered an emergency in the same way as perhaps a diabetic without insulin. The patient should be referred to their own ophthalmic clinic or GP at the earliest opportunity.

There is no danger associated with dilating the eye of a patient who has chronic, open angle glaucoma. Indeed, on each visit to the ophthalmic outpatient department, this procedure will be undertaken to evaluate the optic disc.

Acute glaucoma (angle closure glaucoma)

In acute glaucoma, the outflow of aqueous in the eye is obstructed by the peripheral iris covering the trabecular meshwork at the drainage angle in the anterior chamber. As aqueous continues to be produced, the pressure inside the eye increases rapidly. Patients are usually elderly (it is very unusual to see acute glaucoma in someone under the age of 60) and are likely to be hypermetropic (long-sighted).

A key thing to remember is that patients with acute glaucoma often present with a primary complaint other than their eye. Severe abdominal pain is often the presenting symptom. Nausea and vomiting may also be the main presenting feature.

Any red eye that is noticed may be assumed to be a secondary and unimportant issue unless the clinician keeps a high index of suspicion. Dealing with the eye problem will cure the abdominal pain/nausea/vomiting. Ignoring the eye problems will result in irreversible (and preventable) visual loss.

Signs and symptoms (📖 see Box 13.2)

- Severe pain, (due to the increased intraocular pressure).
- Blurred vision (due to corneal oedema).
- Haloes seen around lights.
- Headache.
- Nausea and vomiting and abdominal pain.

Examination

- Red eye.
- Reflection of light from the cornea will be very diffuse—showing that the cornea is oedematous.
- Semi-dilated oval pupil that responds to light sluggishly if at all.

▶▶ Acute glaucoma is an ophthalmic emergency and the patient should be referred to an ophthalmologist urgently, including emergency ambulance transportation if necessary.

Initial treatment—in emergency care
- Analgesia and anti-emetics may be required.
- Treatment of dehydration if vomiting has been prolonged.
- Reassurance and careful explanation is needed by these ill and often terrified patients.

Box 13.2 Characteristics of acute glaucoma

- Lids normal
- Conjunctiva injected
- Cornea very hazy
- Anterior chamber shallow or flat
- Iris may be difficult to see
- Pupil fixed, oval, semi-dilated
- pain: severe pain in and around eye and head
- Discharge: none
- Photophobia: none
- Systemically:
  - nausea and vomiting
  - severe abdominal pain
  - dehydration

Loss of vision: history

An accurate history of visual loss is crucial to the identification of possible causes. This is especially the case in the emergency setting where specialist examination may not be immediately available.

History—important features

- Are there patches or areas of absolute vision loss or is the vision blurred?
- Sudden or gradual loss? If sudden, is it possible that it has been there for a while but has only just been noticed? If the loss was gradual, over what period of time has it occurred (days, weeks, or even months)?
- Does the loss of vision involve some or all of the vision? Are there sectors of the field of vision that are missing? Is the loss worse centrally or peripherally?
- Was the loss transient—has it come back now or is it recovering (how long was vision affected for) or does it seem to be permanent?
- Is the vision now getting better, or worse, or is it staying the same?
- Are there any other symptoms that the patient is experiencing (such as headache, weakness, or pain elsewhere)?

Monocular versus binocular loss of vision

Ocular pathology, or optic nerve problems, will cause monocular loss of vision. A problem at or posterior to the optic chiasma, in the brain, will cause binocular loss of vision. Conditions include migraine (with visual symptoms, such as fortification spectra, hemianopia, and blurring, that may not be accompanied by headache), vascular lesions, tumour, and stroke.

A generalization, but one that works in practice, is that, if a patient complains of binocular loss of vision, the problem is likely to be of neurological rather than ophthalmic origin and a neurological opinion should be sought. The rare exception to this is in bilateral blurring of vision that has appeared over a small number of days—this is characteristic of papilloedema and can be discovered by eye examination.

Profound monocular loss of vision

This is defined as complete or severely diminished vision affecting the whole of the visual field that may occur suddenly or gradually over a period of days. Sudden, profound loss of vision suggests a vascular cause and the most likely of these are central retinal artery occlusion and vitreous haemorrhage.

Vitreous haemorrhage is the most likely cause if there is an associated history of diabetes.

Signs and symptoms
• The patient may be aware of the haemorrhaging.
• Floaters can be seen by the patient, becoming denser over a short period and resulting in a profound loss of vision.

Any attempt by the clinician to visualize the back of the eye will be unsuccessful due to the haemorrhage between the clinician and the retina.

Management The patient should be referred to an ophthalmologist, although it is unlikely that treatment (laser) will take place until the haemorrhage has cleared sufficiently for the retina to be visualized.

Central retinal artery occlusion

The patient may describe the vision disappearing 'like someone switching the light off'. The loss may be absolute.

Examination
• The retina is likely to be pale due to swelling and the macular area is seen as a 'cherry red spot'.
• An embolus in the central retinal artery may be seen.

▶▶ This condition is an ophthalmic emergency and immediate treatment must start in the emergency setting.

Investigations
• ESR, CRP.
• FBC, lipid, and clotting profile.
• USS of the coronary arteries and ECG—in order to identify the site of the embolus).

Treatment
• IV acetazolamide 500mg increases perfusion of the retina by reducing the intraocular pressure.
• Occular massage to encourage the outflow of aqueous.
• Rebreathing exhaled air by breathing into a paper bag. This increases the carbon dioxide concentration in the body, dilating blood vessels, and perhaps allowing the embolus to move further into the retinal circulation. If the latter occurs, a sector of visual loss, rather than profound loss, may be a good outcome for the patient.

An anoxic retina is irreversibly damaged in 90min and the visual outcome of this condition is often poor.

Segmental loss of vision and loss of central vision

Segmental loss of vision

The most likely causes of the loss of an area of the visual field in one eye are vascular causes such as occlusions of branches of the retinal artery or vein (branch retinal artery or vein occlusions) or retinal detachment.

- If onset is sudden and the loss stable, the cause is likely to be vascular.
- If the area of visual loss changes over time, the cause is more likely to be a retinal detachment.

Branch retinal artery and vein occlusions

These may be seen with an ophthalmoscope.

- A branch retinal artery occlusion will lead to a segment of retina being paler than the rest, all the vessels will appear in the correct location, and an embolus may be seen in one of the vessels.
- There may be multiple retinal haemorrhages if the cause of the loss of vision is a branch retinal vein occlusion. The haemorrhages will be in the area of retina that is served by the blocked vein. Retinal oedema may be seen and an occlusion may be visible.

There is no immediate treatment for either of these conditions, although follow-up by an ophthalmologist will be necessary.

Retinal detachment (RD)

Spontaneous RD affects 1 in 10 000 of the population each year and is more common in males and in short-sighted (myopic) eyes. It most commonly occurs due to collapse of the vitreous gel in middle age resulting in traction on a weak area of retina causing a hole to form. Serous fluid may get between the retina and its basement membrane, pushing them apart and resulting in a retinal detachment.

Signs and symptoms

- Flashing lights. The only way that the brain can interpret movement of the retina is in terms of light so, as the retina moves, the brain interprets and the patient 'sees' flashes of light.
- Floaters. The appearance of a large circular floater is due to the detachment of the vitreous gel from its ring-shaped adhesion to the optic disc. A shower of tiny floaters is due to haemorrhage into the vitreous as a small retinal blood vessel is damaged.
- A sector of loss of vision that tends to enlarge over a period of hours or days may be noticed. The patient may complain of seeing a 'shadow' that tends to move, or a 'curtain' descending over the eye.
- Central vision may be lost due to macular detachment.

The detached retina will appear grey and may seem slightly wrinkled.

▶▶ Patients with retinal detachment need an urgent ophthalmic opinion. Surgery may be almost immediate in order to preserve macular function.

Loss of central vision

Common causes of loss of central vision include age-related macular degeneration (AMD), optic neuritis, central serous retinopathy, and macular burns.

AMD refers to a gradual degeneration of the macula. It is the most common cause of visual loss in the over-75s and affects ~20% of individuals. There is usually a very gradual loss of central vision. Although this is not an acute problem, elderly patients may present in the ED because they have reached a point where they can no longer manage the problems alone. Referral to an ophthalmologist is essential although treatment for this condition is only effective for a very small number of patients. Patients retain navigating vision—their peripheral visual field is not affected.

Optic neuritis is inflammation of the optic nerve. Episodes are usually monocular and it is most common in females aged 20–40 years. It is strongly associated with MS and is the presenting problem in 25% of cases.

The patient is likely to present with loss of central vision that may progress to a generalized loss of vision and can become severe. Other symptoms include pain that is worse on ocular movement (due to the inflamed optic nerve moving as the eye moves) and altered colour perception. The pupil reactions will be abnormal and the optic nerve head may be swollen. Referral to a neurologist or neuro-ophthalmologist for further assessment is required.

Central serous retinopathy (CSR) usually occurs in young adult males. The cause is unknown. Symptoms usually include a unilateral blurring of central vision and a generalized darkening of the visual field with some distortion. Visual acuity is usually only mildly reduced. Referral to an ophthalmologist is necessary although most episodes of CSR resolve spontaneously within 3–6 months.

Macular burns may be caused by MIG (metal inert gas) welding equipment, which produces high intensity white light that the eye transmits rather than absorbs. It can cause macular burns resulting in loss of central vision. The patient may notice a black mark in the centre of the visual field that stays in the same place when they move the eye. Macular burns may be caused by the patient looking at the sun without adequate eye protection.

Blurring of vision and transient loss of vision

Blurring of vision

Blurring of vision may be due to problems anywhere in the visual pathway, between cornea and visual cortex. Many patients will have problems in differentiating between generalized blurring and loss of central vision—therefore careful questioning is required. Some causes of blurring (vitreous haemorrhage, CSR, optic neuritis, vessel occlusion) have already been described.

- Patients with papilloedema often present with blurring of vision. This may be worse in one eye and may be exacerbated by change in position (lying to standing). Patients with bilateral swollen optic discs need urgent neurological referral.
- Opacities in any of the clear structures of the eye will result in blurring of vision as less light reaches the retina.
  - The most common opacity is a cataract—lens opacity. Cataract causes glare and reduction in vision and lens opacities may be seen on examination with a slit lamp or, if severe, with a pen torch. Reassurance and referral to optometrist (for optimization of vision) and GP for referral to an ophthalmologist is appropriate. If the lens opacity has occurred after trauma, or is in a younger person, more urgent referral to an ophthalmologist should be considered.
  - ▶▶ Corneal opacities or irregularities resulting in blurring should be referred to an ophthalmologist urgently.

Transient loss of vision

The most common causes of transient visual loss are vascular and not ophthalmic. Carotid artery disease and giant cell arteritis require referral to a physician.

If transient loss of vision is accompanied by pain in an elderly person, particularly when light levels are low and especially if accompanied by a red eye, intermittent angle closure glaucoma may be suspected and urgent referral to an ophthalmologist is required.

ENT emergencies

Overview

Most EDs see a fair proportion of patients who could be treated in a primary care setting. The proliferation of walk-in centres in recent years, which are mainly nurse led, means that many patients presenting with ENT primary care conditions will be treated by an ENP. This chapter reflects this development and offers advice on when and what to refer on to the GP or the local doctor.

Acute sore throat: assessment

Sore throat is a common presenting complaint and mostly viral in origin. An estimated 30% are caused by bacteria where group A beta haemolytic streptococci (GABHS) are, most frequently the causative organisms. Regardless of cause symptoms will resolve spontaneously in the majority of cases within 1 week of onset. However, a full history is required to exclude other important causes of an acute sore throat.

▶ Any patient having difficulty with breathing or unable to swallow should be referred on to an ENT specialist.

History

Signs and symptoms

- Onset and duration.
- Severity of pain/soreness.
- Ear pain—may be referred.
- Coryzal symptoms.
- Cough.
- Dysphagia.
- Trismus (spasm of pterygoid muscles preventing opening of the mouth).
- Rash.
- Abdominal symptoms.
- Headache.
- Fatigue.

Past medical history

- Diabetes.
- Rheumatic fever.
- Disease causing immunosuppression.
- Asthma—may be relevant if NSAIDs or aspirin gargles are indicated to treat symptoms.
- Immunization history.

Medication

- Combined oral contraceptive pill—may be relevant if treatment with antibiotics is indicated.
- Drugs known to cause neutropenia, e.g. methotrexate, azathioprine, sulphonamides, carbimazole, and sulfasalazine (a sore throat may be the first sign of neutropenia).
- Steroids: oral or inhaled.
- Recent antibiotic use.
- Over the counter medications used to treat symptoms, e.g. use of analgesia (what and when last given).

Ask about allergies with specific reference to:
- antibiotics;
- NSAIDs;
- aspirin.

Examination

- Temperature.
- Pulse.
- Inspect and palpate the cervical lymph glands.
- Inspect the external auditory canal and the tympanic membrane.
- Inspect the oral cavity, buccal mucosa, and oropharynx. Look for exudates or slough, peritonsillar swelling, the position of the uvula, petechiae on the soft palate, and strawberry tongue.
- Check for trismus.
- Inspect the skin for colour and rash and circumoral pallor.

⚠ Do **not** attempt to examine the throat of an individual who has drooling, stridor, or breathing difficulties. They may have epiglottitis.

Pharyngitis and tonsillitis

- Pharyngitis: inflammation of the pharynx and surrounding lymph tissues.
- Tonsillitis: acute inflammation of the tonsils.

Both of these conditions commonly present as an acute sore throat and can be either viral or bacterial in origin. Realistically, it is difficult to determine whether an acute sore throat is viral or bacterial in origin. For most patients antibiotics have little effect on the extent and duration of symptoms. ∴ management is principally focused on advice regarding symptom management. Antibiotics are reserved for those who are most likely to benefit from them.

Viral causes

Caused by adenoviruses, rhinoviruses, and parainfluenzae viruses.

Clinical characteristics

- Sore throat that is reported to be worse on swallowing.
- May be accompanied by fever.
- Possible tender cervical lymphadenopathy.
- Headache and malaise.
- Cough and coryzal symptoms are common.

Bacterial causes

Caused by group A beta haemolytic streptococci. Most common in children of school age; less so in adults and children < 3 years.

Clinical characteristics

- Sore throat that is reported to be worse on swallowing.
- Fever.
- Tender cervical lymphadenopathy (particularly anterior cervical) and slough on inflamed tonsils.
- Headache, malaise, abdominal pain, and vomiting may all occur.

Management

Pain relief and fever management

- Paracetamol and/or ibuprofen should be recommended/prescribed. In children if both preparations are used they should be given simultaneously and not staggered.
- Soluble aspirin gargles.
  - ⚠ For children > 16 years of age only.
  - Anecdotally, gargling with aspirin is reported to relieve pain in some people.
  - Soluble aspirin if used should not be advised in conjunction with ibuprofen.
- Benzydamine gargles: there is some limited evidence to support use. Can be prescribed or obtained over the counter.

Treatment with antibiotics

NICE[1] advise that antibiotics should be reserved for those with one or more of the following criteria.

- Features of marked systemic upset 2° to the acute sore throat.
- Unilateral peritonsillitis.
- History of rheumatic fever.
- Increased risk from acute infection (such as those with diabetes mellitus or immunodeficiency).

When indicated antibiotics should be prescribed or, alternatively, supplied using a Patient Group Direction.

- Phenoxymethylpenicillin (penicillin V).
- Erythromycin (if allergic to penicillin).

▶ Women taking the combined oral contraceptive pill should be advised that additional contraceptive precautions should be taken whilst taking a short course of an antibacterial and for 7 days after stopping. If these 7 days run beyond the end of a packet of OCPs the next packet should be started immediately without a break (in the case of ED (every day) tablets the inactive ones should be omitted).[1]

Other advice

Provide information to patient about the following.

- Prevention of dehydration. Children particularly may be reluctant to drink. Ensure patients or parents understand the importance of maintaining a high fluid intake. Ice lollies can be a useful source of extra fluid for a reluctant child. Adults may find sucking on ice soothing.
- The expected pattern of recovery and duration of symptoms.
- The rationale for providing/not providing antibiotics.
- Signs or symptoms requiring further assessment by a health professional.

Follow-up No specific follow up required in most cases. Patients should be advised to seek further advice from a primary health care professional if they experience: any deterioration in their condition, new symptoms, or if presenting symptoms do not resolve in 5–7 days from onset.

Reference

1 National Institute for Clinical Excellence (NICE) (2001). *Referral guide for patients with acne, acute low back pain, menorrhagia, OA of hip or knee, prostatism, psoriasis and varicose veins; and in children guide for atopic eczema, glue ear and recurrent episodes of acute sore throat.* NICE, London.

Scarlet fever

Scarlet fever is caused by group A beta haemolytic streptococci.

Clinical characteristics

As in bacterial pharyngitis/tonsillitis (📖 see p.432) plus:
- a 'strawberry' tongue;
- an erythematous 'sand paper' rash on trunk and limbs;
- on occasion, Pastia's lines (petechiae in flexor skin creases of joints).

Management

📖 See also Pharyngitis and tonsillitis, p.432.
- Management and follow-up is as for pharyngitis/tonsillitis.
- Antibiotics are indicated and should be provided as for pharyngitis/ tonsillitis but for a duration of 10 days.
- Scarlet fever is a notifiable disease and, as such, the proper officer of the local authority (usually the consultant in communicable disease control) should be notified.
- Children should be excluded from school for 5 days from the start of antibiotic treatment.

Glandular fever (infectious mononucleosis)

Glandular fever is caused by the Epstein–Barr virus. It commonly affects those aged 15–25 years of age. In the early stages it may be difficult to differentiate from bacterial pharyngitis.

Clinical characteristics

- Fetor (bad breath).
- Plummy speech.
- Slough on inflamed tonsils.
- Palatal petechiae.
- Fever.
- Lymphadenopathy (particularly posterior cervical) and general malaise.
- Mild hepato-splenomegaly.

Management

- Pain relief and general advice should be given as for pharyngitis/ tonsillitis (📖 see p.432).
- Antibiotics are not indicated, but in reality may be given due to the difficulty in differentiating glandular fever from other causes of sore throat.

Follow-up The symptoms of glandular fever can persist for some time causing long absences from school/college or university. It is therefore important to advise the child or their parents to see a primary care clinician if the symptoms are not resolving within ~ 7 days so that an FBC and film and Paul Bunnell or Monospot test can be performed to confirm the diagnosis.

In confirmed glandular fever, advice should be given to avoid contact sports for three months.

Coxsackie virus (hand, foot, and mouth disease)

Hand, foot, and mouth disease occurs in children aged 3–10 years.

Clinical characteristics
- Sore throat.
- Vesicles on the oral cavity, the buccal mucosa, tongue, hands, feet, and sometimes buttocks.
- Fever.

Management and follow-up is as for pharyngitis/tonsillitis (see p.432).

Diphtheria

Diphtheria is caused by *Corynecbacterium diphtheriae*. It is uncommon in the UK but quite common in South Africa, Russia, and the developing world.

Clinical characteristics

- Grey adherent membrane on the tonsils, uvula, and pharynx. Bleeding occurs when membrane is removed.
- Fever.
- Severe sore throat.
- Malaise.
- Restlessness.
- Weakness and a thready pulse should raise suspicion when present in an unimmunized individual.

Management Refer to medical practitioner.

Thrush (candidiasis)

Thrush is usually caused by *Candida albicans*. Individuals are likely to have a history of antibiotic or inhaled steroid use or are immunosuppressed.

Clinical characteristics
- Thin, diffuse, or patchy exudates on mucous membranes.
- Afebrile.

Management
- If immunosuppressed refer to medical practitioner.
- Normal immune state. Prescribe nystatin.
- Advise those using inhaled steroids to rinse mouth after inhalation to avoid future problems.

Follow-up No specific follow-up will be required in most cases. Patients should be advised to seek further advice from a primary health care professional if they experience: any deterioration in their condition, new symptoms, or their presenting symptoms are not resolving in 5–7 days from onset.

Peritonsillar abscess (quinsy)

Most common in older children and adults.

Clinical characteristics

- Fever.
- Worsening pharyngitis.
- Increasing unilateral throat and ear pain.
- Dysphagia, drooling, and trismus are common.
- Unilateral peritonsillar swelling and inflammation.
- Uvula may be displaced away from the affected side.

Management

- The airway may become compromised so vigilance is essential.
- IV cannulation and benzylpencillin may be indicated.
- Refer to ENT surgeon for incision and drainage.

Epiglottitis

Usually caused by *Haemophilus influenzae*. Most common in children aged 2–8 years but incidence has diminished since the introduction of Hib immunization. Occurs uncommonly in adults (📖 see p.82).

Clinical characteristics

- Abrupt onset of severe sore throat, fever, and toxicity.
- Usual appearance is a child in a sitting position, leaning forward, head extended, jaw thrust forward, mouth open, tongue protruding, and drooling.
- Voice is muffled.
- Stridor may be present.
- In adults the onset may be slower and severe pain on swallowing may be the only symptom.

Management

❶ Do **not** examine the throat as may cause spasm and obstruction

▶▶ Seek urgent assistance from anaesthetist and ED medical practitioner.

Mumps (epidemic parotitis)

Mumps is an acute, generalized infection caused by the paramyxovirus. It can infect any organ including salivary glands, pancreas, testis, ovary, brain, mammary gland, liver, kidney, joints, and heart. It is highly infectious and spread through respiratory droplets, saliva, and possibly urine. The incubation period is 15–24 days with the period of infectivity extending from about 2–6 days before symptoms appear and for up to 4 days afterwards. Symptoms usually resolve within 7–10 days. There has been a recent increased incidence in older children and young adults who have not received an MMR booster pre-school.

Clinical characteristics

- Non-specific flu-like symptoms followed by development of parotitis.
- Pain near to angle of jaw.
- Fever (40–40.5°C).
- Swelling, often bilateral, that causes distortion of face and neck. The area over the glands may appear hot and flushed.
- In severe swelling, mouth cannot be opened and is dry through blockage of saliva.
- Discomfort usually lasts for 3–4 days.
- May be accompanied by abdominal pain, headache, mild mastitis, and oophoritis in women.

Management

- Management is mainly aimed at pain and fever management.
- Local heat to the inflamed glands may provide some relief.
- Foods and drinks that stimulate saliva production may increase pain and should therefore probably be avoided.
- Mumps is a notifiable disease. The proper officer of the local authority (usually consultant in communicable disease control) should be notified.
- Patients or carers should be informed about the period of infectivity, that mumps is highly infectious, and that contact with those who are most at risk of complications should they contract mumps (see 'Complications of mumps') should be avoided.
- It is recommended that those who have contracted mumps but not yet been immunized should still have the vaccine.

Complications

Orchitis

Orchitis is unusual before puberty but occurs in approximately 1 in 5 cases of mumps in adolescent males. Symptoms usually develop 4–5 days after the start of parotitis. Some degree of atrophy of the testicle is seen in 1/3 of cases but sterility is not as common as often feared.

Clinical characteristics

- Severe, usually unilateral localized testicular pain and tenderness (the 2nd testicle may develop symptoms as symptoms in the first resolve, usually after a few days).
- Swollen, oedematous scrotum with impalpable testicles.
- Fever and sweats.
- Headache and backache.

Management
- Management is mainly aimed at pain and fever management.
- Prednisolone has been suggested for 2–3 days for severe parotitis or orchitis. It may provide good pain relief but does not reduce swelling.
- Reassurance regarding future problems regarding infertility may be required.
- Patients/carers can be directed to the Patient UK website for comprehensive evidence-based information.[1]

Meningitis and encephalitis generally occur without symptoms of parotitis. Patients exhibiting symptoms suggestive of meningitis or encephalitis should be referred to a medical practitioner or the ED (☐ see p.156 and p.158).

Deafness is a rare complication occurring only in around 1:15 000. Individuals with symptoms of hearing loss should be followed up by their GP.

Miscarriage The risk of miscarriage may be increased if mumps is contracted in the 1st trimester of pregnancy (the first 12–16 weeks). Mumps is not, however, thought to increase the risk of fetal abnormality.

Reference
1 ⌁ www.patient.co.uk

Earache/ear pain (otalgia): assessment

Earache is a common presenting problem. It is estimated that in 50% of cases pain or discomfort can be attributed to some pathology within the ear. In the other 50% pain is referred from other structures. The history and examination should be sufficiently comprehensive to ensure that the differential diagnoses of ear pain are considered and that those individuals at risk of developing complications are identified and referred urgently to a doctor or the ED. Fig. 14.1 shows the structure of the ear.

History

Enquire about the following signs and symptoms.
- Onset and duration.
- Location of pain (deep or superficial, radiation).
- Itching.
- Severity of pain/soreness.
- Fever or irritability.
- Ear discharge and quality.
- Dizziness, vertigo, or tinnitus.
- Trauma (includes barotrauma, minor localized trauma with, e.g. a cotton bud in the ear, trauma inflicted by another individual, e.g. a slap or punch to the ear).
- Possible presence of foreign body.
- Hearing loss.
- Sore throat—pain may be referred.
- Coyzal symptoms (Eustachian tube blockage/dysfunction causes earache).
- Dental pain or recent dental treatment (referred pain causes earache).
- Facial numbness or paralysis.
- Nausea or vomiting.
- Previous episodes.
- Recent ear syringing (disturbance of normal environment may precipitate otitis externa).
- Recent ↑ frequency of boils, thrush, or other infections (may be suggestive of diabetes).

Enquire about past medical history.
- Ear surgery or grommets.
- Congenital disorders such as cleft palate.
- Diabetes.
- Immunosuppression
- Cerumen build up.
- Chronic skin disease, e.g. eczema, psoriasis, seborrhoeic dematitis.

Enquire about social history.
- Location and frequency of swimming (increased incidence or otitis externa with frequent swimming).
- Use of a soother/dummy by infants (whether breast of bottle feeding) leads to an increase risk in acute otitis media.
- Passive smoking (↑ risk of ↑ episodes of otitis media).
- Recent use of different hair or facial products (can cause otitis externa).

Specific enquiry should be made about the following medications.
- Combined oral contraceptive pill—may be relevant if treatment with antibiotics is indicated.
- Recent antibiotic use: topical and systemic.
- Over the counter medications used to treat symptoms, e.g. use of analgesia (what and when last given).
- Hypoglycaemic drugs.
- Steroids, both topical and systemic.

Enquire about allergies with specific reference to antibiotics and NSAIDs.

Examination

- Temperature and pulse
- Inspect and palpate the auricular and cervical lymph glands.
- Examine the temporomandibular joint (temporomandibular joint syndrome/pain refers to the ear).
- Inspect and gently move the pinna and tragus.
- Inspect the external auditory canal for inflammation, swelling, discharge, and cerumen.
- Thoroughly inspect the tympanic membrane taking care to identify the following landmarks:
  - the location of the light reflex;
  - the umbo;
  - the annulus.
- Carefully note the position of any perforation.
- Inspect the oral cavity, buccal mucosa, and oropharynx.
- Inspect dentition.

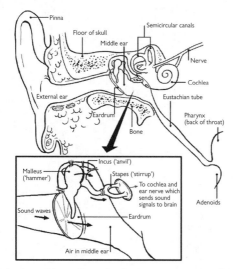

Fig. 14.1 Structure of the ear (Reproduced with permission: diagram © EMIS and PIP (2008) as distributed on ⊕ www.patient.co.uk)

Otitis externa

The term otitis externa (OE) is used to describe any inflammatory condition of the auricle, external ear canal, or outer surface of the eardrum. OE can be classified as localized or diffuse.

- Localized OE is used to describe a furuncle (boil) in the ear.
- Diffuse OE can be acute or chronic; and caused by infections, allergies, irritants, or inflammatory conditions (Clinical Knowledge Summary 2004).[1]
- *Staphylococcus aureus* is the causative organism in the vast majority of cases of localized OE. *S. aureus* and *Pseudomonas aeruginosa* are the bacteria most commonly implicated in cases of diffuse OE. Fungal infection is estimated to be the cause in only 10% of cases of diffuse otitis externa. Otitis externa is common in all ages with the exception of those under 2 years. It is more common in females than males, except in the elderly. There is an increase in incidence at the end of the summer months.
- Chronic otitis externa describes frequent episodes of otitis externa due to long-term damage to the normal ear canal through trauma, chronic skin conditions, or infection. If seen during an acute episode it should be managed as acute otitis externa but an ear swab should ideally be taken before treatment is instigated.

Reference

1 Clinical Knowledge Summaries: ⌘ www.cks.library.nhs.uk

Localized otitis externa

Clinical characteristics

- Earache/pain: sometimes severe.
- May report pain on touching, or lying on, the ear.
- The post-auricular node may be enlarged and tender.
- Pain is experienced on movement of the pinna and tragus.
- Otoscopic examination may be extremely painful.
- A localized area of inflammation and swelling is visualized.
- Little if any discharge is present.
- The tympanic membrane (TM), if visualized, appears normal.
- Pre-auricular and/or post-auricular lymphadenopathy may be present.
- Mild fever < 38°C.

Management

Pain relief

▶ Refer to the BNF for advice on dose, contraindications, and interactions of the following medicines before advising them to patients.

- Paracetamol and/or ibuprofen should be recommended/prescribed. In children, if both preparations are used they should be given simultaneously and not staggered.
- Codeine is the second-line analgesia of choice.
- A combination of codeine, paracetamol, and an NSAID may be required to control severe pain.
- Local heat may be soothing.

Antibiotics

Flucloxacillin (or erythromycin if penicillin allergic) are the antibiotics of choice. Dose and regimen are as follows.

- Flucloxacillin.
- Erythromycin (if allergic to penicillin).

▶ Advise women taking the combined oral contraceptive pill that additional contraceptive precautions should be taken (📖 see p.433).[1]

Other interventions Consider testing the urine or capillary blood for abnormal glucose levels.

Referral criteria Patients who are significantly systemically unwell require assessment by a medical practitioner.

Follow-up

- No specific follow-up will be required in most cases.
- Patients should be advised to seek further advice from a primary health care professional if they experience: any deterioration in their condition, new symptoms, or their presenting symptoms are not resolving in 5–7 days from onset.
- Infrequently, furuncles in the ear may require referral to ENT specialists for incision and drainage.
- Patient information provided by Patient UK is an excellent lay resource.[2]

References

1 British National Formulary (2008): ⌕ www.bnf.org
2 Patient UK ⌕ www.patient.co.uk

Diffuse otitis externa: acute uncomplicated

Clinical characteristics
- There may be a recent history of swimming or visit to a country where climate is hot and/or humid.
- Low grade fever < 38°C.
- Rapid onset (generally within 48h) of ear pain.
- Itch.
- Discharge (usually scant white but occasionally thick).
- Hearing loss (conductive if inflammation occludes canal).
- Pre- and/or post-auricular lymphadenopathy.
- Pain on movement of tragus, pinna, and jaw.
- Tympanic membrane may be inflamed.

Management
Management is focused on pain control, restoration of the normal pH of the ear, and treating the most likely cause, i.e bacterial infection.
- Topical preparations are recommended for first-line treatment unless there is evidence of spreading infection or the individual is systemically unwell.
- If discharge is profuse topical preparations are unlikely to reach the affected tissue. Under such circumstances referral to the ENT team for microsuction and aural toilet should be considered.
- ► Ear syringing should be avoided.

Pain relief
- Paracetamol and/or ibuprofen should be recommended and prescribed/supplied using a PGD.
- The addition of codeine may be required and can be provided as above.

Topical antibacterials and steroids The choice of topical agents is based on probable causative organisms. However, infection is often secondary and dampening down of the inflammatory response may be all that is required. Optimal first-line treatment is a combined antibacterial/steroid preparation. There is little evidence to demonstrate increased efficacy of one preparation over another. The Clinical Knowledge Summary (2004) provides pragmatic advice on selection of treatment.[1] Suggested first-line options are as follows.

> ⚠ If there is suspicion of eardrum perforation the Committee on Safety of Medicines (CSM) has stated that drops containing aminoglycosides (neomycin and gentamicin) are contraindicated due to the risk of ototoxicity

- Flumetasone 0.02% + clioquinol 1% ear drops (Locorten Vioform®).
- Betamethasone 0.1% + neomycin 0.5% ear drops (Betnesol N or Vistamethasone N®).
- Prednisolone 0.5% + neomycin 0.5% ear drops (Predsol N®).

Following should be reserved for use when first-line treatment has failed.
- Hydrocortisone 1% + gentamicin 0.3% ear drops (Gentisone HC ear drops®).

Systemic antibiotics

Reserve oral antibiotics for treating those with evidence of spreading infection or cellulitis. Use in conjunction with a topical preparation.

- Flucloxacillin (or erythromycin if penicillin allergic) are the antibiotics of choice.

▶ Advise women taking the combined oral contraceptive pill that additional contraceptive precautions should be taken (📖 see p.433).[2]

Patient advice

Patients should be advised about the following.

- Application of ear drops.
  - Lie down with the affected ear upwards.
  - Put the prescribed number of drops into the affected ear and remain lying for a few minutes.
  - Depress tragus a few times to allow drops to seep into ear canal.
- Avoid using cotton buds to clean the ears.
- Avoid soaps, shampoos, and chemicals running into the ear. Do this by using cotton wool with petroleum jelly in the ears when bathing.
- Use swim cap or ear plugs when swimming or diving.

Prevention

Prevent otitis externa by avoiding water and moisture build up in the ear canal and maintaining a normal canal environment. Achieve this by:

- use of acidifying ear drops (acetic acid 'EarCalm') before and after swimming;
- using a hairdryer to dry the ear canal;
- using ear plugs when swimming;
- avoidance of ear trauma such as that from use of cotton buds.

Follow-up No specific follow-up required. Patients should be advised to seek further advice/assessment from their primary care practitioner if symptoms fail to resolve within 5–7 days or before then if they should experience any increase in symptoms.

References

1 Clinical Knowledge Summaries: ⌁ www.cks.library.nhs.uk
2 British National Formulary (2008): ⌁ www.bnf.org

Cholesteatoma

A cholesteotoma is a cyst-like tumour made up of a collection of epithelial debris. It usually originates in the attic region. It has erosive properties and requires urgent referral to an ENT specialist. Onset tends to be more gradual than in otitis externa.

Clinical characteristics
- Earache and headache.
- Malodorous (faecal) discharge.
- An attic tympanic membrane perforation may be visible.
- A history of treatment failure for otitis externa.
- Collection of abnormal tissue may be visible, typically in the attic region.

Management Refer to an ENT specialist for further assessment.

Malignant (necrotizing) otitis externa

This is a rare condition that occurs mainly in the elderly, the immuno-suppressed, or those with diabetes. Infection extends into the bone surrounding the ear canal (i.e. mastoid and temporal bones).

Clinical characteristics

- Severe pain.
- Headache.
- Discharge.
- Intensely inflamed ear canal.
- Cellulitis of the pinna and surrounding tissue.
- There may be unilateral facial palsy.

▶ This may be difficult to differentiate from a severe otitis externa. If in doubt refer.

Management ▶▶ Refer urgently to medical practitioner or ENT specialist.

Ramsay Hunt syndrome

Ramsay Hunt syndrome is often used to describe herpes zoster infection of the facial nerve.

Clinical characteristics
- Ear and mastoid region pain.
- Phonophobia.
- Loss of taste.
- Facial paralysis (Bell's palsy).
- Vesicular eruption around the external auditory meatus.
- Vertigo.
- Deafness.

Risk groups The elderly and immunosuppressed are at greater risk of complications.

Management Refer to medical practitioner for further assessment. Aciclovir is the drug of choice.

Acute otitis media

Acute otitis media (AOM) describes fluid in middle ear in association with signs and symptoms of acute infection. It is one of the most frequent diseases in early infancy and childhood. Peak incidence is 6 months–3 years. Most cases resolve without antibiotic treatment. ∴ 'watchful waiting' with fever and pain control is treatment of choice for 1st 72h in most cases. Lower threshold for providing antibiotics is necessary when child is < 2 years or there is perforation with otorrhoea, bilateral AOM, or systemic symptoms, including high temperature (> 38.5°C) or vomiting.

Clinical characteristics

- Earache/pain.
- May be worse on swallowing.
- Preceding or current upper respiratory tract infection.
- Fever often > 38.5°C.
- Nausea and/or vomiting.
- Distorted tympanic membrane (TM) light reflection.
- Handle of malleus flush.
- Bulging TM with loss of landmarks.
- Changes in membrane colour (typically red or yellow).
- Perforated TM with discharge of pus (which may alleviate symptoms); TM may not be visible.

Management 1st line management largely aimed at fever/pain control.

Pain relief and fever management

- Paracetamol and/or ibuprofen should be recommended/prescribed.
- When prescribed or provided together they should be given at the same time rather than staggered (Clinical Knowledge Summary 2006).[1]
- Fluid intake should be encouraged.
- Advice regarding management and prevention of febrile convulsions should be provided. The Clinical Knowledge Summaries website provide comprehensive advice for parents on the prevention and management of febrile convulsions.[1]

Antibiotics

- Amoxicillin (or azithromycin if penicillin allergic) are antibiotics of choice.

▶ Advice for women taking the combined OCP 📖 see 'p.433.

Follow-up

- Further assessment is indicated if pain has not resolved in 72h from first consultation. Antibiotic treatment is then required.
- Advise those with discharging ears to seek further assessment if discharge has not resolved in 7 days. If so consider antibiotic treatment.

Advice Smoking, bottle feeding, and use of dummies or soothers are risk factors for increased episodes of AOM. Parents of children who use soothers or dummies should **not** be advised to stop use until the child reaches the age of 1 year.

AOM with perforation Care should be taken to ensure that the perforation has been caused by AOM. Consider and exclude other causes of discharging ears or perforation such as:
- trauma (▶ if the suspected cause of TM perforation is trauma and the patient is a child consider issues of child protection);
- barotrauma;
- otitis externa;
- cholesteatoma.

Follow-up
- The patient or child's parents should be advised that the TM should be reassessed 2 weeks after the acute episode.
- Persistence of discharge for > 7 days also requires further evaluation.

Complications of AOM with or without perforation
Mastoiditis
- Fever.
- Tenderness over the mastoid antrum.
- Displacement of pinna down and forward due to post-auricular swelling.
- Inflamed, bulging, or perforated TM.
- Signs of conductive deafness.

Management Urgent referral to ENT specialist.

Meningitis Urgent referral to emergency medical practitioner.

Conductive deafness due to perforation or debris in middle ear not uncommon, Should resolve after acute episode resolves. Prolonged deafness for > 2 weeks after initial episode needs evaluation by GP.

Reference

1 Clinical Knowledge Summaries: ⌁ www.cks.library.nhs.uk

Epistaxis

Epistaxis is common inasmuch as most people will have had a nosebleed at some time. However, it is an unpleasant and worrying experience and as such a fairly common presentation in the ED. Epistaxis is classified as anterior or posterior, depending upon the source of bleeding.
- Anterior haemorrhage. The source of bleeding is from the nasal septum (Little's area).
- Posterior haemorrhage. Bleeding from deeper structures of the nose; more common in older people.

Causes

Often there is no cause but consider:
- trauma to the nose;
- nose picking;
- vigorous nose blowing;
- platelet disorders;
- drugs: aspirin and anticoagulants;
- abnormalities of blood vessels (especially in the elderly);
- cocaine use: the drug can lead to destruction of the nasal septum;

Most nose bleeds stop spontaneously and patients can be discharged if there is no further active bleeding. They should be given an advice leaflet.

Management of severe epistaxis

⚠ Remember that patients can die from an epistaxis. If concerned get specialist help.

- Ask the patient to sit upright and forward; and to squeeze the nostrils. Offer constant reassurance as patients find this very distressing.
- Give the patient a bowl and encourage them to breath through the mouth.
- Monitor pulse and BP.
- Monitor for signs of hypovolaemia.
- Establish IV access and collect blood for FBC, Group & Save and clotting if patient is on anticoagulants.

If bleeding continues prepare for packing.
- Use a nasal tampon. These are easy to insert and comfortable for the patient. Use Naseptin® cream to lubricate the tampon.
- Pack both sides. Packs are usually left in place for 24h. Use BIPP (bismuth subnitrate and iodoform paraffin paste) or 1cm ribbon gauze impregnated with petroleum jelly if nasal tampons are not available Posterior bleeds, which are much less common (~ 5%), require packing and a balloon catheter to arrest bleeding.
- Patients with posterior packs require admission and are usually commenced on antibiotics.

Nasal foreign bodies (FBs)

Nasal FBs are most common in children 1-5y where anything that can be inserted into the nostril may be there! Common FBs are stones, tissue and beads. Some may have been insitu for a long period of time. If a child presents with a foul smelling nasal discharge always suspect an FB. It is important to remove nasal FBs as those left insitu are at risk of pulmonary aspiration.

Management

The challenge is obtaining the cooperation of the younger child. Usually you only get one attempt, before the child will be less cooperative.

- **Do not** attempt removal with a struggling/uncooperative child. Refer to ENT.
- **Do not** attempt removal if you have not got the right equipment. Refer to ENT.
- **Do not** attempt removal if you do not feel you have a reasonable chance of success, refer to ENT.

If the FB is visible, suction can be applied with a rigid suction catheter and can be successful. Depending on the shape, size and texture of the FB different equipment is needed.

Soft FBs (tissue/peas)—use crocodile forceps to gently grasp the FB.

Round hard FBs (beads/stones)—a blunt ended probe which is slightly bent into a hook shape needs to be inserted behind the FB to 'hook it' out.

- Once removed the nostril should be checked for any further FB or signs of trauma.
- Always check the other nostril for an FB.
- Failure to remove requires referral to ENT.

Ear/auricular FBs

These are common in children and as with nasal FBs, anything can be inserted into the ear. In adults cotton wool is the most common FB.

The same principles and techniques for removal that are used for nasal FBs can be applied to auricular FBs. However, failure to remove does not require urgent ENT referral and an ENT out-patient clinic appointment can be made.

Following removal the ear should be examined. Signs of trauma to the canal or perforation to the drum should be managed appropriately. If a child presents with an auricular haematoma, consider non-accidental injury.

Retained earrings/butterflies

This is most common in young girls who have recently had their ears pierced and have small stud earrings. In some cases the earring/butterfly is partially visible and can be easily removed. If the earring/butterfly is completed embedded removal can be more difficult.

Management

- Inject the lobe with a small amount of lidocaine.
- Grab the visible earring/butterfly with forceps and remove.
- A small 'nick' in the posterior surface of the lobe may be required to ease removal in embedded earring/butterflies.
- Despite the lobe being red and swollen antibiotics are rarely needed.

Auricular haematoma

A bruised, swollen pinna is usually caused by direct trauma from a blunt force e.g. slap/punch or in contact sports most commonly rugby. Failure to correctly treat an auricular haematoma can result in the development of a 'cauliflower' ear. A haematoma to the pinna causes blood to collect between the skin and the cartilage of the ear. Pressure from the hae-matoma can compromise the blood supply to the cartilage and destroy it—giving the characteristic cauliflower appearance.

Management

- Large haematomas should be aspirated using aseptic technique.
- Apply a pressure bandage to prevent further haematoma development.
- Arrange ENT follow-up.

Nose injury

Many adults and children will seek urgent/emergency care following a nose injury. Falls and assaults are the most common causes. If a patient attends after an assault careful documentation is essential to support any report writing for a subsequent legal investigation. Any epistaxsis at the time has usually settled prior to seeking assessment.

Examination

- Swelling and bruising of the nose.
- Deformity.
- Is the nose deviated to one side?
- Inspect the nasal septum using a torch.
  - Is there any evidence of a septal haematoma?
- Is the patient able to breathe through each nostril?
- Feel for tenderness on the bridge of the nose.
- Feel for tenderness around the cheek and infraorbital region.
- Signs of base of skull fracture or CSF leak.

Nasal fracture is a clinical diagnosis and X-rays are not indicated. If there is significant tenderness, bruising, and swelling, then a diagnosis of nasal fracture can be made.

▶▶ Septal haematoma needs immediate ENT referral.

Management

- Refer obvious displaced fractures to an ENT clinic.
- Pain relief.
- Advise patient not to blow nose for 24h.
- Advise patient that 'black eyes' can develop and bruising can track down the face to the jaw line. This is normal.
- Advise patient to avoid contact sports until the tenderness has settled.
- If there are any problems regarding cosmetic result or breathing after approximately 5 days, ENT follow-up is needed.

Maxillofacial and dental emergencies

Overview of maxillofacial injuries

Maxillofacial injuries can be life-threatening and cause significant morbidity. Some of the patients presenting with these injuries have multisystem trauma due to RTCs, assaults, or, in some cases, sporting injuries. These injuries require expert resuscitation and collaborative management between emergency clinicians and surgical specialists in ENT, trauma surgery, plastic surgery, ophthalmology, and oral and maxillofacial surgery.

Many more patients with less life-threatening facial injuries are managed by ENPs. As there is often a forensic component to these cases nurses need to be aware that they may be called on in the future to account for their examination and findings in court. It is essential to adopt a thorough and systematic approach to examining these patients and to maintain comprehensive records on which to rely at a later date.

Trauma to the maxillofacial anatomy is complex as contained within the face are systems that control specialized functions including sight, hearing, smelling, breathing, eating, and speech. Also, vital structures in the head and neck may be at risk and the psychological impact of disfigurement can be devastating for the patient and his family.

Anatomically the face is divided into 3 parts.

- The upper face, where fractures involve the frontal bone and sinus.
- The midface is divided into upper and lower parts. The upper midface is where maxillary Le Fort II and Le Fort III fractures occur and/or where fractures of the nasal bones, naso-ethmoidal or zygomatico-maxillary complex, and the orbital floor occur. Le Fort I fractures are in the lower part of the midface.
- The lower face, where fractures are isolated to the mandible.

📖 See Maxillary fractures and Figs. 15.1–15.3 p.474–5.

Assessment and resuscitation of patients with facial injuries

Resuscitation

- ATLS guidelines should be followed, bearing in mind that the main complication of maxillary fractures is airway obstruction. This may be caused by haemorrhage, oedema, vomit, or facial instability.
- Call for specialist help without delay.
- Look for and treat airway obstruction: jaw thrust, chin lift, and suction. Be mindful of a possible associated neck injury.
- As intubation is often difficult or impossible prepare for a surgical airway and assist anaesthetist.
- Establish IV access with 2 wide bore cannulae and collect blood for FBC, clotting, group and save, and cross-match.
- Give IV analgesia as prescribed and monitor effect.
- Commence IV infusion as prescribed and document fluid regime.
- Record Glasgow coma score (🕮 see p.642 and p.645).
- Record baseline vital signs. Attach patient to monitoring equipment.
- Record ECG.
- Administer antibiotic medication as prescribed.
- Check patients tetanus status.
- Stay with patient during X-rays or accompany to CT.
- Prepare patient for theatre or transfer depending on location for definitive fracture management.
- Reassure and comfort patient and keep family informed as much as possible and as appropriate.

History taking

As in any trauma situation, address all life-threatening injuries first. A systematic approach to the history and physical examination ensures adequate assessment of a maxillofacial trauma. A history is more likely to be obtained from family, friend, or paramedic.

In most emergency situations history taking and initial management occur simultaneously. Enquire about the following.

- Mechanism and time of injury; loss of consciousness at time or since.
- Location, type, and quality of pain and sensation.
- Any symptoms of visual loss, blurred or double vision, photophobia.
- Symptoms of headache, dizziness, tinnitus, nausea.
- Any loss of hearing.
- Past medical history and any relevant previous injury or ENT condition.
- Known allergies.

Examination

Look

- Note any swelling, bruising, lacerations, deformity, flattening, or discoloration of face.
- Inspect open wounds for foreign bodies.
- Look for asymmetry in face.
- Bleeding from nose or around teeth; check position and alignment of teeth. Check for avulsed teeth.

- Inspect the tongue. Look for intraoral lacerations, bruising, or swelling.
- Nasal deviation and flattening of the nasal bridge.
- Inspect the nasal septum for a haematoma or CSF rhinorrhoea.
- Eyes for pupil size and shape and level; corneal surface. Subconjunctival haemorrhage without a posterior border suggests orbital wall fracture; uneven pupil levels may indicate orbital floor fracture.
- Note lacerations that may involve lachrymal duct. Refer appropriately.
- Eye movement: compare bilaterally. Note any restriction of movement.
- Jaw position, malocclusion, side-to-side movement of jaw, mandible protrusion, opening and closing of mouth.
- Examine the external ear for lacerations and auditory canal for injury or CSF leaks, integrity of the tympanic membrane, perforation, or mastoid area bruising (i.e. Battle sign).
- Face movements (scrunch up and close eyes).

Feel
Palpate bilaterally for swelling, depressions, crepitus, and specific tenderness in:
- frontal bone;
- orbital rim;
- zygomatic arch;
- maxilla;
- nasal bones;
- mandible.

Move
- Check the temporomandibular joint for any pain or clicking, locking, with movement.
- Check for any anaesthesia or loss of sensation in face, cheek, side of nose, and upper lip (infraorbital nerve injury).

Neurological Cranial nerve check if you suspect associated head injury (📖 see Box 15.1).

Box 15.1 The cranial nerves

- CN I, olfactory. Smell.
- CN II, optic. Vision.
- CN III, oculomotor. Eyeball movement; innervation of superior, medial, and inferior recti, inferior oblique, levator palpebrae, and smooth muscle pupilloconstrictor, and ciliary muscle.
- CN IV, trochlear. Eyeball movement; innervation of superior oblique.
- CN V, trigeminal. Sensation from face. Innervates muscles of mastication.
- CN VI, abducens. Eyeball movement, innervation of the lateral rectus muscle.
- CN VII, facial nerve. Innervation of muscles of face. Sense of taste. Innervation of salivary glands.
- CN VIII, vestibulocochlear. Equilibrium and hearing.
- CN IX, glossopharyngeal. Taste, salivation, and swallowing.
- CN X, vagus. Taste, swallowing, palate elevation, and phonics.
- CN XI, spinal accessory. Head rotation and shrugging of shoulders.
- CN XII, hypoglossal. Tongue movement.

Specific investigations of facial injuries

Once ATLS guidelines have been adhered to and C-spine has been X-rayed, facial views should be requested. The most frequently required views are:

- lateral;
- occipitomental;
- orthopantomogram (OPG);

The patient should be assessed by a specialist so that appropriate X-rays are requested in a timely way and appropriate management and follow-up is ensured. ENPs managing less traumatic facial injuries where there is clinical suspicion of a fracture but no fracture is identified on X-ray, should refer these patients on for specialist advice and follow-up care.

Frontal sinus fractures

These are due to severe blow to the forehead. The anterior and/or posterior table of the frontal sinus may be involved. A fracture to the posterior wall of the frontal sinus may result in a dural tear. The nasofrontal duct may also be involved. The patient will present with swelling, tenderness, and crepitus to the forehead. There may be loss of sensation and other symptoms associated with head injury.

- Get specialist help.
- Commence neurological observations; monitor and record meticulously.
- Give analgesia and antibiotics as prescribed.
- Prepare patient for admission.

Advise patient not to blow their nose and ensure adequate pain relief. Refer patient to faciomaxillary specialist.

Zygomatic fractures

These are the second most common fractures of the facial bones after nasal bone fractures. Concurrent ophthalmic injuries are common. The zygoma is the main supporting bone between the maxilla and the skull. Although it is strong, its prominent location makes it vulnerable to injury. Fracture is usually due to a blow to the side of the face, or 2° to RTCs.

- Look for flattening of the cheek, any palpable defect in the orbital margin, diplopia, and subconjunctival haemorrhage.
- A direct blow to the zygomatic arch can result in an isolated fracture involving the zygomatico-temporal suture, which will cause pain on jaw movement.
- Fracture of the arch of the zygoma may be identified by a palpable defect over the area involved.
- Pain upon palpation and limitation of movement of the mandible may be found upon physical examination.

Advise patient not to blow their nose and ensure adequate pain relief. Refer patient to faciomaxillary specialist and ophthalmologist if indicated.

Orbital floor fractures

A direct blow to the eye can result in an isolated fracture of the orbital floor. Herniation of the orbital contents into the maxillary sinus is possible. The incidence of ocular injury is common but globe rupture is rare. Periorbital oedema may be visible.

- Check and record visual acuity.
- Check EOMs (extra ocular movements).
- Check for diplopia (Lateral and upward gaze dysfunction may result due to entrapment of the medial and inferior rectus muscles).
- Infraorbital nerve damage can cause paraesthesia of the cheek and upper gum on the affected side.
- Fracture may not be visible on X-ray but may be assumed on the basis of the 'tear drop sign' (soft tissue mass in roof of maxillary sinus).

Advise patient not to blow their nose and ensure adequate pain relief. Refer patient to faciomaxillary specialist and ophthalmologist.

Mandibular fractures

Direct trauma to the mandible is the most common cause of mandibular fracture. Fractures can occur in multiple locations 2° to the U shape of the jaw and the weak condylar neck. Fractures often occur bilaterally at sites apart from the site of direct trauma. The 'ring bone rule' is applicable to mandibular fractures: 'if you see a fracture or dislocation in a ring bone or ring bone equivalent, look for another fracture or dislocation.'

Signs and symptoms

- Facial deformity, malocclusion of the teeth, or loose or missing teeth. Possible bruising or bleeding to the gums and abnormal mobility of portions of the mandible or teeth.
- Paraesthesia to the lower lip suggests injury to the inferior dental nerve where it passes through the ramus of the mandible.

Investigations and management

- Request an OPG and condylar views.
- Give analgesia and antibiotics as prescribed.
- Check tetanus status.
- Refer to faciomaxillary surgeon for definitive management.

Dislocation of the temporomadibular joint

Dislocation of the mandible can occur without fracture, usually spontaneously during a large yawn, but sometimes it may happen while eating, during a dystonic reaction, or during intubation. It is usually an anterior dislocation but it can be uni- or bilateral. The patient presents with considerable pain, is unable to close the mouth, and dribbles saliva because of difficulty in swallowing.

Management

- X-ray is only indicated if there is a history of trauma.
- Reduction is usually easily achieved without sedation or analgesia provided it has only just happened and the process is properly explained to the patient.
  - Sitting in front of the patient place both thumbs (covered by gauze swab) on to lower molars and press down and backwards at the same time lifting chin with fingers.
- Confirm relocation with an X-ray if a first episode.
- Delayed presentation may be more difficult to relocate due to muscle spasm.
- Advise patient to eat soft diet for 24h and to avoid opening mouth wide or yawning.

Alveolar fractures

These fractures involve the teeth and their bony support and can occur in isolation from a direct low-energy force or can result from extension of the fracture line through the alveolar portion of the maxilla or mandible. Clinical findings include gingival bleeding, mobility of the alveolus, and loose or avulsed teeth.

Maxillary fractures

These are classified as Le Fort I, II, or III (🕮 see Figs. 15.1–15.3).

Le Fort I fracture is a horizontal maxillary fracture across the tooth-bearing portion of the maxilla and separates the alveolar process and hard palate from the rest of the maxilla. The fracture extends through the lower third of the septum and there may be facial oedema and mobility of the hard palate and upper teeth. There may be a haematoma of the soft palate and malocclusion.

Le Fort II fracture is a pyramidal fracture starting at the nasal bone and extending through the lacrimal bone; downward through the zygomatico-maxillary suture producing mobility of the midface. Patients may present with pain, facial oedema, subconjunctival haemorrhage, diplopia, telecanthus, mobility of the maxilla, epistaxis, and possible rhinorrhoea.

Le Fort III fracture

Le Fort III fracture or craniofacial disjunction is a separation of all of the facial bones from the cranial base with simultaneous fracture of the zygoma, maxilla, and nasal bones. The entire midface is fractured from the base of the skull.

Clinical features of Le Fort III fractures include extensive oedema, bruising with facial elongation, and flattening. An anterior open bite may be present due to posterior and inferior displacement of the facial skeleton. Movement of all facial bones in relation to the cranial base with altered papillary levels . Epistaxis and pharyngeal bleeding may lead to hypovolaemic shock and and compromise the airway. CSF rhinorrhoea may also be found upon physical examination.

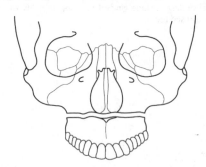

Fig. 15.1 Le fort I (Reproduced with permission from Perry, M. (ed.) (2005). *Head, neck, and dental emergencies*, p. 258. Oxford University Press, Oxford.)

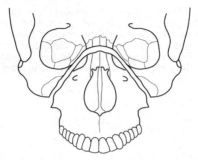

Fig. 15.2 Le Fort II (Reproduced with permission from Perry, M. (ed.) (2005). *Head, neck, and dental emergencies*, Fig. 8.32, p. 258. Oxford University Press, Oxford.)

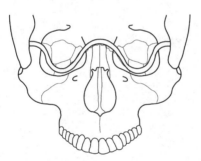

Fig. 15.3 Le Fort III (Reproduced with permission from Perry, M. (ed.) (2005). *Head, neck, and dental emergencies*, Fig. 8.33, p. 259. Oxford University Press, Oxford.)

Nasoethmoidal fractures (NOEs)

These extend from the nose to the ethmoid bones and can result in damage to the medial canthus, lacrimal apparatus, or nasofrontal duct. They also can result in a dural tear at the cribriform plate.

These fractures are characterized by a widened and flattened nasal bridge, epistaxis, rhinorrhoea, periorbital bruising, and subconjunctival haemorrage. There may also be supraorbital and supratrochlear nerve paraesthesia.

Dental anatomy

There are a total of 32 secondary or permanent teeth. These are made up of 4 quadrants of 8 teeth (8 incisors, 4 cuspids, 8 premolars, and 12 molars). Secondary molars erupt behind primary molars. Most secondary teeth are usually present by the age of 14 years.

Trauma to teeth

Chipped teeth do not require emergency treatment. Refer patient to dentist.

Mobile teeth after trauma need urgent dental attention. Advise patient not to handle the tooth and refer to emergency dentist.

Avulsed tooth

The complete displacement of a tooth from its socket is usually due to direct trauma to the mouth area. It is a common occurrence in children because of falls and sporting injuries. In adults it is often due to assault. In a trauma situation, aspiration needs to be considered where there are unaccounted for missing teeth. Check the CXR.

Where the patient has the avulsed tooth it is possible to replant it in the alveolar socket providing it is done within a couple of hours of displacement.
• Advise the patient to bring the tooth in—in milk.
• Gently clean the tooth with saline.
• Position the tooth correctly and apply firm pressure.
• Refer to dentist for definitive care.
• It is not recommended to replant primary teeth and it is contraindicated in patients who have valve disease or those who are immunosuppressed.

Toothache

'Toothache' usually refers to pain around the teeth or gums. The severity of a toothache can range from mild to sharp and excruciating.
• Simple over the counter analgesia such as ibuprofen or paracetamol may give adequate relief.
• If there are symptoms of infection antibiotics are needed. Refer to a dentist.
• In more severe cases where toothache is associated with swelling to the face, difficulty swallowing, and pyrexia, the patient should be commenced on IV antibiotics and referred to a faciomaxillary surgeon.

▶ Remember that pain around the teeth and the jaws can be a symptom of other diseases such as angina, external ear infections, and sinusitis.

Endocrine and metabolic emergencies

Overview

Many patients presenting to the ED may have disordered metabolism due to underlying endocrine disease. These patients are often critically ill and require rapid assessment and intervention to prevent further complication, coma, and death. Emergency care staff need to have an understanding of how these diseases present and their initial management.

Hypoglycaemia

▶ Don't Ever Forget Glucose!

Pathophysiology

A normal glucose range is 3.5–5.5 mmol/L. Hypoglycemia can therefore be defined as a blood sugar < 3.5 mmol/L, although many areas identify that values < 3.0 mmol/L represent clinical significance.

Hypoglycaemia develops when there is an imbalance between the rate of glucose uptake by tissues in contrast with hepatic glucose output and/or glucose intake.

- Patients taking insulin are most at risk, especially in relation to a misjudged dose, insufficient or delayed food intake, exertion that was not accounted for, or infection.
- Oral hypoglycaemics, such as sulphonylureas (e.g. gliclazide) can also lead to hypoglycaemia, whereas metformin does not have this effect.
- Alcohol is also responsible for hypoglycaemia, as alcohol inhibits hepatic gluconeogenesis, whilst patients who are malnourished or have liver disease have ↓ glycogen reserves.
- In addition, although gluconeogenesis occurs mainly in the liver (via substrates such as glycerol and lactate), the renal cortex also has a secondary role in this process. Hence hypoglycaemia can be a feature of profound renal failure.
- Other causes include insulinomas in the pancreas, Addison's disease, pituitary insufficiency, and self-harm/poisoning via insulin or oral hypoglycaemics.
- Hypoglycaemia can also rapidly develop in children in the face of overwhelming physical insult, e.g. sepsis. This leads to a depletion of glucose stores (especially in infants). Thus it is essential that blood sugars are monitored and corrected in such situations.

Clinical features

Early signs of hypoglycaemia relate to the sympathetic nervous system response, and may include sweating, pallor, and tachycardia. Most diabetics are able to identify these early signs and take remedial action. It is particularly noteworthy, however, that β-blockers will inhibit this sympathetic response, and thereby blunt these early warning signs. This is one reason why β-blockers should be generally avoided in diabetic patients. β-Blockers can inhibit gluconeogenesis, which can lead to hypoglycaemia.

Signs and symptoms of hypoglycaemia become particularly notable at < 2.5mmol/L. As glucose levels fall, the neurological impairment becomes more apparent. This reflects that ~ 50% of the body's available glucose is consumed by the brain. Patients can therefore present with a ↓ level of consciousness, seizures, aggression, confusion, and even isolated hemiparesis. Recurrent hypoglycaemic episodes are associated with increased morbidity and mortality 2° to microvascular damage and brain injury.

Assessment/diagnosis In relation to the primary survey, blood sugar monitoring is a vital component of the disability assessment. Diagnosis is based upon presenting signs and symptoms in association with a blood sugar < 3.5mmol/L, initially tested using a blood glucose monitoring meter.

To verify the result, a formal venous blood glucose sample should also be sent to the laboratory. However, treatment should not be delayed whilst awaiting this formal result.

Management

The mode of treatment will depend upon the severity of the patient's signs and symptoms and their compliance. Patients presenting with early signs of hypoglycaemia can be treated with fast-acting oral carbohydrate (10–20g glucose), e.g. a sugary drink with 2 teaspoons of sugar (= 10g) or dextrose sweets. This can be followed by slow-release carbohydrate, such as a sandwich, banana, or milk.

Patients presenting with more profound hypoglycaemia can be treated in a number of ways.

- Glucogel® (formerly known as Hypostop®) is especially useful in the pre-hospital environment and can be rapidly absorbed from the buccal mucosa.
- Glucagon 1mg SC, IM, IV. This is again very useful pre-hospital or when venous access is problematic. Glucagon is unlikely to be effective in hypoglycaemia associated with liver failure or chronic alcoholism, as in these instances there will be limited hepatic glycogen stores for the glucagon to affect. If there is no significant improvement in a patient's condition 10min after administration of glucagon, consider IV glucose.
- Glucose IV infusion. Traditionally, 50mL of 50% glucose would be administered to adult patients with hypoglycaemia via a wide bore cannula sited in a large vein (due to the hypertonic nature of the in-fusion). Increasingly, however, 10% dextrose is used in such situations—either given as 50mL aliquots, or as one 250mL infusion. This reduces the risk of extravasation and subsequent thrombophlebitis. The 50mL aliquots in particular are associated with less rebound hyperglycaemia. The paediatric dose is 5mL/kg of 10% glucose.

With appropriate treatment, most patients show significant signs of improvement within 10–20min and can be discharged home if blood sugar readings remain stable and there are no complications. If neurological signs and symptoms do not improve despite normalization of blood sugars, coexistent pathology should be sought, e.g. stroke or cerebral oedema 2° to hypoglycaemia. Patients presenting with insulin overdose may need prolonged glucose infusion, and potassium levels will need to be closely monitored due to associated hypokalaemia.

Diabetic ketoacidosis (DKA)

Pathophysiology

DKA is almost always associated with type I diabetes, and is only very rarely a feature of type II diabetes. Apart from the first presentation of type I diabetes, DKA is usually precipitated by increased physiological stress, especially infection (e.g. urinary and chest infections), but also MI, stroke, and trauma. This stress increases circulating levels of glucagon, catecholamines, and glucocorticoids, which all increase blood glucose levels. In tandem with this physiological stress, there is insufficient insulin to both homeostatically 'brake' these hormonal processes or to 'drive' glucose into cells. This is especially true if insulin has been either omitted or insufficiently augmented at times of illness. The consequences are as follows.

- Rising blood sugars lead to a hyperosmolar state. This provokes a diuretic response, and ultimately leads to hypovolaemia and electrolyte derangement. Although there is an overall total body potassium deficit secondary to the diuresis, the plasma K^+ is actually raised in a third of cases, and usually normal in the rest. This reflects extracellular shifts in potassium.
- ↑ levels of glucagon (normally inhibited by insulin) lead to ↑ lipolysis, and ↑ production of free fatty acids, from which ketone bodies are derived. This ketone rise results in an acidosis.

Clinical features

Consider metabolic acidosis in any patient who is hyperventilating.

- Hyperventilation (Küssmaul respiration).
- Polydipsia.
- Polyuria.
- Hypotension.
- Tachycardia.
- Acetone breath is virtually pathognomonic of DKA.
- Nausea/vomiting.
- Abdominal pain.
- Altered consciousness.

Diagnosis

Diagnosis is made on the basis of ↑ blood glucose, metabolic acidaemia, and the presence of ketones in the urine. The following tests therefore need to be obtained.

- Bedside and laboratory glucose.
- Urine dipstick checking for ketones, glucose, and signs of infection.
- Arterial or venous blood gas.

Other investigations should include the following.
- CXR (as chest infection may be present).
- ECG (looking for signs of acute coronary syndrome or hypo-/hyperkalaemia);
- U & E, FBC, CRP, and/or blood cultures.

Patients with infection in the context of DKA may be apyrexial.

Nursing interventions

- Ensure airway patency, and administer high flow oxygen.
- Fluid replacement. Refer to local protocols. Fluid is generally 0.9% sodium chloride. In adults the first litre is usually given over 30–60min and the second litre over 60–120min.
- When the blood glucose is < 15mmol/L following insulin therapy, switch from 0.9% sodium chloride to 5% dextrose. This reduces the risk of hypoglycaemia and an overrapid correction of osmolality and cerebral oedema.
- Beware excessive rehydration. Coexisting cardiac pathology may lead to pulmonary oedema, whilst cerebral oedema 2° to rapid fluid shifts (most commonly affecting children and young adults) is associated with high mortality.
- Insulin. Refer to local policies. Sliding scale regimens normally utilize 50 units of Actrapid® added to 50mL 0.9% sodium chloride administered via syringe driver.
- Electrolyte replacement. Fluid and insulin therapy can lead to rapid intracellular movement of K^+. If the plasma K^+ value is < 5.5mmol/L, potassium needs to be added to the replacement fluids.
- Seek and treat any underlying cause, e.g. infection, MI.
- Consider: NG tube if persistent vomiting; urinary catheter (especially if the patient is oliguric or anuric); CVP monitoring in the critically ill patient.
- ⚠ Ensure thromboembolic prophylaxis (patients with DKA have a hypercoaguable state).
- Patients who are profoundly acidaemic/critically ill will need an ITU/HDU opinion.

Hyperosmolar non-ketotic hyperglycaemia (HONK)

Pathophysiology

HONK is associated with type II diabetes. It has a gradual onset of days and even weeks and is associated with a significant mortality rate of ~ 10%. As with DKA, the main precipitating factor of HONK is concurrent illness (especially infection). Glucagon, catecholamines, and glucocorticoids lead to a significant rise in blood glucose levels, and a resultant profound homeostatic imbalance 2° to marked hyperosmolality. Although there may be a small rise in ketones, patients with HONK are by definition not ketoacidotic.

Clinical features

- Hypovolaemic (2° to the hyperosmolar diuresis).
- Hypotensive.
- Tachycardic.
- ↓ level of consciousness, especially in the elderly.
- Electrolyte imbalance.
- Signs and symptoms of thromboembolic disease (such as stroke, MI, PE, DVT) 2° to an underlying hypercoaguable state. This is a major cause of mortality.

Diagnosis

Diagnosis is made on the following basis.

- ↑ bedside and laboratory glucose (often > 30mmol/L).
- ↑ urine and blood osmolality.
- There may be a coexistent lactic acidaemia 2° to hypoperfusion, but ketones are absent or minimally present.

Nursing interventions

- Ensure airway patency, and administer high flow oxygen.
- Full set of vital signs including ECG.
- Establish IV access. Collect blood for FBC, U & E, clotting glucose, CRP, cultures if pyrexial.
- Commence IV fluid resuscitation cautiously.
- Rapid dilution of the blood and a rapid drop in osmolality increase the risk of rebound cerebral oedema.
- If not shocked fluid replacement needs to be gradual. A rate of 200mL/h of 0.9% sodium chloride is often appropriate.
- If plasma sodium is very high, use 0.45% sodium chloride slowly.
- Urinalysis and monitor urine output.
- A general guide is that a half dose of the insulin usually required for DKA should initially be infused, e.g. 3 units/h of Actrapid® rather than 6 units/h.
- Give low molecular weight heparin as prescribed to minimize risks associated with hypercoaguable blood.

Acid–base disorders

The normal blood pH is 7.35–7.45, and a number of homeostatic mechanisms ensure that this narrow normal range is maintained. For example, respiratory and renal adjustments alter the plasma levels of carbon dioxide (CO_2) and bicarbonate (HCO_3), respectively, and thereby ensure an optimal pH. Variations away from these normal values can have a deleterious effect upon cellular and organ function. For example, cardiac function deteriorates in the face of profound acidaemia.

Terminology

- Acidaemia relates to a plasma pH < 7.35 (H^+ > 45nmol/L). This is 2° to an acidotic process (respiratory, metabolic, or mixed) that leads to a rise in H^+ concentrations. Such acidotic processes, however, do not always lead to an acidaemia, as respiratory or metabolic compensation can occur.
- Alkalaemia relates to a plasma pH > 7.45 ((H^+ < 35nmol/L). This is 2° to an alkalotic process (respiratory, metabolic, or mixed) that leads to a fall in H^+ concentrations. Again, such alkalotic processes do not always lead to an alkalaemia, as metabolic or respiratory compensation can occur.

Respiratory and metabolic acidaemia

Respiratory acidaemia

CO_2 combines with water to form carbonic acid, and hence an ↑ $PaCO_2$ leads to a more acid environment, and a ↓ pH. For example, patients with acute ventilatory failure develop ↑ $PaCO_2$ (> 6.0kPa) 2° to insufficient alveolar gas exchange, and hence a respiratory acidaemia ensues. Renal compensation, via the ↑ renal retention and secretion of HCO_2 and ↑ renal excretion of H^+, takes time.

Normal values
- pH = 7.35–7.45.
- H^+ = 35–45nmol/L.
- $PaCO_2$ = 4.5–6.0kPa.
- HCO_3 = 22–26mmol/L.
- Base excess = −2 to +2mmol/L.

However, it is often notable that patients with chronic hypercapnia have a coexisting raised HCO_2 to maintain homeostasis. Short-term management of respiratory acidaemia relates to treating the underlying cause, e.g. BIPAP for ventilatory failure 2° to an exacerbation of COPD.

Metabolic acidaemia

A metabolic acidaemia is characterized by a pH < 7.35, and HCO_3 < 22mmol/L (base excess < −2), and is caused by a gain of acid and/or a loss of base. A number of processes can lead to these results.
- ↑ acid intake, e.g. poisoning with salicylates (aspirin) or ethylene glycol (antifreeze).
- ↑ acid production, e.g. lactic acid 2° to hypoperfusion, and ↑ ketones in DKA.
- ↓ acid excretion, e.g. in acute renal failure.
- ↑ base excretion, e.g. diarrhoea and fistulas.

A falling HCO_3 level therefore most commonly reflects the increasing utilization of HCO_3 in its attempts to neutralize excess acid.

Respiratory compensation may fully or partially counteract a metabolic acidosis. The respiratory centre in the brainstem detects ↑ H^+ and provokes ↑ alveolar ventilation to lower the $PaCO_2$ (e.g. Küssmaul respiration in DKA). This drop in $PaCO_2$ leads to ↓ production of carbonic acid and therefore ↑ pH.

Hypokalaemia

Hypokalaemia (serum K^+ < 3.5mmol/L) may occur due to ↓ dietary intake, or ↑ gastrointestinal and renal losses (e.g. diarrhoea and vomiting, DKA, diuretic use).

Clinical signs

- Skeletal muscle weakness.
- Constipation.
- Parylitic ileus.
- Hypotension and arrhythmias (e.g. SVT and VT).
- ECG. T wave flattening, ST segment depression, and U waves.

Nursing intervention/management

Based on treating the underlying cause of the hypokalaemia.

- Full set of vital signs and ECG; commence continuous cardiac monitoring.
- Mild cases can be treated with oral supplements (e.g. Sando-K®).
- IV replacement may be necessary: 20mmol/h.
- An accelerated regimen has been proposed by the Resuscitation Council (UK)[1] (e.g. 20mmol over 10min) for life-threatening arrhythmias. Central access is preferable in such circumstances, and full ECG monitoring is required, as well as expert help.

Reference

1 Resuscitation Council UK (2006). *Advanced life support*, 5th edn. Resuscitation Council, London.

Hyperkalaemia

Hyperkalaemia (serum K$^+$ > 5.5mmol/L) may occur due to renal failure, cell injury (e.g. rhabdomyolysis and burns), and endocrine diseases such as hypoadrenalism and DKA. Hyperkalaemia can ensue due to the body's attempt to correct an ion imbalance. Thus, one should always consider acidosis as a primary cause before attempting to treat the hyperkalaemia.

Features

- Muscle weakness.
- Abdominal cramps.
- Paraesthesia.
- Hypotension and arrhythmias (e.g. heart blocks, VT).
- ECG may show changes such as peaked, tented T waves, prolonged PR intervals, and widened QRS complexes.

Nursing intervention/management

- Full set of vital signs and commence continuous cardiac monitoring.
- In severe cases (K$^+$ > 6.5mmol/L and ECG changes) administer 10mL of 10% calcium gluconate IV over 5min as prescribed to give immediate cardioprotection.
- Administer by salbutamol 5mg nebulizer (may be repeated). This shifts potassium into cells.
- Correction of metabolic acidaemia with 50mL 8.4% sodium bicarbonate IV over 5min.
- 10 units of Actrapid® insulin in 50mL 50% dextrose IV over approximately 15–30min shifts potassium into cells.
- Polystyrene sulphonate resins (e.g. Calcium Resonium®) can also be either rectally or orally administered to promote gastrointestinal excretion.
- Diuretics (e.g. furosemide) can be administered to increase renal excretion of potassium.
- The underlying cause should be sought and treated, e.g hydrocortisone for an Addisonian crisis; dialysis for renal failure.

Hyponatraemia

Hyponatraemia (serum Na^+ < 135mmol/L) is often associated with a low osmotic pressure. Caution is therefore required to avoid overly vigourous sodium correction, as the rapid intravascular rise in osmotic pressure can lead to rapid fluid shifts from tissues, especially the brain (pontine demyelination). Rates of correction of 0.5mmol/L/h may be appropriate.

Features of hyponatraemia

- Nausea, vomiting.
- Headache.
- Fatigue.
- Seizures and coma.

Causes of hyponatraemia

- Too little sodium intake (depletional hyponatraemia).
- Too much water (dilutional hyponatraemia), e.g. 2° to fluid overload, SIADH, nephrotic syndrome.
  - If symptomatic, diuretics such as furosemide can be used and hypertonic saline (e.g. 1.8% sodium chloride) can be given in judicious aliquots to replace urinary sodium losses.
  - Fluid restriction can be utilized in asymptomatic patients.
- Loss of both sodium and water (but Na^+ > water), e.g. diarrhoea and vomiting, overdiuresis.

Management

- If symptomatic, emergency treatment includes the judicious use of hypertonic 1.8% sodium chloride.
- Asymptomatic patients can receive 0.9% sodium chloride to gradually raise the sodium levels.

Hypernatraemia

Hypernatraemia (serum Na^+ >145mmol/L) is often associated with a high osmotic pressure. Caution is therefore required to avoid an overly vigorous reduction in sodium levels, as the rapid reduction in intravascular osmotic pressure can lead to rapid shifts of fluid into the tissues, especially the brain (cerebral oedema).

Features of hypernatraemia

- Thirst.
- Lethargy.
- Seizures and coma.

Causes of hypernatraemia

- Too much sodium, e.g. excess IV sodium chloride.
- Cushing's and Conn's syndromes.
- Too little water, e.g. diabetes insipidus.

Management

- If hypovolaemic, emergency management consists of fluid resuscitation with either colloid or 5% dextrose. Thiazide diuretics can be utilized in conjunction with these fluids to promote renal sodium excretion.
- Loss of both sodium and water (but water > Na^+), e.g. HONK. Consider judicious use of 0.9% sodium chloride, or 0.45% sodium chloride in severe cases (both sodium and water need to be replaced, but water is proportionately more necessary).

Anion gap

When aiming to determine which metabolic process is responsible for a metabolic acidaemia, the calculation of the anion gap can prove valuable.

Anion gap = plasma (sodium + potassium) – (bicarbonate + chloride)

Normal range = 8–16mmol/L.

To maintain electroneutrality, cations (positive ions, such as sodium and potassium) and anions (negative ions, such as bicarbonate and chloride) need to balance. The differential which therefore exists when calculating the anion gap represents those anions not routinely measured in the laboratory, e.g. phosphates, lactic acid, and ketones. A widening anion gap suggests increasing numbers of these anions, and is especially associated with increased acid ingestion or production, or decreased acid excretion, as represented in the following mnemonic.

A MUDPILE CAT

- Alcohol.
- Methanol.
- Uraemia.
- DKA.
- Paraldehyde.
- Iron/isoniazid
- Lacticacidosois.
- Ethyleneglycol.
- Carbamazepine.
- Aspirin.
- Toluene.

Respiratory and metabolic alkalaemia

Respiratory alkalaemia

A respiratory alkalaemia is characterized by a pH > 7.45, and ↓ $PaCO_2$ (< 4.5kPa) 2° to hyperventilation (which leads to a corresponding reduction in carbonic acid production). Causes of hyperventilation leading to alkalaemia include:

- anxiety
- pain
- drugs, such as the early stages of salicylate poisoning
- hypermetabolic states, e.g. fever
- hypoxia, e.g. pulmonary embolus or anaemia.

The cause of the hyperventilation needs to be sought, and treatment initiated, e.g. rebreathing exhaled CO_2 in cases of anxiety (via paper bag) or oxygen therapy if hypoxic.

Metabolic compensation for respiratory alkalaemia occurs via the kidneys, as both HCO_3 excretion and H^+ secretion increase. This process, however, takes time. Hence it may take a couple of days for full compensation to be achieved.

⚠ Never dismiss hyperventilation as hysterical—you may miss serious underlying pathology.

Metabolic alkalaemia

A metabolic alkalaemia is characterized by a pH > 7.45, and a raised plasma bicarbonate (> 26mmol/L, base excess > 2mmol/L), and is caused by a loss of H^+ (acid) and/or a gain in bicarbonate.

The underlying cause needs to be sought and treated, e.g. fluid and electrolyte replenishment. Respiratory compensation may also be noted. Hypoventilation leads to ↑ $PaCO_2$ and, as a result, ↑ carbonic acid levels. Such compensation, however, is limited by hypoxia, which ultimately restimulates ventilation.

Hypoadrenal crisis

Pathophysiology

Primary hypoadrenalism (Addison's disease) is most commonly caused by autoimmune processes that lead to the destruction of the adrenal cortex. These patients therefore require long-term steroid replacement therapy (e.g. hydrocortisone, which has both a glucocorticoid and mineralocorticoid effect). A hypoadrenal ('Addisonian') crisis may therefore ensue if there is either a sudden withdrawal of steroid therapy; or if there is an insufficient increase of steroid therapy at times of physiological stress (e.g. infection, trauma, MI).

In contrast, patients develop secondary hypoadrenalism when the whole hypothalamus–pituitary–adrenal axis is suppressed, most commonly due to long-term steroid use for non-endocrine disease, e.g. COPD, or to avoid transplant rejection. These patients are also prone to hypoadrenal crisis if steroid therapy is suddenly curtailed (hence the necessity for weaning such patients off steroid medication).

Clinical features

- Glucocorticoid deficiency can lead to weakness, vomiting, hypoglycaemia, weight loss, abdominal pain, and coma.
- Mineralocorticoid deficiency can lead to dehydration, hyponatraemia, hyperkalaemia, postural hypotension, and hypovolaemic shock.

Diagnosis These patients are treated on clinical suspicion, as formal diagnosis is based upon plasma cortisol and ACTH levels, and synacthen tests.

Nursing intervention/management

- Ensure airway patency and oxygenation. Full set of vital signs and ECG.
- Fluid replacement. If shocked, consider colloid; otherwise utilize 0.9% sodium chloride.
- Give hydrocortisone 100mg IV stat as prescribed
- Manage hypoglycaemia and hyperkalaemia.
- Seek and treat any underlying co-morbidity, e.g. infection, MI.

Thyrotoxic crisis

Pathophysiology

This is a rare condition, sometimes known as a thyroid storm. Patients tend to have pre-existing hyperthyroidism, most notably 'Graves' disease' (thyroid stimulating auto-antibodies lead to ↑ levels of T3 and T4). The crisis itself is usually precipitated by ↑ physiological stress, including infection, trauma, surgery, and diabetic emergencies. However, cessation of anti-thyroid therapy and thyroxine overdose can also provoke a crisis.

Clinical features

Features include:
- hyperpyrexia;
- tachycardia and arrhythmias (especially AF);
- cardiac failure;
- irritability, agitation, confusion, and coma.

Deterioration can be rapid. Mortality is ~ 10%.

Diagnosis

The diagnosis is confirmed by standard thyroid function tests (i.e. T3, T4, and TSH). Treatment, however, should not be delayed whilst awaiting formal test results. Hence the clinical history (especially a history of existing hyperthyroidism) and signs/symptoms should initially guide management.
    The following investigations can aid diagnosis.
- ECG (for identification of arrhythmias).
- CXR (for identification of heart failure or chest infection).
- U & E, FBC, blood cultures, glucose, and urinalysis.

Nursing intervention/management

These patients may be very agitated and frightened and need a competent reassuring response.
- Ensure airway patency and oxygenation.
- Full set of vital signs.
  - Capillary blood glucose.
  - ECG once more settled.
- Commence continuous cardiac monitoring.
- IV access and gradual fluid replacement (initially with 0.9% sodium chloride).
- Maintain strict fluid balance.
- Routine bloods including TFTs.
- Acute agitation can be treated with titrated IV or oral benzodiazepines.
- Consider antipyretics for hyperpyrexia: but avoid aspirin as it increases circulating thyroxine levels.
- Give corticosteroids (e.g. hydrocortisone 100mg IV) as prescribed. These suppress many of the features of hyperthyroidism.
- Give other medications as prescribed (potassium iodide and carbimazole are used to inhibit T4 synthesis).
- Be aware of possible underlying co-morbidity, e.g. infection, DKA.

Myxoedema (hypothyroid) coma

Pathophysiology

This is a rare condition, associated with profound hypothyroidism. Precipitating factors include infection, surgery, MI, stroke, and cold weather. The elderly are predominantly affected, especially in the context of pre-existing hypothyroidism.

Clinical features

The usual clinical features associated with hypothyroidism are profoundly exacerbated. These include:

- hypoventilation;
- bradycardia and cardiac failure;
- confusion and coma;
- metabolic and respiratory acidaemia;
- hypothermia.

Diagnosis TFTs lead to a definitive diagnosis, but management should initially be based upon clinical suspicion 2° to history and examination.

Nursing interventions

- ITU involvement may be necessary from the outset.
- Ensure airway patency and oxygenation.
- Full set of vital signs, capillary blood glucose, ECG.
- Ensure continuous cardiac monitoring.
- Establish IV access and collect routine bloods including TFTs, CRP, and blood cultures if pyrexial.
- Observe for hypotension, cardiac failure, bradycardia, and seizures.
- Use warming blanket to gradually re-warm the patient.
- Give low dose T4 replacement as prescribed.
- Give corticosteroids (e.g. hydrocortisone 100mg IV) as prescribed. These may be necessary as co-existing hypoadrenal crisis may be masked by myxoedema.
- Ensure patient has one to one continuous nursing as these patients are highly dependent and very unwell.

Heat illness

Pathophysiology

The hypothalamus regulates temperature to ensure homeostasis, utilizing mechanisms such as sweating and vasodilatation to achieve temperature control. At times, however, these homeostatic processes are inadequate to ensure thermoregulation, especially when ambient temperatures and humidity rise, prolonged activity is undertaken (e.g. intense physical exertion), and fluid and electrolyte intake does not match losses. Children and the elderly are particularly at risk of heat illness, but other risk factors include coexistent alcohol use, cardiac disease, and recreational drugs, such as ecstasy and cocaine. More recently, marathon runners have been brought to the ED suffering from heat illness.

- Heat cramps and heat exhaustion signify mild to moderate heat illness (temperature < 40.5°C). Cramps occur 2° to electrolyte deficiencies following hypotonic fluid replacement, whilst exhaustion occurs 2° to both water and electrolyte losses. Both forms of presentation are eminently treatable.
- Heat stroke, however, signifies severe heat illness (core temperature > 40.5°C). The physiological response to the ↑ body temperature is completely overwhelmed and, as a result, there is a derangement in fluid and electrolyte balance, as well as multiorgan damage, e.g. cerebral oedema, renal failure, and coagulopathies. The overall mortality rate approaches 10%, but is higher in the elderly population.

Clinical features of heat cramp /exhaustion

- Core temperature < 40.5°C.
- Muscle cramps.
- Fatigue.
- Headache.
- Nausea and vomiting.
- Collapse (often 2° to postural hypotension).

Clinical features of heat stroke

- Core temperature > 40.5°C.
- Circulation: hypotension, tachycardia, arrhythmias, and signs of disseminated intravascular coagulation (DIC), such as petechial and purpuric rashes.
- Neurological: confusion, seizures, and coma.
- Metabolic: acidaemia, hypoglycaemia, and signs of jaundice.
- Renal: features of rhabdomyolysis, such as haematuria and myoglobinuria may be present.

Diagnosis

Diagnosis is based upon the accurate measurement of temperature (e.g. rectal), in conjunction with underlying signs and symptoms.

⚠ If the patient's clinical condition is more severe than would be expected for a given temperature, remember that cooling may have occurred in transit to the ED. Failure to take this into account may lead to a significant underappreciation of the multiorgan damage that has already ensued, with a corresponding delay in initiating emergency treatment.

Nursing intervention/management

Heat cramp/exhaustion Simple cooling techniques (e.g. removing clothing, cooling ambient temperature) in conjunction with oral rehydration/electrolyte solutions are usually sufficient. IV fluid replacement may be required if signs/symptoms are more significant.

Heat stroke

- Ensure airway patency, and administer high flow oxygen. Seek ITU assistance as appropriate.
  - Full set of vital signs.
  - Capillary blood glucose.
  - ECG.
- IV fluids (e.g. 0.9% sodium chloride) should be commenced, but judicious fluid replacement is required to avoid precipitating cerebral/pulmonary oedema. Invasive monitoring may be required to assist with clinical decision-making.
- Urinary catheter and strict fluid balance initiated.
- Collect blood for FBC, U & E, coagulation, glucose.
- Request CXR.
- Seizures should be managed with benzodiazepines first line.
- Cooling. All clothing should be removed, and a cooling rate of 0.1°C/min should be aimed for. This is best achieved with evaporative cooling, e.g. cool water is sprayed on to the patient, and fans are utilized to blow air over the patient. In addition, ice packs over areas such as the groin, axillae, and neck can directly cool circulating blood, but caution is required to avoid direct thermal injury to the skin. In the face of refractory hyperthermia more aggressive management may be required, such as gastric, peritoneal, pleural, and/or bladder lavage with cold water or cardiopulmonary bypass if available.
- Antipyretics, such as paracetamol, are not indicated as the pathophysiological processes of fever and heat illness differ.
- Adjuncts to the resuscitation process should include a urinary catheter so that an accurate fluid balance can be determined.

Frostbite

Pathophysiology

Frostbite occurs when tissue temperatures fall < 0°C. This leads to extra-cellular ice crystal formation which directly results in cell membrane damage, but also leads to an increase in osmotic pressure. This can ultimately lead to cell dehydration and death. In tandem, peripheral vaso-constriction decreases blood flow and encourages the development of microthrombi—this leads to tissue ischaemia and, ultimately, tissue necrosis. As with any ischaemia, a penumbral region surrounds the necrotic core, and this can potentially be salvageable. Treatment is therefore directed at limiting further damage to this area, and restoring perfusion.

Clinical features

- Symptoms usually relate to the severity of the exposure. Paraesthesia and anaesthesia are the most common presenting features,
- Initial sensory deficits, such as in light touch and pain, are replaced by complete sensory loss as ischaemia and neuropraxia progress.
- Distal extremities are most at risk, including toes, fingers, ears, nose, and penis. Tissues may initially appear mottled or white.
- Rewarming is associated with the development of reperfusion erythema even in the most severe cases as well as the development of an aching, throbbing pain that may last for a significant period (even months).
- Rewarming may also lead to blister and oedema formation. Their presence is often a better prognostic indicator in severe cases than their absence.
- In the most severe cases, black necrotic tissue develops, reflecting irreversible ischaemic damage.

Diagnosis

There is often a poor correlation between initial presentation and eventual outcome. For this reason, the extent of the cold injury is often based upon retrospective analysis.

- Superficial frostbite = no eventual tissue loss.
- Deep frostbite = tissue loss.

In the initial management phase, however, diagnosis is based upon a sound assessment of the patient. This includes a thorough history, especially the time of exposure, and a thorough clinical examination, including an assessment of sensation, colour, function, and the development of erythema and blisters on rewarming.

More long-term diagnostic and prognostic perspectives can be gained from comparison X-rays, angiography, and MRI. In severe cases the final assessment and demarcation of viable from non-viable tissue can take up to 3 months to determine. For this reason there is often a corresponding delay prior to any surgical intervention.

Intervention/management

- If rewarming can be successfully undertaken pre-hospital then it should be attempted.

- Immersion of the injured body part in water at 40–42°C leads to rapid rewarming, which has been shown to be more efficacious than gradual rewarming.
- Friction massage should be avoided, as it worsens tissue damage.

Emergency department

- Treat concurrent hypothermia if present.
- Immerse the affected body part in water maintained at 40–42°C until distal erythema is noted (may take up to 30min).
- Subsequently dry the injured area, and elevate where possible to limit post-thaw oedema.
- Any open wounds should be dressed appropriately.
- The vast majority pf patients will require hospital admission. Therefore refer to the appropriate speciality (perhaps orthopaedics or specialist plastics/burns unit where available).
- Ongoing monitoring will be required to determine the extent of the injury and for the management of complications, e.g. compartment syndrome and infections.

Hypothermia

Pathophysiology

The term hypothermia relates to a core body temperature < 35°C. The following classification is often used in practice.
- Mild hypothermia—temperature 32–35°C.
- Moderate hypothermia—temperature 30–32°C.
- Severe hypothermia—temperature < 30°C.

Hypothermia most commonly occurs 2° to environmental exposure to cold conditions (such as poorly heated housing in winter, exposure to wet and windy conditions when undertaking outdoor pursuits, or cold water immersion). Added risk factors include immobility (e.g. following injury, decreased level of consciousness 2° to alcohol or drug use, and co-morbidity in the elderly) and thermoregulatory/metabolic impairment (e.g. infants, the elderly, and those with hypothyroidism). The elderly are at further risk in the presence of cognitive impairment, such as dementia, leading to decreased cold awareness.

As the body cools, both brain and cardiovascular function begins to fail—essentially the body begins to 'shut down'. Paradoxically this can provide some protection to both the brain and other vital organs in the face of profound hypothermic insult. The ultimate sequelae, however, are complete cardiovascular collapse and death, often 2° to arrhythmias.

Clinical features
- Hypotension and arrhythmias.
- Sinus bradycardia is followed by AF, VF, and asystole sequentially.
- Respiratory depression.
- Lethargy, confusion, and coma.

Diagnosis A low reading rectal thermometer is required to confirm diagnosis. In cases of profound hypothermia signs of life should be sought for up to a minute before declaring cardiac arrest, e.g. via palpation of the carotid artery in conjunction with ECG trace and signs of breathing. The pulse may be very slow, irregular, and small in volume.

Management

Patients with cardiac output
Patients with profound hypothermia should be handled carefully, as undue movement can precipitate arrhythmias and cardiac arrest.
- A. Ensure airway patency and ITU involvement as required.
- B. Warmed, humidified oxygen should be utilized where available.
- C. Ensure ECG monitoring and IV access. Warmed fluids should be given if the patient is hypotensive, but caution is required to avoid precipitating pulmonary oedema.
- D. Hypoglycaemia should be sought for and corrected where necessary.
- E. Wet clothing should be removed, and the skin dried.
- Passive rewarming is appropriate for mild/moderate hypothermia, and includes a warm clinical environment, blankets, bonnets for the head, and the use of warm air delivery systems such as the Bair Hugger where available.

- As a general rule patients who have cooled slowly need to be warmed slowly, especially if elderly. In such cases 0.5°C/h is probably appropriate and helps to limit the development of cerebral/pulmonary oedema.
- Active rewarming is required in cases of severe hypothermia or cardiac arrest. Warmed fluids (40–45°C) can be instilled into the bladder, stomach, and peritoneal and pleural cavities. The fluid is left in situ for 10–20min, and then replaced to ensure that warming is optimized.
- Cardiopulmonary bypass, however, is the mode of choice where available, and can lead to very rapid rewarming.
- Adjuncts should include blood investigations, ABG, CXR, and NG tube and urinary catheter as required.
- An ECG should be obtained, both to seek arrhythmias, but also to determine whether J waves are seen at the junction of the QRS complex and ST segment. These waves may appear at temperatures < 32°C.

Patients in cardiac arrest

Once cardiac arrest has been diagnosed in a hypothermic patient, the following factors should be considered in conjunction with the standard approach to resuscitation.

- Warmed, humidified oxygen, and active rewarming techniques should be used.
- IV drugs should be withheld until the temperature is > 30°C, and, subsequently, time intervals between doses should be doubled until the temperature is > 35°C, in order to reflect slower drug metabolism associated with hypothermia, and hence the ↑ potential for toxic drug dosages.
- VF/pulseless VT should be initially treated with defibrillation. If 3 shocks have not been effective, and the temperature is < 30°C, further attempts should be withheld until the temperature is > 30°C.
- Prolonged resuscitation may be necessary. Death should not be confirmed until either the patient has been rewarmed (e.g. > 32°C), or attempts to raise the core body temperature have failed.
- If resuscitation has been successful, aim to maintain the patient's temperature at 32–34°C.

Drowning

Pathophysiology

Drowning incidents involve respiratory impairment 2° to submersion or immersion in a liquid. This liquid, normally water, prevents the victim form breathing air. ∴ the ultimate sequela of drowning incidents is death 2° to suffocation. Almost a half of deaths involve children < 4 years old.

Specific patterns of drowning have been noted.

- 'Wet drowning'. Fluid is aspirated into the lungs, leading to pulmonary damage, such as alveolar–capillary membrane dysfunction and surfactant loss. Survivors often develop acute respiratory distress syndrome (ARDS) 2° to such damage, which has been termed 'secondary drowning'.
- 'Dry drowning'. Post-mortem studies have revealed that ~ 10–20% of drowning deaths are 2° to intense laryngospasm following a small amount of water entering the larynx. Minimal lung aspiration is therefore found.

Hypothermia may occur concurrently with a drowning incident, and this may offer some protection to vital organs, especially if the hypothermia develops rapidly, e.g. submersion in water < 5°C. In addition, young children can gain neurological protection after prolonged immersion (even > 60min) 2° to the diving reflex, especially in combination with hypothermia. Cold water and hypoxia lead to a reflex bradycardia and peripheral vasoconstriction, with subsequent redistribution of blood to the brain and heart.

There is no evidence that drowning in either fresh or salt water alters initial presentation or management. However, there is evidence that prolonged immersion in water leads to a 'hydrostatic squeeze' on the body. On removal from water, this pressure is alleviated, intravascular pressures drop, and hypotension and cardiovascular collapse ensue. Removing such patients from the water in a horizontal position rather than a vertical position helps to lessen such cardiovascular consequences.

Clinical features

Patients involved in drowning incidents may present with a wide range of signs and symptoms, which may range between cardiac arrest, hypoxic coma, or a normal clinical examination.

Patients presenting with a significant history of a drowning incident should be closely monitored for signs of developing ARDS, e.g. dyspnoea, hypoxia, or pulmonary oedema.

Nursing intervention/management

In the presence of cardiorespiratory arrest, full ALS should be implemented. Consider also concurrent neck injury and hypothermia.

For patients who are spontaneously breathing and with a cardiac output, the following management should be considered.

- A. C-spine injury. Immobilization should be considered and the patient treated accordingly, and the airway maintained. Suction may be required to remove fluid and debris from the upper airway.

- B. High flow oxygen should be utilized. CPAP may be required if ARDS develops.
- C. IV fluids should be administered if the patient is hypotensive, but caution is required to avoid fluid overload.
- D. Hypoglycaemia should be considered and treated if necessary.
- E. Wet clothing should be removed, and a core temperature obtained. Rewarm as indicated.
- Adjuncts include blood investigations, CXR, and ECG.
- An NG tube will assist with gastric decompression if water has been swallowed.
- Antibiotics may be required if the water was contaminated with sewage or other waste.
- Consider also tetanus status if there are cuts or abrasions to the skin.

Outcome depends upon a number of factors. Patients with a brief submersion/immersion time and who receive prompt medical assistance have the best prognosis. Patients who are asymptomatic in the ED should be closely observed for at least 6h prior to discharge, and only then discharged if ABGs and clinical examination remain normal.

Diving emergencies

Barotrauma

Barotrauma relates to injury to air-containing body systems following changes in atmospheric pressure or, in the case of diving, water pressure.

On descent, the water pressure increases and hence air is compressed or 'squeezed'. As a result the middle ear in particular is prone to trauma from these compressive forces, especially if the Eustachian tube is congested, thereby limiting pressure equalization. As a consequence the tympanic membrane can perforate, with resultant conductive hearing loss and/or the development of a nystagmus and vertigo if cold water reaches into the middle ear itself. In such instances prophylactic antibiotics are often indicated to avoid otitis media. Similarly, pressure changes in the inner ear can lead to vestibular damage and resultant tinnitus, vertigo, and hearing loss.

Barosinusitis leads to pain over ethmoid, frontal and/or maxillary sinuses. This is more common in those with polyps, mucosal thickening, or other history of sinus problems.

Facial barotraumas with resultant facial bruising, swelling, and subconjunctival haemorrhage can result if the negative pressure in a diver's facemask is not equalized during a dive by occasional nasal exhalation.

Pulmonary barotrauma

This is typically a complication of ascent, as the volume of air in the lungs will expand as the diver comes to the surface. Exhalation on ascent will usually overcome this issue, but rapid ascent with breath holding (e.g. in an emergency) or air trapping 2° to asthma or other lung pathology can result in trauma. Pulmonary barotraumas can thus result in the following conditions.

Arterial gas embolism (AGE) Complications include cardiac ischaemia, arrhythmias, and stroke, as oxygenated blood is mechanically obstructed by the air, and therefore doesn't reach the tissues. AGE should be suspected in any patient who develops neurological, cardiac, or breathing symptoms on or shortly following ascent (typically < 10min). Management centres upon hyperbaric treatment.

Pneumomediastinum and subcutaneous emphysema

Air from alveolar rupture travels into the neck, mediastinum, and/or pericardium. Features include:
- hoarse voice
- retrosternal chest pain;
- crepitus may be felt subcutaneously at the neck.

High flow oxygen is usually sufficient to deal with this clinical situation.

Pneumothorax Air from alveolar rupture can pass into the pleural cavity. Further air volume expansion on ascent can lead to a tension pneumothorax. Standard treatment is advocated.

Alveolar haemorrhage Haemoptysis 2° to alveolar rupture may occur independently, or in conjunction with the other conditions listed here.

Decompression sickness (DCS)

Diving at depth leads to an accumulation of dissolved nitrogen in tissues and blood. On ascent this dissolved nitrogen comes out of solution, and begins to form small nitrogen bubbles. In a controlled dive these bubbles are transported to the lungs, and exhaled before significant problems ensue. DCS, however, arises when nitrogen comes out of solution faster than it can be excreted and hence larger bubbles form in the tissues and blood. These can lead to ischaemia and tissue hypoxia.

- Type I DCS affects the musculoskeletal system and skin, and produces the classic aching joints associated with 'the bends', especially in the shoulders and elbows. This pain is aggravated by movement.
- Type II DCS involves other organs and tends to be more serious. In such cases signs and symptoms can be very similar to those of AGE and it can be very difficult to differentiate between the two pathological processes. Typically, however, DCS develops > 10min following ascent. Management is with hyperbaric treatment.

Risk factors for the development of DCS include increased duration and depth of dive, rapid ascent, frequent dives without full excretion of nitrogen between dives, obesity, heavy exertion on a dive, and air travel soon after diving. In addition, if one diver develops DCS, it is advisable to fully assess any fellow diver who may have been with them as a 'buddy'.

Hyperbaric treatment

Hyperbaric therapy is the only definitive treatment for both DCS and AGE. Speed is of the essence—recompression within 5min of surfacing for patients with AGE carries a mortality rate of 5%, whereas recompression delayed to 5h or more carries a mortality rate of 10%. Hyperbaric treatment relieves mechanical obstruction by reducing the size of air or nitrogen bubble volume, increases nitrogen excretion, and increases oxygen delivery to the tissues. The pressure and duration of recompression is calculated using predetermined charts.

Nursing interventions

Whilst waiting for hyperbaric treatment to commence, 100% oxygen should be administered. This speeds the excretion of nitrogen.

- Entonox® should *never* be used.
- Intubated patients need to have the ETT cuff inflated with water, and not air—otherwise the cuff will deflate on recompression.
- Ground transportation is preferable to air transportation for patients requiring hyperbaric treatment as altitude increases gas bubble size.

Altitude-related illness

Those at risk of developing altitude-related illnesses are people who do not normally live at altitude, but who have recently ascended to mountainous areas without gradual acclimatization (especially over 3000 metres). At high altitude, the atmospheric partial pressure of oxygen is lower. As a result, people arriving at high altitude become hypoxic, with a decreased partial pressure of oxygen in arterial blood (PaO_2). This causes a hypoxic ventilatory response (HVR). The HVR for any individual can vary depending upon a number of factors such as genetics, comorbidity, and even alcohol and caffeine intake. Patients most at risk of developing altitude illness have a poor HVR, resulting in hypoxaemia, and this in turn can lead to acute mountain sickness (AMS), high altitude cerebral oedema (HACO), and high altitude pulmonary oedema (HAPO).

Acute mountain sickness and high altitude cerebral oedema

Hypoxaemia can result in ↑ cerebral blood flow and volume and ↑ vascular permeability leading to the development of cerebral oedema. Patients with AMS may have early signs of rising intracranial pressure (ICP), and present with headache, nausea ,vomiting, and fatigue.

- AMS often develops within a few hours, is fairly common, and begins to resolve in most cases within a few days as acclimatization ensues. Management involves halting any further ascent. More severe cases can be treated with oxygen, simple analgesics (not opiates as these can further depress the HVR), and acetazolamide (which speeds the acclimatization process).
- The most severe form of AMS is HACO, which reflects a significant rise in ICP. Cerebellar ataxia may be an early indicator, followed by seizures, focal deficits, and coma. Management involves immediate descent where possible, oxygen, dexamethasone, diuretics (e.g. mannitol), and hyperbaric therapy.

High altitude pulmonary oedema

Hypoxaemia can also lead to pulmonary artery hypertension and increased vascular permeability in the lungs with resultant pulmonary oedema. Features include dyspnoea at rest, cough, and haemoptysis in severe cases.

▶▶ Early recognition is vital, as death can rapidly ensue. Management involves immediate descent where possible, oxygen (with CPAP if available), diuretics, and hyperbaric therapy in severe cases.

Haematological emergencies

Overview

Patients with haematological disease may be immunocompromised due to their condition or to the treatment prescribed for their condition. These patients are usually treated in outpatient clinics or have chemotherapy as day cases and are often advised to attend their local ED if they develop new symptoms. Patients may be neutropenic as a result of treatment and thus vulnerable to infection. It is not uncommon for patients with haematological disease to present in the ED with life-threatening complications of their disease. In addition to recognizing shock (☐ see p.246), it is also important for the nurse to understand haemostatic mechanisms.

Haemostasis is the process of clot formation in the walls of damaged blood vessels to prevent blood loss while at the same time maintaining blood in a fluid state within the vascular system. Blood disorders occur when haemostasis falls out of balance.

- If blood becomes too thin, it loses the ability to form the blood clots that stop bleeding.
- When blood becomes too thick, the risk of blood clots developing within the blood vessels rises creating a potentially life-threatening condition such as disseminated intravascular coagulation (DIC).

Abnormalities of haemostasis

People with bleeding disorders bleed easily, and may lose excessive amounts of blood from injuries, surgery, or dental surgery. Severe bleeding disorders may even cause spontaneous bleeding without any injury. Injury to a blood vessel initiates a series of events that forms a clot (haemostasis). The ability of the blood to clot is a vital part of the body's natural defence. This process of forming a clot is referred to as coagulation. Further chemical interactions are required to dissolve the blood clot as the body heals. A shift in haemostasis can result in coagulation that is either too slow or too fast. Blood disorders result from imbalances in haemostasis. Haemostatic disorders can be inherited or acquired. Acquired disorders are by far the most common, particularly thrombocytopenia. Bleeding is to be expected where there has been blunt or penetrating trauma but a clotting disorder should be considered if bleeding is excessive and not responding to conventional pressure or if it is evident from uninjured sites.

Von Willebrand's disease

- Von Willebrand's disease is the most common bleeding disorder.
- It affects up to 1% of the population and may be found in both sexes.
- Symptoms of Von Willebrand's are usually mild, and many people may not even be aware that they have a clotting deficiency.
  - People with Von Willebrand's disease bruise easily, and may suffer from frequent nosebleeds.
  - Women with Von Willebrand's disease may have heavy periods.
- Treatment is usually with factor VIII concentrate.

Haemophilia

Haemophilia, perhaps the best known of the bleeding disorders, is a genetic disease caused by mutations of genes on the X chromosome.

- Because the mutated gene is recessive, the majority of haemophiliacs are male.
- Patients with haemophilia A may present with haematuria or bleeding into large joints.
- Intracranial bleeding is a major cause of death in this patient group.

Disseminated intravascular coagulation (DIC)

DIC is a syndrome of widespread intravascular coagulation. It may be a serious complication of septicaemia (□ see p.247), extensive tissue injury, or other diseases where fibrin is deposited in the vascular system and many small- and medium-sized vessels are thrombosed. The increased consumption of platelets causes bleeding to occur at the same time. The overall picture is one of widespread tissue ischaemia due to clot formation and bleeding due to consumpti\on of clotting factors and platelets.

Causes of DIC

These include the following.
- Infection (especially Gram-negative infection).
- Vascular, e.g. aortic aneurysm.
- Trauma, especially burns and head injuries.
- Obstetric: placental abruption, severe pre-eclampsia, intrauterine death.
- Malignancy: carcinoma of the prostate, ovary, lung, pancreas.
- Others: drug reactions, incompatible blood transfusions.
- Massive blood transfusion (□ see p.518).

Signs of DIC

The signs of DIC are complex.
- Clotting problems:
  - venous thromboembolism;
  - skin necrosis or gangrene;
  - coma due to cerebral infarction;
  - multi-organ failure.
- Bleeding problems:
  - spontaneous bruising;
  - bleeding from venepuncture sites;
  - bleeding from gastrointestinal system;
  - post-operative bleeding.

Nursing assessment and intervention for patients with bleeding disorders

▶▶ If the patient is known to have a bleeding disorder and presents with haemorrhage or history of trauma get senior help.

- Initial assessment of the patient should be guided by the principles of ABC, remembering that any traumatic bleeding into the neck or pharynx may rapidly compromise breathing.
- Obtain a brief medical history at the same time as assessing the patient. Consider:
  - allergies;
  - medication, both prescribed and over-the-counter;
  - herbal remedies and supplements.
- Undress and record temperature remembering that hypothermia aggravates any bleeding disorder, while a raised temperature may indicate sepsis.
- Pain score.
- Record respiration rate and O_2 saturation and give high flow oxygen.
- Record and monitor BP and pulse. A tachycardia and hypotension are indicative of shock.
- Attach to cardiac monitor if complaining of chest pain.
- Obtain 12-lead ECG.
- Record blood sugar.
- Record neurological vital signs and consider intracranial haemorrhage in any patient with headache or altered level of consciousness.
- Obtain a urine sample and test for haematuria.
- IV access needs to be established but this should be done by a clinician skilled in this procedure to avoid further bleeding.
- Central line insertion should only be considered in extremis since uncontrollable haemorrhage may occur.
- IM injections should be avoided.
- Blood samples should be collected for FBC, group and save, and cross-match.
- Before giving any drug check whether it may aggravate the condition or interfere with any other medication the patient is having.
- Ensure patient comfort and privacy and give emotional support to family.

Sickle cell disease

Sickle cell disease occurs in Afro-Caribbean, Middle Eastern, and some Mediterranean people. It is an inherited disorder of haemoglobin synthesis. The resulting abnormality produces a normocytic, haemolytic anaemia with multiple diversely shaped red blood cells that are susceptible to morphologically changing into a sickle shape. The sickle cells produce thrombosis and obstruction in small vessels, leading to ischaemia and necrosis of distal tissue causing severe pain. Patients with sickle cell anaemia have chronic anaemia (Hb 8–10g/dL) and are particularly prone to infection.

Sickle cell crisis may occur for no apparent reason or as a result of infection or dehydration. The crisis may involve thrombosis, haemolysis, marrow aplasia, or acute splenic or liver sequestration. Cerebral sickling may present with strange behaviour, confusion, or fits. Because of these different processes patients may complain of severe pain anywhere in the body with some symptoms resembling acute medical or surgical emergencies. They may also present with jaundice or priapism.

- Joint pain. Osteomyelitis and septic arthritis occur more frequently in sickle cell disease.
- Acute chest syndrome presents as chest pain, hypoxia, tachypnoea, and wheezing. This may be severe and is a leading cause of death in sickle patients.
- Acute splenic sequestration: large numbers of red blood cells aggregate in the spleen causing enlarged spleen, hypovolaemia, and thrombocytopenia. The patient may present in a state of shock. This presentation is more common in young children.

Nursing assessment and intervention specific to sickle cell disease

Follow the general assessment approach described above (☐ see p.515) bearing in mind that the priorities for these patients are as follows.

- Pain relief. As pain is always severe it needs to be managed with titrated opiate analgesia.
- Oxygen.
- IV access if dehydrated and not drinking.
- IV fluids.
- FBC, coagulation studies, U & E, and CRP.
- Give medication as prescribed.
- Transfusion should be commenced promptly if the patient has severe chest syndrome with hypoxia, has had a CVA, or has priapism.

▶ It is very important to be understanding and provide emotional support to sickle patients who are usually young and disadvantaged because of their condition. It is especially important not to dismiss their pain, which can be unremitting and severe.

Blood transfusion

Resuscitation of patients in the ED often involves blood transfusions and in many cases, especially trauma or a GI bleed, it may be necessary to activate the major haemorrhage protocol (📖 see Fig. 17.1).

Patients suffering a major haemorrhage will be very frightened and very unwell and it is essential that the nurse caring for such patients appears calm, knowledgeable, and in control. Do not wait till you have a patient with a large GI bleed to read and understand the protocol. Familiarize yourself with it right away.

Many trusts have specific care plans for patients undergoing transfusion and these should be used to minimize risk of incorrect transfusion or a transfusion reaction.

The following should be strictly adhered to.

- All blood products should be administered through a giving set with an integral filter to trap aggregates.
- All patients receiving a blood transfusion must wear an identity bracelet that documents their name, date of birth, and hospital number.
- Rigorous checking of blood and blood products must be done as per hospital policy to ensure patient safety.
- Ensure that the blood has been prescribed with reasons for transfusion clearly documented in the patient's notes.
- Transfusion must be commenced within 30min of blood being collected from the hospital fridge.
- Record baseline temperature, pulse blood pressure, and respiratory rate immediately before starting the transfusion.
- Document the transfusion start time and date on the compatibility form and drug chart.
- Record temperature, pulse, blood pressure, and respiratory rate 15min after commencement of transfusion.
- If vital signs within normal range at 15min, subsequent observations can be recorded at hourly intervals
- Vital signs should be recorded at the end of the transfusion and the finish time documented on the compatibility form.
- Urine output must be monitored throughout the transfusion.
- All medications should be given as charted and in a timely way.
- If any transfusion adverse reaction occurs, stop the transfusion immediately, record vital signs, and ask the medical team to urgently review the patient.
- Transfusion should be completed within 4 hours.
- For further details on the Blood transfusion procedure 📖 see p.586.

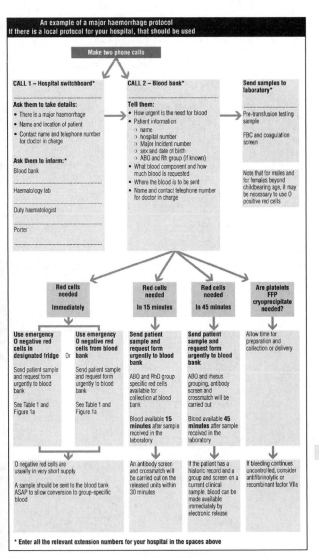

Fig. 17.1 Major haemorrhage protocol. (Reproduced with permission subject to Crown copyright from UK Blood Transfusion and Tissue Transplant Services (2007). *Handbook of Transfusion Medicine*, 4th edn, Fig. 1a. UK Blood Transfusion and Tissue Transplant Services, London. Available at ⏚ *http://www.transfusionguidelines.org.uk*)

Overdose and poisoning

Overview

Acute and chronic poisoning by drugs, chemicals, traditional remedies, plants, and animal/snake/insect bites is a common presentation in the ED. Poisoning may be accidental or intentional. Accidental poisoning is more common in children, whereas intentional poisoning is more common in adolescents and young adults. Poisoning can also affect all the members of a household, workplace, or community due to multiple exposures from a common source. This may occur through ingestion from a contaminated food or water supply or through inhalation of toxic gases or sprays.

Poisoning in children

Accidental poisoning is the term used when a child becomes exposed due to natural exploratory behaviour or from imitating adults without knowing the possible consequences. This type of poisoning occurs from the ages of 6 months to 5 years with a peak at 18 months to 2 years. Frequently, this type of ingestion is of minimal toxicity, but the incident causes great concern to the parents.

The other types of poisoning that may occur in small children are iatrogenic and non-accidental.

- Therapeutic poisoning occurs especially in premature infants and neonates, where a small error in dose can cause life-threatening toxicity (especially with drugs such as chloramphenicol, theophylline, and digoxin).
- Non-accidental poisoning (i.e. intentional) may range from a carer's attempt to sedate a child in order to quieten them, to Munchhausen's syndrome by proxy.

Poisoning in teenagers and adults

- In teenage children, deliberate self-harm and substance misuse are the commonest causes of poisoning.
- In early adult life, deliberate self-harm in the form of parasuicidal gestures is common.
- All through adult life poisoning can occur in industrial settings.
- Serious suicidal attempts become more common and are more likely to be successful especially in males > 45 years old. There may be underlying factors such as mental or physical illness, alcohol or substance misuse, unemployment, and marital separation.

History taking

Obtaining a history may be difficult especially if the patient is drowsy. Note that the information obtained may be unreliable. A history from family or friends may be more accurate.

The diagnosis of poisoning is most often apparent from the history and circumstances, but the nurse may need to consider poisoning when the patient presents with unexplained symptoms, collapse, or coma without any apparent cause. Intentional poisoning of a child or an adult by another person may present with a misleading history and clinical findings that do not fit with a medical illness. The patient who insists they have been poisoned must be listened to carefully to decide whether their suspicions are justified and if the symptoms are consistent with poisoning. A minority of these may have actually been poisoned, while some are suffering from a paranoid delusion of poisoning. In these cases the alleged source of the poisoning is vague and the symptoms are ill-defined.

It is common practice to measure salicylate and paracetamol levels when it is known or suspected that these drugs have been ingested. It is especially important with paracetamol since there may be no symptoms even in a potentially fatal overdose.

As in all history taking the nurse needs to ask the following.

- What drugs or chemicals have been taken? The time, the amount, and whether they were ingested, injected, or inhaled?
- Has the patient vomited since taking the poison?
- What other medications are being taken?
- Does the patient have any known allergies?
- Does the patient have any other medical conditions?
- Any previous history of depression, mental illness, or attempted suicide?

Nursing assessment/interventions

The overall aim of the nursing assessment is to identify the cause; maintain the safety of the patient in terms of airway, breathing, and circulation; and minimize the risk of further absorption while providing supportive measures both physical and emotional to the patient who may be very distressed.

General assessment/intervention

Airway

- Establish and protect airway.
- Airway adjuncts or intubation may be necessary.
- Suck out any secretions and remove dentures.
- If the patient's gag reflex is reduced or absent they will need intubating.
  - ▶▶ Call the anesthetist.
- Once the airway has been secured, high flow oxygen should be administered.
- Record oxygen saturations. Assess respiratory rate and effectiveness.
  - Respiration may be slowed by opiates, barbiturates, or tricyclics.
  - Wheezing may be evident after inhalation of chlorine gas.

Circulation

- Establish venous access using wide bore cannula and collect blood samples for FBC, group and save, U & E, coagulation studies, toxicology screening, and also prescribed medication screening.
- Observe skin for cyanosis or fresh needlemarks.
- Observe any burns or swelling around the mouth and throat.
- Serum glucose should be established on arrival in the ED and corrected if abnormal.
- Attach the patient to a monitor.
- Commence meticulous recordings of BP, HR, RR, oxygen saturations.
- Record a 12 lead ECG.
  - Tricyclic antidepressants can cause tachycardia and tachyarrhythmias and hypotension.
  - Cocaine can also cause tachyarrythmias and even MI.
  - Bradycardia may be caused by organophosphate insecticides or β-blocker medication.
- If patient is hypotensive give IV fluids as prescribed.

Neurological monitoring

- Record GCS and make sure neurological status is frequently reassessed. Meticulous monitoring and frequent reassessment are crucial to detecting any further deterioration in level of consciousness.
  - ▶ Remember that changes in the GCS may be more significant than the overall score.
- Observe pupil size and reaction.
  - Pinpoint pupils may be due to narcotics.
  - Dilated pupils may be due to cocaine, amphetamines, atropine, or tricyclic antidepressants.
- Seizures may be due to withdrawal from drugs/alcohol but also may be due to poisoning from overdose. Seizures are dangerous because they cause hypoxia and acidosis and can lead to cardiac arrest. Drugs that

may cause seizures in overdosage include mefenamic acid, theophylline and tricyclic antidepressants.

Specific interventions

- Hypothermia can occur with any drug causing coma especially barbiturates and phenothiazines. Check rectal temperature using low reading thermometer Use warming blanket and warm fluids IV to warm the patient.
- Hyperthermia may occur with amphetamines, cocaine, ecstasy, MAOIs, and theophylline. Convulsions/seizures are common.
  - ▶▶ Get help (📖 see p.499.)
- When the eyes and/or skin have been contaminated by corrosives or pesticides, the eyes must be attended to first and washed out continuously with clean water for 10–15min. The skin should be washed with soap and water paying particular attention to thinner areas of the skin (axillae, groins, and face).
- Ingested corrosives, acids, or alkalis should be treated by immediately giving the patient a few cups of water to drink in order to dilute and so prevent damage to the tissues. However after 10 or 20 minutes this action may well be too late and the patient may be unable to swallow.
- Contacting the National Posion Information service will give detailed information about signs and symptoms, toxication and management ⌁ www. toxbase.org.

Gastric lavage (📖 see p.620)
Emptying the stomach by gastric lavage should only be carried out on the advice of the poisons unit. If the ingestion was < 1h ago, activated charcoal may be given as a suspension in water. This is specially prepared charcoal with a large surface area giving it a high adsorbent capacity, which adsorbs most drugs and poisons in a ratio of about one part poison to ten parts charcoal. The dose is 25–50g for an adult and 1g/kg body weight in a child. Exceptions include iron, lithium, alcohol, methanol, ethylene glycol, corrosives, acids, and alkalis and where oral antidotes or medication need to be given.

Whole bowel lavage is another method of decontaminating the intestine. This involves giving isotonic fluid, using solutions normally used to prepare the bowel for X-ray procedures. The adult dose is 500mL/h to 2L/h, given until the effluent is clear. It can be used to clear the gut of sustained release preparations, iron, lithium, heavy metals, and illicit drug packets.

Ipecacuanha has been widely used in the past but there is no evidence to suggest it reduces drug absorption. It is now contraindicated as it may lead to prolonged vomiting, drowsiness, and aspiration pneumonia.

Psychosocial care Serious overdoses need medical admission. Less serious overdoses are usually managed in the observation ward of the ED. Admitting these patients allows some time for more pastoral care and assessment by the psychiatric team Every deliberate self-poisoning should be assessed in an objective and sympathetic way to ensure that every effort is being made to help these patients, hopefully preventing a further occurrence.

Poisoning from therapeutic drugs

Paracetamol

Paracetamol is the most widely available analgesic worldwide. It is safe in therapeutic use, but overdose of > 300mg/kg can cause liver failure and sometimes kidney failure. It is important to note that during the first few hours the patient remains conscious and there may be few or no symptoms apart from malaise, nausea, and vomiting. More advanced signs such as jaundice and elevated LFTs may take 2–3 days to appear.

- Treatment is usually indicated if the patient has taken > 150mg/kg.
- Fatal liver damage can be prevented by giving an antidote within 10–12h of ingestion so every case needs to be carefully assessed and blood taken for measurement of blood paracetamol levels once 4h have passed since ingestion.
- Some patients are at ↑ risk of liver damage, e.g. those taking enzyme-inducing agents (e.g. phenytoin, rifampicin, heavy alcohol users) and those who are malnourished or who have been fasting recently.
- If the patient presents within 1h of ingesting a potentially toxic amount, give activated charcoal and collect blood for paracetamol/salicylate levels and a clotting screen.

Salicylates Common features of toxicity from aspirin and other salicylates include vomiting, dehydration, tinnitus, deafness, sweating, warm extremities, and hyperventilation. Severe poisoning is likely to cause coma, convulsions, pulmonary oedema, and cardiovascular collapse. If any of these occur the outcome is likely to be fatal. However, the patient is likely to remain conscious and alert for many hours even after a large overdose. Repeated measurements of drug levels are needed, as drug levels can rise for many hours after a large ingestion.

Tricyclic antidepressants

- Symptoms of overdose include tachycardia, dilated pupils, cardiac arrhythmias and widened QRS complex, hypotension, hot dry skin, and dry mouth.
- Cardiac monitoring should be continued for at least 6h after ingestion.
- Convulsions, respiratory depression, and coma can occur.
- If the patient presents within 1h of ingesting a potentially toxic amount give activated charcoal.

Selective serotonin reuptake inhibitors (SSRIs) may cause few or no symptoms even after large overdoses. However, many patients experience gastrointestinal upset and drowsiness, while some develop tachycardia, muscle stiffness, and hypertension. Convulsions may occur. If the patient presents within 1h of ingesting a potentially toxic amount give activated charcoal.

Benzodiazepines

These are relatively safe when taken in overdose, although they can cause life-threatening problems particularly in older people and patients with severe chronic obstructive airways disease.

- Symptoms of overdose range from drowsiness, ataxia, and nystagmus to hypotension, respiratory depression, and coma, particularly if taken with alcohol or other CNS depressants.
- The effects of benzodiazepines can be reversed with flumazenil, but it is safer to protect the airway and to let the patient recover.

Iron tablets

- Early symptoms of iron overdose include nausea, vomiting, abdominal pain, and diarrhoea. The patient's vomit and stools may be grey or black.
- Haematemesis and rectal bleeding may occur and, in severe cases, coma and shock.
- Most patients, especially children, will need measurement of serum iron, possibly gastric lavage and desferrioxamine treatment, even if their symptoms have resolved within a few hours.
- AXR may show location of tablets.

Cardiac glycosides

Chronic therapeutic toxicity with the drugs e.g., digitoxin, digitalis (foxglove: *Digitalis purpurea* or *Digitalis lanata*) or oleander plants (*Nerium oleander* or yellow oleander: *Thevetia peruviana*) may be involved in self-poisoning.

- Nausea, vomiting, cardiac arrhythmias, hypotension and death may result.
- The patient should be given activated charcoal if able to swallow with subsequent close observation of ABCs.
- A plasma potassium concentration > 5.3mmol/L is an indication of severe poisoning.
- If available (and they should be ordered at once), digoxin-specific Fab antibodies should have sufficient cross-reactivity to bind with all the cardiac glycosides.

Drug misuse

Alcohol Alcoholic drinks cause the typical signs of intoxication (slurred speech, ataxia, confusion, and aggression). Larger amounts can cause vomiting, coma, and hypoventilation, with the risk of aspiration of vomit. If the patient is unconscious on arrival, assess and manage as for the comatose patient. This subject is treated in more detail (☐ see Alcohol misuse, p.534.)

Opioids

- Features of opioid poisoning include a progressive depression of the CNS leading to drowsiness, coma, respiratory depression, and, ultimately, respiratory arrest.
- The patient will usually have pinpoint pupils and a slowed respiratory rate.
- There may also be hypotension and tachycardia.

Initial management depends on the patient's level of consciousness.

- If the patient is conscious and presents within 1h of ingesting a potentially toxic amount of an opiate, give activated charcoal.
- If respiration appears inadequate, call the anaesthetist.
- In respiratory depression or impaired consciousness, consider prescribing naloxone 0.8–2.0mg IV and repeating the dose every 2–3min up to a maximum 10mg (this can be given by IM or SC injection if the IV route is not feasible). Give naloxone as prescribed.

The duration of action of some opioids (e.g. dihydrocodeine, dextropropoxyphene, and methadone) can outlast that of an IV or IM dose of naloxone and deterioration may later occur despite initial reversal. Repeated doses, or an infusion, of naloxone may be required. Naloxone may not reverse the effects of buprenorphine so improvement may be delayed. Such patients need very close monitoring and frequent reassessment.

Illicit drugs

Illicit drugs are an increasing problem in every society. Many different substances can be misused, from glue or petrol sniffing, to cannabis to 'hard' drugs. The popularity of a substance varies with age and social scene.

Heroin causes the largest problem, and poisoning can occur due to an excessive dose in a naive user as well as to a 'regular' dose in a person who has lost their tolerance. It is important to remember that 10mg of heroin IV could be fatal for a non-user, but the average user who presents to an addiction centre for help is taking 750mg daily. Tolerance starts to be lost within a couple of days of abstinence, and toxicity can then occur from the user's normal dose. Management of toxicity is described under ☐ see Opioids. Abscesses and infectious illnesses are a further problem apart from toxicity.

Cocaine causes massive surges in BP due to widespread constriction of blood vessels, and chest pain is the commonest complication requiring medical attention. It usually resolves within a few hours without causing any apparent long-term damage. Every patient with symptoms following cocaine use should be given IV diazepam in relatively large doses, and those with chest pain should be given aspirin as for any patient with acute cardiac chest pain. Hallucinations, aggression and convulsions, and CVAs may also follow cocaine use. Long-term users can develop accelerated atheroma.

Hallucinogens (LSD, some types of mushrooms, some plants) can lead to a sought after hallucinatory experience in which visual images are distorted and pleasant. However, the experience may be disturbing or frightening and physical restraint may be necessary. If possible, try to 'talk down' the patient one to one in a quiet dimly lit place. If this fails, IV diazepam is the best drug to calm the patient.

Ecstasy (MDMA) is now popular as a 'dance drug'. Some people may develop hyperthermic collapse due to dancing for too long without replacing fluid, and the urgent treatment is IV fluid, which should bring down the pulse rate and enable normal temperature regulation. Rarely, some people drink too much fluid and become confused or develop convulsions, because this drug causes a surge in levels of antidiuretic hormone. Most patients will recover naturally provided no more fluid is given.

Poisoning from other substances

Lead

- In children, lead poisoning most commonly results from pica due to ingestion of lead paint from old buildings. Surma (black eye cosmetic made from lead sulphide) is another cause.
- In adults, lead poisoning may arise from contaminated water supplies or from occupational causes—painting or manufacturing.
- Children usually present with anaemia and failure to thrive.
- Adults present with abdominal pain, constipation, muscle weakness (wrist or foot drop), and, in the most severe cases, encephalopathy with convulsions.
- The diagnosis may be suspected by finding punctate basophilia on a blood film and confirmed by measuring blood lead concentrations.

Caustic chemicals

Ingestion of caustic chemicals may cause severe burns and oedema of the mouth, pharynx, upper airway, and upper GI tract.

- If the patient is conscious and able to swallow, give water or milk (3 cupfuls) immediately to dilute the acid or alkali.
- Do **not** give neutralizing chemicals as the heat released can cause further injury.
- If vomiting occurs, the oesophagus may be damaged.

Carbon monoxide

Carbon monoxide is produced when carbon-containing fuels burn in air, and more is produced when insufficient oxygen reaches the fire leading to poisoning. Motor exhaust fumes are an important cause of poisoning.

- Immediate features of exposure include headache, weakness, tachypnoea, dizziness, nausea, and agitation (🕮 see p.536).
- Vomiting, impaired consciousness, respiratory failure, MI, and cerebral oedema may occur in severe cases.
- If several people experience symptoms such as headache and vomiting, it is important to consider carbon monoxide poisoning as a possible cause.
- Give oxygen at a high concentration while assessing the patient. If patient is vomiting use nasal cannulae.

Organophosphates and carbamates

Organophosphorus and carbamate insecticides are used to control insects in homes and gardens. They can cause serious poisoning, which may be fatal through inhalation, skin contact, or ingestion. The amount that causes toxicity varies between chemicals. Some products contain petroleum distillate which can cause pulmonary oedema if aspirated.

- The onset of symptoms may be delayed for up to 12h.
- Symptoms include confusion, exhaustion, nausea, vomiting, diarrhoea, wheezing, sweating, salivation, and fasciculation of the muscles.
- The patient may have miosis, bradycardia, incontinence, and seizures.
- Pulmonary oedema and loss of consciousness are serious signs.
- After clearing the airway of secretions, the most important treatment is to give atropine in large doses (2mg at a time) until the mouth is dry.
- Diazepam can be given to relieve anxiety and control seizures.

Prognosis and long-term care

The long-term outlook following acute poisoning is generally good. The great majority of poisonings leave no permanent damage. The main limitation is when the poisoning has been due to deliberate self-harm, and the patient may be suffering from depression or schizophrenia, sometimes with alcoholism as another complicating factor. In these cases, there is a risk of further episodes of self-poisoning or of suicide by another method, and long-term antidepressant or antipsychotic medication may be indicated.

Where a patient has been poisoned in the course of their occupation, one needs to decide whether the exposure has been intentional, whether carelessness has been involved, and whether the safety practices are deficient or absent. The practitioner can then advise the patient and the employers appropriately.

Poisoning due to substance misuse carries the risks associated with the substance and the mode of use (e.g. IV injection, which may lead to bacterial or viral infections). Long-term contact with an addiction centre or agency may help to minimize the dangers and improve prognosis.

In a small number of poisonings, there may be long-term morbidity. Carbon monoxide and organophosphates (see p.530) are important examples. Lead poisoning in children may lead to developmental delay and permanent mental impairment, whereas in adults eventual full recovery is the rule even after severe poisoning.

Food poisoning

Food poisoning is caused by the ingestion of foods that contain bacteria or toxins. Salmonella is a type of bacteria, which is usually found in poultry, eggs, unprocessed milk, and in meat and water. It may also be carried by pets such as turtles and birds.

The salmonella bacterium affects the stomach and intestines. In more serious cases, the bacteria may affect the blood itself. The bacteria attack all age groups and both sexes. Children, the elderly, and people who already have medical problems are likely to be more adversely affected.

Symptoms

Symptoms include the following:
- Diarrhoea or constipation, possibly blood in faeces.
- Abdominal pain.
- Nausea/vomiting.
- Fever, headache, exhaustion.

In the case of less serious infections there are fewer symptoms—usually only diarrhoea 2 or 3 times a day for a couple of days. Most mild types of salmonella infection will resolve on their own in a few days without requiring any intervention other than rest and plenty of fluid.

Severe infection may cause excessive diarrhoea, stomach cramps, and general malaise. In such situations stool samples should be sent for investigation as treatment with antibiotics may be indicated.

Alcohol misuse

Alcohol misuse is a worrying problem for EDs. About 14 million people are treated in EDs in the UK every year. It is estimated that a significant number of these have consumed alcohol before attendance and this figure rises after midnight. The number of alcohol-related deaths in the UK has more than doubled from 4144 in 1991 to 8758 in 2006.[1] In addition the UK has the third highest rates for binge drinking in Europe.[2]

Emergency presentations associated with or caused by alcohol may be physiological, psychological, social, or all three. ED nurses should bear in mind that alcoholics are more vulnerable to heart attacks, strokes, and injury and therefore maintain a high level of suspicion during assessment. Accurate assessment of patients and helping those whose conditions are complicated by alcohol are challenging but essential aspects of practice.

History taking and assessment

- Taking an alcohol history should be standard wherever possible.
- Never label a patient as 'drunk' as such labels are not only judgemental but can obscure serious pathology and delay urgent intervention.
- Patients who are perceived as being under the influence of alcohol and are being disruptive should not be removed by the police before being medically examined.
- Basic vital signs and a capillary blood glucose should be obtained at the very least.

A sound understanding of the pathophysiological impact of alcoholism is essential for ED nurses and should be a powerful impetus to intervene with hazardous or binge drinkers by referring them to appropriate services. It is significant and of concern that hazardous drinkers continue to miss the opportunity of effective interventions, often because of their behaviour, but also because of staff inaction in this area.

Acute intoxication

Acute alcohol intoxication occurs after the ingestion of a large amount of alcohol. Inexperienced drinkers, or those sensitive to alcohol, may become acutely intoxicated and suffer serious consequences after ingesting smaller amounts of alcohol.

Signs of acute intoxication

These include:
- slurred speech;
- nystagmus;
- incoherence/confusion;
- facial flushing;
- unsteady gait.

Careful assessment is essential as these signs may mask other pathology or coexist with other pathology such as head injury. These patients are vulnerable and need close observation.

Alcohol withdrawal

Alcohol withdrawal fits are grand mal seizures that occur hours or days after the last alcoholic drink. These patients are often known to the ED.

Nevertheless, it is essential to check the patient's capillary blood glucose and exclude head injury as another possible causes of fitting. Fitting is controlled by IV or PR diazepam.

Alcoholic ketoacidosis is a metabolic complication of alcohol use and starvation characterized by hyperketonaemia and anion gap metabolic acidosis without significant hyperglycaemia. It may present in chronic alcohol misusers following a sudden cessation or reduction of alcohol consumption. It is often confused with diabetic ketoacidosis.

Wernicke's encephalopathy is a neurological disease caused by thiamine deficiency. It has two components: Wernicke's encephalopathy and Korsakoff's psychosis. Wernicke's encephalopathy is a potentially reversible but severe condition, whereas Korsakoff's psychosis is a chronic and debilitating condition. Wernicke's encephalopathy presents as acute confusion, nystagmus, ophthalmoplegia, ataxia and polyneuropathy. The signs of WE may be misinterpreted as head injury. This patient group, who can be abusive and obstructive, often walk out without treatment. As Wernicke's encephalopathy is a treatable and reversible condition, it is imperative that clinical staff act in the patients' best interest and encourage them to stay for treatment. Treatment is by parenteral thiamine (Pabrinex®) IV over 30min. Patients should be given oral thiamine and multivitamins on discharge.

Korsakoff's psychosis Some alcoholic patients with Wernicke's encephalopathy may also develop Korsakoff's psychosis. This is a chronic, irreversible condition characterized by severe memory loss. These patients may confabulate or lie in response to their acute confusion and memory loss. The patient may also have abnormality of gait due to polyneuropathy. Visual disturbance with eyelid drooping and abnormal eye movements may also be evident.

Delirium tremens This is a severe manifestation of alcohol withdrawal, which is characterized by hallucinations, delusions, disorientation, and confusion. This is a most distressing condition where the patient is vulnerable to arrhythmias, which may be the result of infection, acidosis, electrolyte imbalance, or cardiomyopathy. Treatment initially is by IV diazepam to control fitting.

Alcoholic cirrhosis is the most advanced form of alcohol-induced liver disease. It also impacts on other organs, e.g. brain and kidneys. Signs and symptoms reflect this involvement but also include portal hypertension, splenomegaly, ascites, renal failure, confusion, and even liver cancer (☐ see Alcoholic liver disease (ALD), p.338.)

References

1 ONS (2006). *Alcohol related deaths*. Office for National Statistics, London. Available at ⌁ http://www.statistics.gov.uk/downloads/theme_health/Alcohol_related_deaths_UK_1991_2005.

2 Anderson, P. and Baumberg, B. (2006). *Alcohol in Europe. A public health perspective*. A Report to the European Commission. Institute of Alcohol Studies, London.

Carbon monoxide poisoning

Pathophysiology

Carbon monoxide (CO) is produced by the incomplete combustion of carbon-containing materials, and may therefore be emitted from car exhausts, blocked central heating vents, and house fires. CO has a very strong affinity to haemoglobin, and therefore preferentially binds with this to form carboxyhaemaglobin (COHb). As a result, the oxygen-carrying capacity of blood is diminished, as is the release of oxygen from blood to the tissues. In severe cases this can lead to tissue hypoxia and cell death.

Clinical features

Initial features include:

- headache;
- nausea and vomiting;
- dizziness and signs of confusion.

Severe CO poisoning leads to coma, seizures, hypotension, and a metabolic acidaemia, all of which can lead to cardiac arrest and death. The classic cherry red skin colour is most likely to be seen post mortem rather than in live patients (except in the immediate periarrest period).

Diagnosis is based upon clinical suspicion, history, examination, and COHb levels measured on ABG. COHb in non-poisoned healthy patients is usually < 5%, but may be up to 8% in smokers. A value > 10% certainly suggests CO poisoning. ▶▶ Pulse oximetry values will be meaningless, as the COHb levels will contribute to the percentage reading.

Nursing intervention/management

- Ensure removal from the CO source.
- Ensure that the airway is patent, and administer high flow oxygen (100%).
- The half-life of CO is approximately 5h on breathing air, 1h on 100% oxygen, and 40min with hyperbaric therapy. If hyperbaric therapy is not locally available its value is debatable as COHb levels may already be significantly decreased with high flow 100% oxygen by the time a transfer is arranged. Those most likely to benefit from hyperbaric treatment include patients with a history of unconsciousness, a COHb > 20%, pregnancy (due to fetal haemaglobin levels), and cardiac complications such as MI and arrhythmias.
- Managing the critically ill patient in a hyperbaric chamber, however, presents its own problems, and may not actually be practicable.

Patients presenting with carbon monoxide poisoning will feel confused and unwell and need support and reassurance.

Nursing interventions for patients with alcohol-related problems

Apart from the standard physical assessment, the nursing role in relation to patients with alcohol-related problems is to deliver care in a non-judgemental way. Nurses are in an optimum position to use the 'teach-able moment' in the ED when patients are more receptive to advice. It is imperative that nurses as health promoters use each opportunity as it presents to highlight hazardous drinking and counsel patients. Nurses may be reluctant to intervene with abusive or violent patients, but some patients may be receptive to intervention. A number of screening tools are currently used for assessing hazardous drinking and dependency. These include the Paddington Alcohol Test (PAT) and the CAGE screening tool.

Useful information

Drinkline—National Alcohol Helpline, Tel: 0800 917 8282.

Alcoholics Anonymous UK, PO Box 1, 10 Toft Green, York YO1 7NJ. Helpline: 0845 769 7555 Web: ⌂ www.alcoholics-anonymous.org.uk.

Al-Anon Family Groups, 61 Great Dover Street, London SE1 4YF. Tel: 020 7403 0888. Web: ⌂ www.al-anonuk.org.uk

British Liver Trust, 2 Southampton Road, Ringwood BH24 1HY. Tel: 0800 652 7330. Web: ⌂ www.britishlivertrust.org.uk

Alcohol Education and Research Council (AERC), May 2005. Web: ⌂ http://www.aerc.org.uk/documents/pdf/insights

Further reading

Henry, J.A. and Wiseman, H. (eds.) (1997). *Management of poisoning. Handbook for healthcare workers.* World Health Organization, Geneva.

Poisons Information Centres in the UK

Mental health emergencies

Overview

Patients suffering from mental illness may turn to the ED in times of crisis or when their behaviour is of concern to their family or other health care professionals. However it is increasingly recognized that EDs often fall short in the care they offer this vulnerable group. The management of such patients often causes anxiety among emergency nurses as they may be unsure of how to assess and manage patients who are withdrawn or disturbed. Many EDs now have a dedicated psychiatric liaison service but ED nurses will still have a major part to play in their care, especially at triage or in generally looking after the patient. Patients presenting with mental health problems often have complex needs and ED nurses need much greater understanding to be skilled and competent in assessing and caring for them.

Assessing the patient with mental health problems

The initial assessment of the patient is of vital importance in ascertaining the extent of the patient's condition and determining the risk of harm to self or others.

- On assessing a patient presenting with a mental health problem, the nurse should ensure that there is another member of staff present if there are concerns about a patient's behaviour.
- Triage areas should have alarms and be designed so that an easy escape route is available.
- The nurse should greet the patient in a calm and welcoming manner, in an attempt to put the patient at ease. They should maintain eye contact throughout.
- Skilful questioning by the triage nurse is important so that relevant and pertinent information is obtained on the patient's condition.
  - ▶ Do not be afraid to ask questions that probe into the patients current mental state, e.g. 'how is your mood today?' or 'what was your intention when you harmed yourself?'
- Visual assessment of the patient is also important and can assist greatly in determining the extent of the patient's condition. The nurse should observe the following.
  - Patient's appearance. Look for any signs of self-neglect, e.g. poor hygiene.
  - Posture. Is the patient adopting a poor posture or displaying abnormal movements such as rocking or twitching? If so, note if the patient is maintaining eye contact.
  - Speech. Is it difficult to engage the patient in conversation, or is the speech quick and hurried (pressurized speech)? The content of conversation is also important to ascertain any delusions or hallucinations.
- Another possible aspect of the initial assessment is speaking with friends and family to find out about previous or current psychiatric care.

Many emergency nurses are unsure how to assess the risk of further self-harm or suicide attempts. As discussed, questioning is an important part of the initial assessment and staff should not be wary of asking questions such as those related to the self-harm act and the intentions of this.

Deliberate self-harm

Deliberate self harm (DSH) is an increasingly common presentation to the ED. It can be in the form of self-inflicted injury such as cuts, burns, or scratches or due to the ingestion of poisons or overdose (📖 see p.526).

While DSH and suicide are apparently increasing due to various social and psychological issues, many of those who engage in DSH may have a treatable mental disorder or substance abuse/dependence at the time of presentation to the ED.

Identifying the risk of further self-harm is an important component of the assessment. The triage nurse must ensure that their concerns are not only clearly documented but communicated to the team so all relevant staff are aware of the patient's vulnerability. Using a scoring system such as the Modified SAD PERSONS score is useful (📖 see Table 19.1).

- All DSH patients need to be in an area where they can be safely observed.
- Some patients may need persuading to stay for psychiatric assessment. If a patient is unwilling to stay but has obvious mental illness or diminished capacity, then urgent mental health assessment is indicated and appropriate measures should be taken to prevent the patient leaving.[1]

Treatment

- Many of the superficial injuries inflicted can be treated easily with simple first aid and wound care but some of the deeper lacerations and stab wounds, e.g. wounds to the face or those involving underlying structures such as nerves or tendons, need to be fully assessed and may need specialist opinion.
- If objects have been swallowed or inserted (into anus or vagina), the patient may also need referral to the appropriate specialty.
- Self-poisoning may be treated by the administration of activated charcoal, which reduces absorption of the substance. Treatment though is dependent on the substance and route of ingestion and advice should first be sought from the local poisons information centre (🖰 www.toxbase.org) (📖 see p.530).
- Attempted asphyxiation is traumatic for all those involved. Attempted hangings can cause injury through cerebral hypoxia as a result of asphyxiation and, less commonly, spinal cord injury, though the latter requires a strong noose and high drop height.
  - Patients on arrival should undergo usual ATLS procedures and may require respiratory assistance.
  - C-spine fractures should be considered and the patient should be C-spine immobilized until a fracture is ruled out (📖 see, p.260).
  - Injury to the neck can cause soft tissue swelling and airway obstruction so close observation of patient's respiratory rate, colour, and oxygen saturation is required.

General principles

- Unless patient is unconscious or has reduced GCS treatment should take place in a private and secure part of the ED in an area free of any sources for further self-harm (e.g. sharps bins, oxygen tubing, etc.).

- As far as possible the patient should not be left alone and should be in an area where maximum observation is possible.
- Wounds and self-poisoning should be treated by the emergency physician or ENP and a basic mental health assessment performed to assess the risk of further self-harm and the patient's desired outcome from self-harming.
- Security staff may be required to assist clinicians.
- The patient should then be reviewed by a mental health professional who will conduct a full mental health assessment and recommend admission or follow-up care.

Table 19.1 Modified SAD PERSONS score. Guide for referral and admission

	Score
Sex male	1
Age < 19 years or > 45 years	1
Depression/hopelessness	2
Previous suicide attempts or psychiatric care	1
Excessive alcohol or drug use	1
Rational thinking loss (psychotic or organic illness)	2
Separated, widowed, or divorced	1
Organized or serious attempt	2
No social support	1
Stated future intent (determined to repeat or ambivalent)	2

Interpretation of total score:

- < 6. May be safe to wait for psychiatric assessment in majors
- 6–8. Urgent psychiatric assessment
- > 8. Constant vigilance necessary while awaiting urgent assessment

Reference

1 National Institute for Clinical Excellence (NICE) (2004). *Self-harm: the short-term physical and psychological management and secondary prevention of self-harm in primary and secondary care*, Clinical Guideline CG016. NICE, London.

Obsessive compulsive disorder

Obsessive compulsive disorder (OCD) is characterized by the presence of obsessions or compulsions or both.

- **Obsessions** are defined as an unwanted intrusive thought, urge, or image that repeatedly enters a person's mind. Often they are perceived by the person to be excessive or unreasonable. Some common obsessions are contamination, fear of harm, obsession with order and symmetry, urge to hoard useless possessions.
- **Compulsions** are repetitive behaviours or mental acts that the individual feels driven to perform.
  - A compulsion can be seen by others, e.g. checking a door is locked or a tap has been turned off: this is commonly referred to as 'ritual'.
  - A compulsion may also be a more covert or mental act that is not obvious to others, e.g. repeating a certain phrase in the mind (this is often known as 'rumination').

Patients are unlikely to present to EDs exclusively with OCD but this may be related to other conditions such as depression, acute anxiety, eating disorder, drug and alcohol addiction, and schizophrenia. Nurses, therefore, should bear in mind that OCD may just be a symptom of a more serious underlying mental health problem.

Patients with such ideas need to be cared for in a quiet environment free from excessive stimuli. Nurses should adopt a calm and understanding approach when dealing with patients with such symptoms.

The most important fact for emergency nurses to remember is that these obsessions and compulsions are real to the patient.

Post-traumatic stress disorder

After any traumatic event it is usual to experience a range of symptoms including anxiety, depression, and dramatic recollections of the event and a heightened sense of awareness and arousal. Most individuals find that these symptoms will reduce after a period of a few weeks.

Some patients though find that symptoms persist over a longer period of time. It is important that as emergency nurses we realize that some patients who present to EDs may go on to experience symptoms of post-traumatic stress disorder, particularly victims of sexual assaults, RTCs, and episodes of violence.

Anxiety and panic attacks

Patients who experience acute episodes of anxiety or panic are common presentations in the ED. A panic attack can be described as an episode of extreme fear and is usually combined with a multitude of symptoms that have a rapid onset and can occur spontaneously or be associated with certain stimuli such as crowded places.

- Common symptoms associated with anxiety are tachycardia and palpitations, chest pain, shortness of breath and hyperventilation, dizziness and faint, shaking, and numbness to limbs.
- These symptoms may be associated with other conditions such as cardiac and respiratory conditions, drug misuse, thyroid dysfunction, and diabetic conditions.
- Basic investigations should be performed to rule out a physical cause (e.g. CBG, routine set of bloods, and basic observations).
- Performing simple observations is often therapeutic and is reassuring to patients who often feel there is something seriously wrong with them. The basic treatment in the ED, while excluding a medical cause, should be supportive and reassuring.
  - Try to care for the patient in a calm environment.
  - In severe cases, benzodiazepines may be of use in relieving the acute anxiety and fear.
- Referral to the psychiatric liaison service may be useful in managing the condition in the longer term.
- Organic causes for the symptoms must be ruled out before the diagnosis of a panic attack is reached. This is a high risk area for missing an acute physiological problem.

Phobias and phobic disorders

A phobia is an unreasonable fear of a certain situation or presence of certain object. This causes increased anxiety in the patient often to a high level.

These disorders can be divided into three categories.

- **Agoraphobia** is an unreasonable fear of specific places or events and is commonly described as fear of open spaces. It can also include fear of crowds, fear of being left outside, and fear of travelling, especially alone.
- **Social phobia**. The patient suffers increased anxiety in social situations and may find themselves unable to speak or interact in even the smallest social gatherings.
- **Specific phobias**. Anxiety is increased in specific situations, e.g. response to a certain object (animate or inanimate), place, or procedure. Examples include spiders, cars, hospitals, X-rays, and needles.

The symptoms and treatment will be similar to those of acute anxiety, although the patient may require longer-term help to rationalize and conquer their fear.

Acute psychosis

This will be one of the main psychiatric conditions that emergency nurses will encounter.

- Acute psychosis can be a result of certain psychiatric conditions such as schizophrenia, bipolar disorder, and depression.
- It can also be caused by recreational drugs such as crack cocaine.
- It may also present in some physical illnesses such as HIV and AIDS, alcohol withdrawal, and even in elderly patients with sepsis or altered renal function.

Evaluation of symptoms of psychosis in the ED should focus on excluding underlying organic causes for the symptoms and includes recording of vital signs, ECG, CXR, and blood and urine analysis.

Features of psychosis

Hallucinations

Hallucinations are false sensory perceptions that occur while a person is awake and conscious.

Common types of hallucination include the following.

- Hearing voices when no one has spoken (auditory). The patient often blames the auditory hallucinations for telling them to self-harm or harm others or carry out acts that they would not normally perform.
- Seeing objects or beings that are not there (visual).
- Feeling a crawling sensation on the skin (tactile).

Less common are hallucinations related to taste or smell (olfactory).

> Whether the hallucinations are caused by psychiatric or physical causes it is important to remember that the patient may become agitated and frightened and should not be left unattended.

Delusions

Delusions are false beliefs in something untrue. They are irrational and defy normal reasoning and remain firm in the mind even when overwhelming proof is presented to dispute them.

Delusions are a common feature of several psychiatric conditions including schizophrenia and bipolar disorder. They can also feature in illnesses with an organic or physical cause such as dementia.

Delusions fall into five categories.

- Persecutory. The patient experiences feelings of paranoia and has an unshakeable belief that a person or persons are plotting against them or attempting to harm them.
- Grandiose. These delusions centre around an over-inflated sense of self-worth. The patient may believe that they have a unique mission in life or are of extreme importance.
- Jealousy. Usually centres on fidelity of partners with belief that their partner has been unfaithful.
- Erotomanic. Individuals hold the belief that another person is in love with them. Often this is someone famous or important.
- Somatic. These involve the belief that something is wrong physically and that the patient is suffering from a serious medical problem.

Management

Whatever the reason for a patient presenting to the ED with psychotic symptoms the patient is clearly going to be upset and frightened and they may exhibit aggressive or violent behaviour. Emergency nurses must be competent and able in dealing with these patients, ensuring their own safety as well as that of the patients.

• Many trusts offer training in managing violence and aggression. These teach de-escalation techniques, which can be extremely useful in these situations.
• Patients should, where possible, be cared for in an environment that is calm and has minimal external stimuli.
• The same people, where possible, should care for the patient as this is important in developing a relationship of trust with the patient.

Dementia and delirium

Dementia is a syndrome with many causes characterized by progressive decline in cognitive function, personality and behavior. Although dementia is more common in the older patient population, it may occur in a younger patient. Higher mental functions are affected first in the early phase of the disease. As the disease progresses the patient may become more disorientated and present in an acute confusional state not knowing where they are or what day of the week, month or even what year it is. They may also not recognize their carers'. It is very important for ED staff to understand that patients with existing cognitive impairment are at 5 times the risk of having episodes of delirium. Some mental illnesses, such as depression and psychosis, may also produce symptoms which must be differentiated from both delirium and dementia.

Delirium (acute confusional state)

Delirium is essentially reversible brain failure and is a medical emergency. It is a rapidly developing disorder of disturbed attention that fluctuates with time. Delirium is largely unrecognised and untreated in the acute setting as it is often confused with dementia. 20% of older patients in hospital will develop delirium but it can occur at any age.

Causes

- Infection.
- Pain.
- Dehydration/constipation.
- Recent injury/surgery.
- Admission to hospital.
- Prescribed Medication.

Although the signs and symptoms of delirium vary from patient to patient, there are several characteristic features that help make the diagnosis

- Fluctuating conscious level typically worse as the day progresses and at night.
- Disorientation more marked than ususal.
- Hallucinations/psychosis.
- Ataxia.
- Incontinence.
- Dysarthria.
- Withdrawn/listless but can be hyperactive and/or disruptive.

ED staff need to be aware that the ED is a frightening and disorientating place for patients who have any level of confusion. It is also very stressful for carers. It is imperative therefore that these frail elderly patients are prioritised and transferred to quieter more conducive environments as soon as clinically safe.

Relatives are key in the safe and effective management of these patients so engaging them at the outset is essential.

Sedation and restraint of patients

Sedation is often a contentious issue in EDs as it is often difficult to balance the need for sedation against the need for a patient to be able to undertake a full psychiatric assessment.

Restraint

This is another area that emergency nurses find difficult.

- Only those who have received training in restraint techniques should undertake this task as wrongly applied restraint can lead to injury of the patient and the staff members involved.
- Some trusts offer training in control and restraint techniques and often combine this with de-escalation techniques that may reduce the need for restraint. All emergency nurses should undertake such training.
- Patients do not have to be under arrest or section to be restrained. Common law allows restraint if a person is assessed by trained staff to be a risk to themselves or others.
- Restraint should use a level of force that is reasonable and appropriate and for the minimum amount of time.
- One member of staff should lead the team and also be responsible for the patient's head and neck and for observing the airway, etc.[1]
- Rapid tranquillization or restraint should only take place when all other efforts to calm the patient have failed and it is obvious that harm will come to the patient or others if measures are not taken.

It is important for ED staff to recognize the signs of impending disturbed or violent behaviour in a patient as measures can be taken to diffuse the situation, thus eliminating the need for restraint or medication.

- Common features of impending violence in an individual may be restlessness, anger, increase in respiratory rate and blood pressure, and increase in rate of speech.

Methods of chemical restraint

- Before sedation is given to a patient the nurse must ensure that resuscitation equipment is nearby in the event of any adverse reaction.
- Risks associated with sedation include loss of consciousness, airway obstruction, and cardiac or respiratory problems.
- Use of anaesthetic drugs in restraint is rare and should only be carried out in the resuscitation area in the presence of an anaesthetist.
- NICE have produced guidelines into the rapid tranquillization of violent patients.[1]

Oral tranquillization

This is the preferred option.

- Nonpsychotic: 1–2mg lorazepam.
- Psychotic: 1–2mg lorazepam + antipsychotic such as haloperidol.

Intramuscular tranquillization

Use IM tranquillization where oral tranquillization has failed or has been refused.

- Nonpsychotic: 1–2mg lorazepam (maximum of 4mg in 24h).
- Psychotic: 1–2mg lorazepam + 0.5–10mg haloperidol.

IV tranquillization

IV tranquillization is used where immediate tranquillization is essential.
- 2mg lorazepam or 0.5–10mg haloperidol.
- The BNF recommends that lorazepam be diluted with a similar amount of water for injection.

Reference

1 National Institute for Clinical Excellence (2005). *Violence: the short-term management of disturbed/violent behaviour in in-patient psychiatric settings and emergency departments*, Clinical Guideline CG05. NICE, London.

Depression

Patients suffering solely with depression are unlikely to present to the ED However, depressive symptoms may be part of a wider picture.

- Patients who are severely depressed may present to the ED as a result of self-harm or poisoning as in overdose or as a result of self-neglect, e.g. not eating or drinking.
- Depression may also be the result of an increase in alcohol consumption or drug addiction.
- On occasion depression may be due to a serious physical illness such as HIV/AIDS or any chronic illness.

Depression can be a debilitating condition. People often say 'I am so depressed' and everyone feels sadness from time to time, but this is very different to someone suffering major or chronic depression who may experience feelings of worthlessness, low self-esteem, and lack of purpose or achievement in their life. They may also experience disturbed sleep and feel constantly tired.

Major depression

- Symptoms of depression include:
  - feelings of gloom and doom;
  - loss of interest in work, home, family, leisure activities;
  - weight loss or weight gain;
  - changes in sleep pattern (early morning wakening is common);
  - constant tiredness;
  - suicidal thoughts.
- Recreational drugs such as cannabis and cocaine can also cause the symptoms of depression and depression can be a side-effect of some prescription medicines.
- Depression can also be the reaction to an event or environmental factor, e.g. the death of a loved one, losing employment, financial and personal problems.
- **Seasonal affective disorder** (SAD) is a reaction to the change from summer to winter and is usually prevalent in autumn months when the clocks change and the nights become longer. SAD is characterized by an increase in levels of anxiety, overeating, and extreme fatigue.
- Postnatal depression affects some women following childbirth.
- Manic depression as part of bipolar disorder is discussed in 📖 see 'Bipolar disorder' p.555.

Bipolar disorder

Bipolar disorder is characterized by two phases of the illness, the depressive phase and the manic phase. EDs are more likely to encounter patients with bipolar disorder in the manic phase of the illness.

The symptoms of the depressive phase are detailed in 📖 see Depression p.554. The manic phase is thought to present after 2–4 episodes of the depressive phase. Symptoms may include the following.

- Insomnia.
- Pressure of speech.
- Feeling of all being well and full of new ideas, delusions, and hallucinations.
- Grandiose delusions are prevalent.
- Patients may also change their appearance in this phase and resort to garish colours in clothing and make-up.

Treatment of the manic phase in the ED will centre on calming the patient and ensuring a safe environment. In extreme cases hospital admission is often necessary.

Admission to hospital with a psychiatric illness

Admission to hospital for mental health conditions is less common now due to the increase of care in the community. Many acutely ill patients may be cared for in their own homes by community psychiatric nurses or separate teams who manage the acute episode of the illness, e.g. crisis teams.

Occasionally admission to an inpatient ward is necessary. Patients suffering mental illness in the ED may be admitted to hospital via informal admission, where the patient agrees voluntarily to admission to hospital, or be admitted under a section of the Mental Health Act 1983.

Admission under a section of the Mental Health Act 1983
▶ Note that mental health legislation is different in Scotland.

The Mental Health Act is a long and complicated document and outlines the conditions for application for and detention of patients suffering mental illness. It also sets out the rights of patients detained under the act and the appeals process if a patient disagrees with detention.

Where a patient is acutely unwell and is considered a danger to himself or herself or another person then the law allows for compulsory admission to a mental health facility. The Mental Health Act has many different parts but the main areas that ED staff will encounter are the following.

Section 2
- This is a compulsory admission for assessment or for assessment and treatment.
- In the ED the usual procedure is that the patient is assessed by a mental health practitioner and, if it is felt that admission may be required and the patient is unwilling, a team of 2 doctors and a social worker will come and assess the patient. If compulsory admission is necessary then an application for admission to hospital under the Mental Health Act is made.
- In the ED the application for admission is normally made by a social worker, known as an 'approved social worker', i.e. a social worker who is specially trained in mental illness and approved by the borough they are working for to assess mentally ill patients.
- The patient's nearest relative can also make the application.
- Two doctors, one of who must be approved by the Secretary of State or health authority as being experienced in assessing the mentally ill, must also examine the patient. Both must give a recommendation for admission and treatment and this must be recorded on the section forms.
- Section 2 can last up to 28 days.

Section 3
- This is a compulsory admission to undertake treatment.
- The procedure for application and implementation is the same as for Section 2. This section can last up to 6 months and can be renewed after this.

Section 4
- This is a section for admission in case of emergency and lasts up to 72h to allow full assessment and examination to take place. After this a further, longer section may be applied.
- This section is similar to Sections 2 and 3 but only one doctor need make the medical recommendation.

Section 136 (Place of Safety Order)
- The police apply this when someone in a public place is acting in a manner that suggests they may harm themselves or others.
- The Police may apply a Section 136 to allow removal of the person to hospital for examination.
- Some EDs are not a place of safety and in this case the place of safety could be the nearest mental health unit.

Management of compulsory admission

Compulsory admission may be very upsetting for the patient and their families and sensitivity is required in dealing with these cases.

Often admissions from EDs to mental health facilities may involve patients being transferred to another site.
- Where a section has been applied the patient should be escorted by a nurse and the approved social worker, who will bring the Section papers to the admitting facility.

Transport to the admitting hospital must be carefully planned and the patient should be in a stable condition and safe enough to travel.

Skills reminder

Introduction

This chapter aims to provide a quick reference guide to the numerous skills that are used every day in emergency care settings. It is not meant to be a definitive guide for the uninitiated but a quick clinical reminder that can be used in practice. Where relevant you will find information about the following: rationale for the skill/procedure; equipment needed; nursing role; how to perform the procedure; patient assessment and monitoring; and any special considerations.

This chapter aims to provide a quick refresher for skills not routinely used. It could also be used by the experienced nurse when teaching junior/inexperienced staff unfamiliar with various procedures.

❶ An assumption has been made that safe sharps disposal and the correct level of infection prevention and control will be undertaken when any clinical skill is performed. For this reason the repeated mention of sharps disposal, handwashing, eye protection, and sterile gloves, gowns, and aprons has been omitted from each of the skills in this chapter.

There are many skills in emergency care that are transferrable between adults and children. Where there are specific 'paediatric considerations' (📖 see symbols and abbreviations, p.xxv) to a particular skill, this is denoted by the following ⊕.

Airway management

Ensuring that all patients have an adequate and secure patent airway is, in most cases, the highest priority of care and an essential life-saving procedure. All nursing assessments should start with the 'ABC' of cardiopulmonary resuscitation. Without a patent airway any further patient assessment is futile and irreversible brain damage will occur within minutes.

The talking and fully conscious patient with a GCS of 15 is demonstrating the following.

- A patent airway.
- Ventilation is intact.
- The brain is being adequately perfused.

▶ Remember that a conscious patient with GCS 15 may still have debris or secretions in the airway that must be assessed.

- Any reduction in GCS will reduce airway muscle tone; this can cause the tongue to partially or completely occlude the airway and allow secretions to gather with a risk of aspiration.
- Following facial trauma there may also be blood, swelling, and/or foreign bodies such as teeth in the airway.

Nursing role

- Assess the airway for patency.
- Use manual methods to open an obstructed airway.
- Use basic airway adjuncts to intervene if the airway is compromised, e.g. suction, oral airway.
- Assist in the maintenance of the airway using advanced airway adjuncts, e.g. intubation, surgical airway.
- Deliver oxygen when required using appropriate methods.
- Continually assess airway patency and ventilatory status of the patient using clinical observation and relevant monitoring.
- Explain procedures clearly to the patient and any family members.

Look, listen, feel

This is the standard assessment approach that should be used when assessing the airway of any unresponsive patient.

- Look for chest rise and fall.
- Listen for breathing and any abnormal airway sounds.
- Feel for breath.

Manual airway opening manoeuvres

Any patient who is not able to open their mouth when asked should have it manually opened and inspected for actual or potential obstruction. Any abnormal finding following the 'look, listen, feel' assessment (📖 see Airway management, p.561) also requires further intervention. The tongue is the most common cause of airway obstruction in a patient with a reduced GCS. Manual airway opening techniques are a simple and effective way of lifting the tongue from the oropharynx in many situations.

Head tilt/chin lift (Fig. 20.1)
- Place the palm of one hand on the patient's forehead.
- Gently extend the neck by lifting the chin in an upward direction with thumb and/or fingers of the other hand.

❶ Not to be used following trauma in case the C-spine is injured. In these instances a jaw thrust is required.

Jaw thrust (Fig. 20.2)
Must be used in injured patients and is also an alternative if a head/tilt, chin/lift is unsuccessful.
- Stand behind the patient.
- Place the tip of the index fingers of each hand on the angle of each mandible (the heel of the hand can rest of the patients cheek if there is no sign of facial injury).
- Lift the jaw upwards, towards the ceiling.

▶ Following any airway intervention, the patient must be reassessed for signs of airway patency and/or effective breathing. Continuous monitoring of vital signs is mandatory at all stages of airway management.

Airway opening manoeuvres in children
❹ The upper airway anatomy in infants and children differs from that of the older child and adult. ∴ there are some slight differences in management.

Head tilt/chin lift
- In an infant: neutral position with slight chin lift.
- In a small child: slight head tilt chin lift.

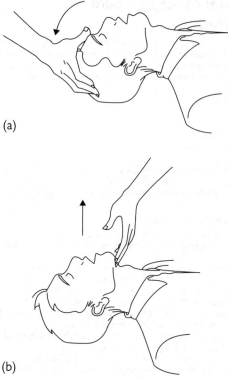

Fig. 20.1 (a) Performing a head tilt. (b) Performing a chin lift (Reproduced with permission from Thomas, J. and Monaghan, T. (eds.) (2007). *Oxford Handbook of Clinical Examination and Skills*, p. 576. Oxford University Press, Oxford.)

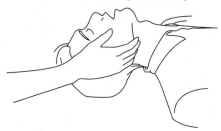

Fig. 20.2 Performing a jaw-thurst. (Reproduced with permission from Thomas, J. and Monaghan, T. (eds.) (2007). *Oxford Handbook of Clinical Examination and Skills*, p. 597. Oxford University Press, Oxford.)

Removal of foreign bodies/ secretions

Once the tongue has been manually lifted from the oropharynx the airway needs further assessment for the presence of foreign bodies. The airway is at risk of aspiration if protective reflexes are lost.

The airway must be assessed for the presence of the following.

- Vomit.
- Secretions.
- Blood.
- Teeth.
- Foreign bodies.
- Swelling.

- Gurgling suggests liquid foreign bodies.
- Snoring suggests tongue obstruction.
- Stridor suggests foreign body obstruction.

Removal of foreign bodies

- Liquid foreign bodies (blood, saliva, vomit, secretions) should be removed by gentle suction under direct vision using a rigid Yankauer sucker.
  - ⚠ Care must be taken to ensure the Yankauer is not advanced to the back of the throat, which may stimulate the gag reflex or cause laryngospasm spasm and compromise the airway further.
  - Fine-bore flexible suction catheters can also be used and are ideal when an airway adjunct is in situ as they can be fed though the airway to reach secretions in the oropharynx.
- Solid foreign bodies should be removed from the mouth/oropharynx under direct vision using suitable forceps.
  - 🔧 ⚠ Care must be taken not to push the object further into the trachea as this may result in the need for a surgical airway. This is of particular relevance in children who have a 'cone-shaped' larynx so that FBs are most likely to become wedged.

Simple airway adjuncts

Simple airway adjuncts should be inserted to relieve airway obstruction by the tongue. When inserted properly the health care professional may no longer need to manually maintain the airway through head/tilt, chin/lift, or jaw. However simple airway adjuncts are not a definitive means of airway protection as the aspiration of blood, vomit, and other secretions can still occur.

Oropharyngeal airway

An Oropharyngeal airway (also known as an OPA, Guedel airway, or oral airway) is a curved and flattened plastic tube with a reinforced flange at the outer end. OPAs come in four adult sizes (5, 4, 3, 2) and three (1, 0, 00) for children. They must be measured to ensure the correct size is inserted.

- Indications. Patients with tongue obstruction and an absent gag reflex.
- Contraindications. Presence of a gag reflex as the patient may vomit or develop laryngospasm. in this case a nasopharyngeal airway is preferred.

Sizing Place the OPA along the side of the face with the flange at the incisor. The tip should end at the angle of the mandible.

Insertion

For adults do the following.

- Open the patient's mouth
- Insert the OPA upside down into the mouth (the tip should point to the roof of the mouth).
- Once the tip reaches the end of the hard palate rotate the OPA 180°.

▶ This method of insertion ensures that OPA does not push the tongue further into the oropharynx.

Alternatively, the OPA can be inserted under direct vision using a tongue depressor to anchor the tongue forward allowing the OPA to be inserted the right way up.

⊛ ▶ This alternative method is the advised method in children and infants.

Considerations

- Improper sizing may cause trauma and bleeding in the airway.
- If the OPA is too large it may close the glottis and thus occlude the airway.
- A patient having a seizure with clenched teeth will not tolerate an OPA.

Nasopharyngeal airway

A nasopharyngeal airway (also known as an NPA) is a flexible tube designed to be inserted into the nasal passage to secure an airway. It has a bevel at the insertion end and a flanged end to which a safety pin is attached prior to insertion. The NPA is also curved along its length to allow easy placement within the nasal passage. An NPA can be used when a gag reflex is present and is often used in the post-ictal patient. NPAs come in several pre-set sizes (6.0–9.0). (Smaller sizes are available for children.)

- Indications. Patients with airway obstruction ± a gag reflex.
- Contraindications. Suspected base of skull fracture.

Cautions

- Known history of nasal polyps.
- Known history of epistaxis.

Sizing

There are several approved methods for sizing.

- Measure from the tip of the patient's nose to the tragus of the ear.
- Does the tip easily insert into the nostril without causing it to blanch? This will be the right size.
- The diameter of the tube is the same as the patient's little finger; this will be the right size.

Insertion

- Insert a safety pin into the flanged end.
- Lubricate the NPA with a water-based gel.
- With the concave aspect facing upwards, the NPA is inserted posteriorly into the nostril using a gentle rotating motion (a small clockwise motion followed by a gentle anti-clockwise motion) until the flange rests against the nostril.

If there is difficulty inserting the NPA, consider using the other nostril. Do **not** force the NPA into the nasal passage. If well lubricated and the right size it should slide fairly easily into place.

Considerations

- Improper sizing can cause trauma and bleeding to the nasal passage.

▶ Following any airway intervention, the patient must be reassessed for signs of airway patency and/or effective breathing. Continuous monitoring of vital signs is mandatory at all stages of airway management.

Laryngeal mask airway (LMA)

A LMA provides an alternate airway adjunct for use with bag–valve–mask ventilation. It comprises a tube with an inflatable cuff that is inserted into the pharynx and, when inflated, sits tight over the larynx. Although not the gold standard for airway management in cardiac arrest, LMA insertion is increasingly used when there is no one immediately available with intubation skills. An LMA may not fully protect the airway from aspiration. In difficult intubation situations when the C-spine is not at risk LMA can be a useful airway adjunct.

- Indications.
  - GCS of 3/15 to ensure absent gag reflex.
  - Inability to maintain a patent airway with simple airway opening manoeuvres.
  - Can be used as a temporary alternative in difficult endotracheal intubation.
- Contraindications.
  - Trauma.

Sizing

An LMA can be selected based on the size and weight of the patient requiring airway support (Table 20.1). Clinical studies have shown that a better seal is obtained by using a larger size LMA with less air volume inserted into the cuff. Therefore, start by choosing the largest size you think will fit and inflate with the smallest volume required to obtain an adequate seal. Using too small a mask and overinflating the cuff will decrease compliance and may result in a poor fit within the laryngeal space.

Equipment required

- Bag–valve–mask (BVM).
- Selection of LMAs
- Lubricating jelly.
- Syringe with adequate volume for LMA cuff.
- Pulse oximeter.s
- Catheter mount and ventilator if required.

Inserting

- Oxygenate patient prior to insertion.
- Lubricate the cuff.
- Push the apex of the mask with the open end pointing downwards toward the tongue into the back of the mouth. The tube follows the natural bend of the oropharynx and rests over the larynx.
- Once you are unable to push the tube further back, inflate the cuff to achieve a good seal
- Connect BVM and auscultate the lung fields to ensure good air entry.
- Connect catheter mount and ventilator if required.
- Check SpO_2.

❸ Table 20.1 Sizing an LMA

LMA size	Suitable patient	Maximum cuff inflation volume
1	Neonates/infants < 5kg	4mL
1.5	Infants 5–10kg	7mL
2	Infant/child 10–20kg	10mL
2.5	Child 20–30kg	14mL
3	Child 30–50kg	20mL
4	Adult 50–70kg	30mL
5	Adult 70–100kg	40mL
6	Adult > 100kg	50mL

Endotracheal intubation

Endotracheal intubation involves the insertion of an endotracheal tube (ETT) into the trachea. It is the definitive method of airway control as the airway is protected from aspiration and the ETT provides a means of mechanical ventilation. In emergency situations an ETT is usually passed through the oral route. Prior to transfer the nasal route may be used.

During cardiac arrest intubation is performed without the need for anaesthetic drugs. However, in most other situations it will be performed as part of a rapid sequence induction (RSI) where induction agents, muscle relaxants, and anaesthetic agents are required.

Indications for intubation

- High aspiration risk.
- Apnoea.
- GCS < 9.
- Sustained seizure activity.
- Unstable mid-face trauma.
- Airway injuries.
- Large flail segment.
- Respiratory failure.
- Inability to otherwise maintain an airway or adequate oxygenation.
- Ventilation.

ETT sizes

- 7.0, 7.5, or 8.0 for women.
- 8.0, 8.5, or 9.0 for men.
- Term babies: 3.0 or 3.5.
- ⊕ For other children use the calculation (age/4) +4.

Nursing role

The nurse must assemble and check the equipment (📖 see Box 20.1)
▶ The patient must receive full monitoring before, during, and after the procedure.

Cricoid pressure will be required in all intubations using RSI and may also be requested during cardiac arrest intubations. The correct and sustained application of downward pressure supplied by the thumb and forefinger over the cricoid cartilage will protect the airway from aspiration. This technique can also assist in the visualization of the vocal cords and increase the ease of inserting the ETT. Cricoid pressure must be applied and removed only following the instruction of the intubating clinician.

▶ Cricoid pressure should only be undertaken by clinicians trained and experienced in its application.

Box 20.1 Endotracheal intubation: equipment needed and checks required

- ETT with 10mL syringe of air and lubricating gel.
  - Inflate ETT cuff with 10mL of air and check for leaks.
  - Deflate cuff.
  - Lubricate with gel.
- Laryngoscope
  - Check that it is correct blade as requested.
  - Use straight blades in children: size 1, infant; size 2, older children.
  - Check that light bulb is working.
- Suction. Check that it is turned on and working effectively
- Bag–valve–mask with connecting catheter mount, filter, and oxygen.
  - Check that oxygen turned on at 15L/min and reservoir full.
  - Prior to intubation a face mask will be used.
- Ribbon gauze to tie in the ETT. Check that it is of suitable length.
- Bougie or stylet (for difficult intubation; acts as a guide through narrow airways). Ensure that it is clean and the type requested
- Stethoscope. Use to check bilateral air entry.
- SpO_2 monitoring. Check that there is good placement and signal strength.
- Waveform capnography. Connect to monitor.

Paediatric considerations

- ❶ Children are more difficult to intubate than adults due to different upper airway anatomy. Specific equipment is required and an intubating clinician who has experience in managing children's airways.
- Uncuffed ETT should be used in pre-pubescent children to reduce the development of subglottic stenosis.

Considerations prior to/during intubation

- The patient must be pre-oxygenated with high flow oxygen delivered by bag-valve mask for at least 15sec.
- The intubation should take no longer than 30sec. After 30sec (which the nurse should time) the intubation should stop and pre-oxygenation should resume.

Checking tube placement following intubation

- Observe for bilateral chest rise and fall.
- Observe oxygen saturations.
- Attach to capnography and observe recordings.
- Chest auscultation for bilateral air entry.
- Auscultation over the epigastrium for gurgling indicating oesophageal intubation.

Surgical airway

A surgical airway is described as 'the technique of failure' as it should only be used in situations where all other methods of securing the airway have been attempted and failed. All techniques require knowledge of the regional anatomy and should only be performed by or under the instruction of an experienced and skilled clinician.

Cricothyroidotomy

This procedure provides a temporary emergency airway in situations where there is obstruction at or above the level of the larynx, such that oral/nasal, endotracheal intubation is impossible. It is a relatively quick procedure, taking < 2min to complete.

There are two main techniques (for more information 📖 see p.574).

- Percutaneous needle cricothyroidotomy punctures the cricothyroid membrane and enables oxygenation through a fine bore cannula.
- Surgical cricothyroidotomy creates a surgical incision through which a tracheostomy tube is passed.

Indications

Need for an emergency airway when:
- standard endotracheal or nasotracheal intubation cannot be achieved or failed attempts;
- need to avoid C-spine manipulation;
- severe facial trauma;
- excessive haemorrhage obscuring the view of the vocal cords;
- oedema of throat tissues preventing visualization of cords;
- foreign body in upper airway.

Contraindications

- Inability to identify landmarks.
- Underlying anatomical abnormality.
- Tracheal transection.

⊕ In young children needle cricothyroidotomy followed by a tracheostomy is the preferred method.

Complications of a surgical airway

- Aspiration.
- Cellulitis.
- Haemorrhage/haematoma.
- False passage.
- Mediastinal emphysema.
- Subglottic stenosis.

Percutaneous needle and surgical cricothyroidotomy

Percutaneous needle cricothyroidotomy (Fig. 20.3)

- This technique can result in significant hypercarbia and should only be used for 30–40min.
- Needle cricothyroidotomy will provide oxygenation but will not ventilate; there will be no chest rise and fall.
- ABG sample should be monitored.

Equipment

- 12–14 Fr cannula
- 'Y' connector.
- Syringe.
- Oxygen delivery at 15L/min.
- Vital observation monitoring.

Procedure

- The skin over the cricothyroid membrane is pierced by the cannula which is then inserted into the trachea.
- The cannula is aspirated to confirm its position.
- The oxygen supply is connected via the Y-connector
- Deliver 15 L/min for an adult. In a child set the gas flow to the age of the child in years.
- Oxygenate by covering the patent port of Y-connector with a thumb to allow oxygen to flow for 1sec (transtracheal insufflation). Remove thumb to allow expiration for 4sec via the upper airway. Jet insufflation devices are also available to deliver the oxygen.

Surgical cricothyroidotomy (Fig. 20.4)

Equipment

- Skin cleansing solution
- Scalpel
- Curved forceps
- Plastic cuffed tracheostomy tube or cuffed ET tube (size 6-8 in the adult)
- Gauze
- Syringe to inflate cuff
- Tracheal suction catheter
- Catheter mount
- Ventilating device
- Securing device

Procedure

- The skin is dissected overlying the cricothyroid membrane and an incision made in the membrane so that the tracheostomy tube can be inserted.
- Once inserted the cuff should be inflated and the tube secured and attached to a ventilating device.

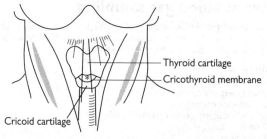

Fig. 20.3 Percutaneous needle cricothyroidotomy. (Reproduced with permission from Wyatt, J., et al. (2005). *Oxford Handbook of Accident and Emergency Medicine*, 2nd edn, p. 319. Oxford University Press, Oxford.)

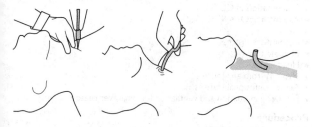

Fig. 20.4 Surgical cricothyroidotomy (Reproduced with permission from Wyatt, J., et al. (2005). *Oxford Handbook of Accident and Emergency Medicine*, 2nd edn, p. 319. Oxford University Press, Oxford.)

Arterial blood gas sampling

Arterial blood gas (ABG) sampling allows for immediate analysis of the patient's acid–base balance by sampling arterial blood. Most resuscitation rooms and critical care areas have an ABG machine.

Equipment
- Two tier trolley—cleaned.
- Sterile gloves and apron.
- Skin cleansing equipment.
- Appropriate blood gas syringe and needle.
- Gauze and tape.
- 1% local anaesthetic.

Indications
- Post cardiac arrest.
- Shock.
- Suspected PE.
- Exacerbation of COPD.
- Asthma if SpO_2 < 93%.
- DKA.
- Respiratory distress.
- Multiple trauma.
- Head injury.
- Hypoxia from any cause.
- Acute confusional state.
- Following intubation and ventilation for whatever reason.

Procedure
- Identify that you have the correct patient.
- If the patient is conscious explain the procedure to them and obtain consent. Explain to relative if appropriate.
- Assemble equipment needed for procedure and place on the bottom level of two tier trolley at the patient's bedside.
- Assemble appropriate equipment on the cleansed top level of the trolley.
- Select the appropriate site for arterial blood sampling. Most commonly the radial artery is used but femoral and to a lesser extent brachial can also be used.
- Perform an Allen's test to ensure patency of the ulna artery.

Allen's test
1 The hand is elevated with the fist closed for 30sec.
2 The ulnar and radial arteries are occluded by pressure.
3 The elevated hand is opened. It should appear pale (pallor can be observed at the finger nails).
4 Pressure over the ulnar artery is released and the colour should return in 7sec. This suggests that ulnar artery supply is sufficient and it is safe to puncture the radial artery.

If colour does not return or returns after more than 7sec, then the ulnar artery supply to the hand is not sufficient and ∴ the radial artery cannot be safely punctured.

- Expose the selected site and palpate for radial pulse. This is helped by hyperextending the wrist and resting it on a pillow.
- Palpate radial artery and cleanse skin with appropriate swab.
- Administer 1% local anaesthetic (LA) to subcutaneous area to reduce the pain. This is rarely done routinely in emergency care settings but reduces the amount of pain experienced by the patient considerably. LA also enables the patient to remain still during the procedure.
- Expel any bubbles and the heparin from the blood gas syringe.
- Introduce the needle at an angle of 60°, passing through the artery.
- Withdraw the needle whilst simultaneously pulling the plunger back slightly; carry on until blood begins to fill the syringe.
- When the syringe has filled to the appropriate level, withdraw the needle and apply pressure over the puncture site with gauze for 5min.
- Remove the needle from the syringe and apply the cap provided in the packaging. Label the syringe with trust approved identification. Send the sample for ABG analysis.
- Dispose of the all equipment.

Risks

- Introduction of infection.
- Leakage of blood and formation of haematoma.
- Pain.
- Needlestick injury.
- Contamination to the clinician.

Arterial line insertion and invasive blood pressure monitoring

▶ This should only be carried out in a closely monitored environment, such as critical care, ED resuscitation area, or theatre.

Indications

- When continuous BP monitoring is required in critical injury or illness.
- An arterial line also allows easy convenient access to the arterial circulation for ABG analysis.

Equipment

- Monitoring equipment.
- Pressure bag.
- 500mL bag of normal saline or heparinized saline.
- Transducer cable, arterial giving set (with red stripe running through to indicate arterial if available).
- Appropriately sized arterial catheter, long for femoral or short for radial. Smaller sizes for young children.
- Sterile dressing field, gloves, and apron.
- Suture pack.
- Appropriate sutures.
- 1% lidocaine.
- Variety of syringes.
- Skin cleansing equipment.
- Transparent dressing, arterial catheter label.

Procedure

- If the patient is not unconscious or sedated explain the procedure to the patient and/or relatives.
- Place the saline/heparinized saline bag into the pressure bag.
- Run the saline/heparinized saline through the arterial line set using the flush device to prime the line and ensure there are no bubbles.
- Inflate pressure bag to 300mmHg. This ensures that the infusion is under higher pressure than the patient's systolic BP and the fluid maintains the patency of the arterial catheter.
- Prepare the equipment ensuring that there is a sterile field around the chosen arterial insertion site.
- Following insertion of the arterial catheter connect the arterial line set aseptically. **Ensure** that all cannula connections are securely fastened.
- Secure cannula with transparent dressing and label the line.
- Connect the transducer cable to the arterial line set.
- Zero the transducer device.
- Turn the three-way tap distal to the patient 'off' to the patient and then open the port to air.
- Zero the monitoring equipment.

- Once zeroed, close the port and turn the three-way tap 'off' to the port.
- Secure the transducer device (level with the right atrium) with tape to the upper arm.
- The arterial line should produce a waveform on the monitor and the patient's BP and mean arterial pressure are displayed on the monitor screen. A mean arterial pressure of > 65mmHg indicates adequate perfusion.

Complications

- Massive blood loss.
- Infection.
- Loss of blood supply to hand.
- Injection of medications directly into the artery by mistaking it for venous access.

Bag–valve–mask ventilation

A BVM or 'Ambu' bag is a hand-held device that provides mechanical ventilation. A BVM consist of a self-inflating bag, a one-way valve, and a face mask. When a reservoir and supplemental high flow oxygen is attached 80–90% oxygen concentrations can be delivered. When the self-inflating bag is squeezed, the device forces air via a one-way valve into the patient's lungs. When the bag is released, it self-inflates, drawing in ambient air and any supplied oxygen, whilst the patient's lungs deflate through the one way valve.

Indications
- Respiratory arrest.
- Inadequate respiratory rate.
- Inadequate respiratory effort.

Complications
- Overinflating the lungs can damage delicate tissues.
- Air leak into the stomach causes gastric distension and possible vomiting.

Equipment
- Correct size BVM with reservoir.
- ☻ Appropriate sized face mask (0, 1, 2 for children; 3, 4, 5 for adults).
- Suction.
- Airway adjunct if required.
- Pulse oximeter.

Ventilating with a BVM
- The correct size BVM needs to be selected. An adult BVM can be used for any age but if the BVM is too small there will be inadequate ventilation.
- Ensure an adequate jaw thrust is employed.
- A good face mask seal must be achieved; this may require a 'two-person' technique (Fig. 20.6). One person uses both hands to secure the face mask. The second person operates the self-inflating bag.
- ☻ In children, a one person technique should use the following hand position (Fig. 20.5). The thumb and index finger form a 'C' shape and provide anterior pressure over the mask; the middle, ring, and little fingers form an 'E' on the line of the jaw and create the seal.
- Airway opening manoeuvres or an airway adjunct may be required.
- ☻ A self-inflating bag should be squeezed to deliver 5–6mL/kg of air (e.g. 50mL in a 10kg child; ~ 500mL in an adult).
- The patient's chest should visibly rise with each ventilation.
- A rate of 10–12 ventilations/min should be adequate for an adult.
- ☻ A rate of 20–30 ventilations/min is adequate for a child and 30–40 ventilations/min for an infant.

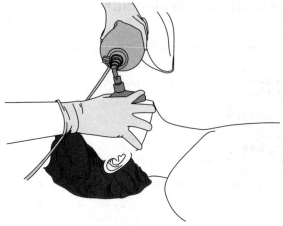

Fig. 20.5 ❺ One person BVM technique.

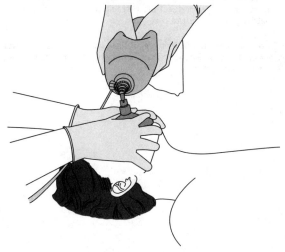

Fig. 20.6 Two person BVM technique.

Basic life support—adult

📖 See Fig. 20.7.
- Unresponsive?
  - Shake shoulders and ask loudly into both ears "are you alright?"
- Shout for help.
- Open airway.
  - Use head tilt and chin lift technique.
  - If possibility of C-spine injury use a jaw thrust.
- Not breathing normally?
  - Look, listen, and feel for up to 10sec.
  - Feel for a carotid pulse.
  - If breathing, place in recovery position.
- Call 999 if out of hospital
- In hospital pull emergency buzzer/put out cardiac arrest call.
- Give 30 chest compressions
  - Place the heel of one hand in the centre of the chest and the other hand on top, interlocking fingers.
  - Press down on the sternum 4–5cm, keeping arms straight.
  - Repeat at a rate of approx 100 times a minute.
- 2 rescue breaths: 30 compressions
  - Use bag and valve mask or pocket mask if available with highflow supplemental oxygen.
  - If not, take a normal breath and place lips around the patient's mouth ensuring a good seal. Blow steadily into the mouth whilst watching for the chest to rise.

▶ Stop to recheck the patient only if they start to breathe normally. Otherwise do not interrupt resuscitation. Continue until medical help/ advanced life support arrives.

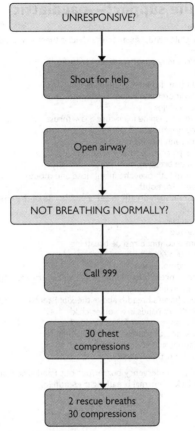

Fig. 20.7 Adult basic life support. (Reproduced with permission from The Resuscitation Council (2005). *Resuscitation guidelines*. Resuscitation Council, London. Available from ⏚ www.resus.org.uk)

Basic life support—paediatric

- Unresponsive?
  - Shake the child gently; speak to the child. Is there any age-appropriate response?
- Shout for help—in hospital get senior help.
- Open airway.
  - Use head tilt and chin lift technique.
  - Neutral position for an infant.
  - Sniffing for a child.
  - If possibility of C-spine injury use a jaw thrust.
- Not breathing normally?
  - Look, listen, and feel for up to 10sec.
  - If breathing place in recovery position.
  - Give 5 rescue breaths.
  - Infant, your mouth over the infant nose and mouth
  - Child, mouth to mouth
  - Deliver just enough breath to see a visible rise of the chest
- Feel for a pulse
  - Infant – brachial
  - Child – carotid
- Pulse >60bpm – continue rescue breathing
- No pulse or rate <60bpm
- Give 15 chest compressions
  - Infant – one fingers breadth above the xiphisternum, place 2 fingers, or hands encircling
  - Child – one fingers breadth above the xiphisternum, place the heel of one hand/two hands in an older child
  - Press down on the chest 1/3 of its depth.
  - Repeat at a rate of approx 100 times a minute.
- Give 2 ventilations and continue 15:2 ratio.
- Give CPR for 1min; then call 999.

▶▶ In hospital pull emergency buzzer/put out Paediatric Cardiac Arrest Call as soon as lack of normal breathing is identified.

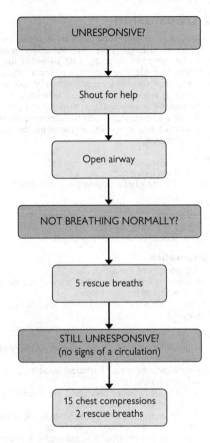

After 1 minute call resuscitation team then continue CPR

Fig. 20.8 Paediatric basic life support. (Health care professionals with a duty to respond) (Reproduced with permission from The Resuscitation Council (2005). *Resuscitation guidelines*. Resuscitation Council, London. Available from www.resus. org.uk)

Blood transfusion

The transfusion of blood and blood products is a fairly common occurrence in emergency settings. In the resuscitation room the procedure usually has to be carried out urgently, a full patient history may not be known, and there may not have been time to order fully cross-matched blood. In less critical situations cross-matched blood will have been ordered and the transfusion can be administered in a planned way. Whatever the method of administration the following principles must be followed as transfusion errors can have serious consequences. The administering clinician must also be familiar with local policies and procedures that relate to transfusion.

Indications
- Replacement of red blood cells.
- Replacement of clotting factors/other blood products.

Equipment
- Blood/blood product.
- Blood giving set with integral filter.
- Blood warmer should be used if > 50mL/kg/h.

Patient preparation
- Explain the procedure to the patient.
- Ensure the patient is wearing an identity bracelet that documents their name, date of birth, and hospital number.
- Ensure all patient identification checks have been carried out according to local policy.

Procedure
- Collect the blood/blood products, ensuring all the checking processes are completed correctly.
- When in the clinical area ensure the blood/blood products are checked again according to hospital policy.
- Ensure that the blood has been prescribed with reasons for transfusion clearly documented in the patient's notes.
- Transfusion must be commenced within 30min of the blood/blood product being collected from the hospital fridge.
- Record baseline temperature, pulse, blood pressure, and respiratory rate immediately before starting the transfusion.
- Document the transfusion start time and date on the compatibility form and drug chart.
- Record temperature, pulse, blood pressure, and respiratory rate 15min after commencement of transfusion.
- If vital signs within normal range at 15min, subsequent observations can be recorded at hourly intervals.
- Vital signs should be recorded at the end of the transfusion and the finish time documented on the compatibility form.
- Urine output must be monitored throughout the transfusion.
- Transfusion should be completed within 4 hours.

- All medications should be given as charted and in a timely way.
- If any transfusion adverse reaction occurs stop the transfusion immediately, record vital signs, and ask the medical team to urgently review the patient.
- Notify lab.
- Keep bag and giving set to which reaction has occured and return to lab. Keep IV line patient with saline.
- No meds to be given through the blood giving set/line.

Cannulation

▶ Cannulation is a routine emergency care skill. However there is a danger, because it is done so frequently, that important assessment steps are not taken.

Prior to cannulation considerations should be given as to why the cannula is being inserted and what it will be used for. This will allow the clinician to decide if a cannula is even needed and then to select the right sized cannula and the right site (📖 see Table 20.2).

Equipment
- One appropriately sized cannula.
- Skin cleaning product (as per Trust policy).
- One adhesive cannula dressing (check patient allergies).
- 10mL syringe with 5mL normal saline.
- Personal protective equipment, i.e. gloves and apron.
- Tourniquet.
- Kidney dish and sharps bin.

Procedure
- Introduce yourself to the patient, explain the procedure, and gain informed consent.
- Select a site for the cannula based on why it is being inserted.
  - If rapid transfusion of large amounts of blood/fluid is anticipated a large vein is needed . The antecubital fossa (ACF) is widely used for this purpose.
  - If a cannula is needed for medication or maintenance fluid a smaller vein can be used and is often better tolerated by the patient. The dorsum of the hand or cephalic vein as it runs over the radial aspect of the wrist can be used for this purpose.
  - The veins of the ankle/foot should be avoided due to the risk of DVT development.
  - Ideally the patient's non- dominant arm should be used.
- Look for a suitable vein and apply a tourniquet to assess it further.
  - Palpate the selected vein to assess its suitability. It should be bouncy, prominent, refill easily when depressed, and fairly straight to accommodate the length of the cannula.
  - ❸ Several sites should be assessed, particularly in children. This will ensure that the best vein has been selected and will minimize the number of attempts required.
- Clean skin with an appropriate agent/product according to Trust policy.
- Anchor the chosen vein by applying traction to the skin distal to the cannulation site so it becomes taunt. Do not release traction until cannula is in situ.
- Puncture the skin over the vein at a 30–45° angle. Observe for blood in the flashback chamber—the cannula is in the vein. Decreasing the angle, guide the cannula a little further into the vein 1–2mm. Gradually slide the cannula off the needle all the way into the vein.
- Discard the needle in a sharps bin.

- Apply cap to cannulae end or other appliance as per local policy.
- Secure with adhesive dressing.
- Flush cannulae as per local policy.

Risks associated with cannula insertion include:
- introduction of infection (including MRSA);
- haematoma formation;
- thrombosis of the vein;
- pain;
- allergy to device/dressing;
- phlebitis;
- cellulitis.

⊕ **Table 20.2** Cannula sizes and uses

Colour	Gauge	Indications
Yellow	24	Paediatric
Blue	22	Paediatric
Pink	20	Paediatric, 2–3 litres of fluid/24h
Green	18	Larger volumes
White	17	Rapid infusion, viscous solution
Grey	16	Rapid infusion, viscous solution
Brown	14	Rapid infusion of blood

Capnography

Capnography is the measurement of end tidal CO_2 and should be measured in all intubated and ventilated patients. Capnography measures the CO_2 content in the expired breath. The establishment of an end tidal CO_2 measurement confirms that the ETT is in the airway. A continuous trace enables the clinician to optimize the ventilator settings and tailor them to the patient's condition.

There are two principal ways of monitoring end tidal CO_2. The CO_2 level can be transduced through an airway adapter and then via a cable out to monitoring equipment, giving a continuous trace. Alternatively, a disposable device can be attached to the breathing circuit. This will change colour confirming the presence of CO_2. The disposable device will not give a continuous trace.

Equipment

- CO_2 airway adapter and transducer cable compatible with monitoring equipment.
- Disposable CO_2 detector.

Procedure

- After intubation ensure the ETT is held securely
- Connect the airway adapter between the ETT filter and breathing circuit (it usually will only fit one way round)
  - Disposable end tidal CO_2 detector. The colour of the detector changes according to CO_2 levels. If using these devices refer to the manufacturer's instruction about the interpretation of the colour change.
  - Transduced end tidal CO_2 monitors. Attach the transducer cable to the airway adapter; it will only attach one way. Connect the cable to the appropriate monitor (some machines need to be warmed up before use).
- With transduced end tidal CO_2 monitoring, a continuous waveform will be present on the monitor and give a numerical reading in either kPa or mmHg.
- With the disposable devices there will be a colour change in the presence of CO_2

Caution If the patient has drunk carbonated drinks or ingested antacids before intubation there can be CO_2 in the oesophagus. This could lead to a false reading if a misplaced oesophageal intubation occurs. Ordinarily CO_2 should not be detected in the oesophagus.

Cardiac pacing

Temporary transcutaneous cardiac pacing is an emergency procedure that is required when a patient has a symptomatic bradycardia. Transcutaneous pacing enables the patient's condition to be stabilized until a temporary pacing wire can be inserted.

Indications

- 3rd degree heart block.
- Ventricular standstill.
- Symptomatic bradycardias: hypotension; altered level of consciousness; chest pain; breathlessness. See ◌ www.resus.org.uk

Equipment

- Defibrillator with pacing facility.
- Pacing pads.
- Razor.
- Alcohol skin prep if the patient is clammy.
- Sedation.

▶ It is vital that the operator has a detailed knowledge of the defibrillator to be used—machines vary in their pacing capabilities and parameters.

Patient preparation

- Explain the procedure to the patient and family. There will be some discomfort felt as the machine delivers each paced beat and the patient may 'jolt'.
- Explain that this is a temporary procedure and that pain relief and sedation can be given.
- Ensure adequate pain relief.
- Ensure sedated if appropriate.

Procedure

- Prepare the chest skin and clip hair if there is time. If not, shave chest hair, taking care not to cause skin abrasions. If the skin is clammy wipe with alcohol skin prep.
- Ensure the patient is monitored through lead II via the 3 chest leads.
- Disconnect the defibrillator paddles if not already and connect the pacing cable.
- Connect a set of multifunction electrodes.
- Apply the pads (there is a diagram on each pad indicating where it should be placed). One pad to the right of the sternum just below the clavicle; the other to the 5th/6th intercostal space in the left anterior axillary line. ▢ See Fig. 20.9.
  - This pad position is quick and easy to perform. However, the anterior/posteriorly (front and back of the patient's chest) may be more effective in obtaining mechanical and electrical capture.
- Ensure the pads are well adhered.
- Plug the pacing pads into the pacing cable.
- Turn the pacer on.

- Using the other pacing buttons select the required:
    - mode ('demand' or 'fixed'). Demand is usually used;
    - paced pulses per minute (ppm). Start at 70ppm;
    - milliamps (mA). Start at the lowest setting.
- Your selection will be displayed in the pacing dialogue box on screen.
- When ready to start pacing press the start/stop button once. (Pressing this button again will stop pacing.)
- Establish electrical capture (a QRS complex should immediately follow a pacing spike). The mA will need to be slowly increased until electrical capture is achieved.
- Establish mechanical capture (check the patient's pulse).
- Once pacing is established monitor BP and heart rate and palpate a pulse every 5min.
- Prepare for transfer to coronary care for immediate transvenous cardiac pacing.

▶ If patients are symptomatic and an external pacing machine is not available you can perform external cardiac percussion using a clenched fist. With blows (more gentle than a precordial thump) delivered at a rate of 100/min you can produce a QRS complex.

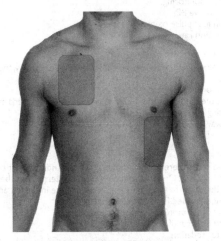

Fig. 20.9 Correct position of the gel pads or AED electrodes on the patient. Ensure that they are not touching or overlaying any wires, oxygen tubing or any other conducting maaterial. Ensure that the patient's chest is dry and shaved if particularly hairy. (Reproduced with permission from Thomas, J. and Monaghan, T. (eds.) (2007). *Oxford Handbook of Clinical Examination and Skills*, p. 639. Oxford University Press, Oxford.)

Cardioversion

Cardioversion is a procedure that delivers a synchronized electrical current at a specified moment in the cardiac cycle. It is used to terminate an abnormally fast heart rhythm in an unstable patient, e.g. ventricular tachycardia. Cardioversion should be carried out by an appropriately trained clinician and only when indicated. The nurse has a vital role in monitoring the patient and preparing them and their relatives for the procedure, which often has to be carried out rapidly.

▶ The nurse and clinician delivering the cardioversion ***must be*** familiar with the defibrillator and how to operate it for cardioversion and defibrillation.

Equipment
- Defibrillator.
- Adhesive conductive pads.
- Razor.
- Appropriate sedation.
- Full monitoring:
  - cardiac monitoring;
  - non-invasive BP;
  - continuous pulse oximetry;
  - respiration rate.

Patient preparation
- Explain the procedure to the patient and, where necessary, their relatives.
- Obtain informed consent.
- Connect the patient to the defibrillator using the 3 standard cardiac monitoring chest leads.
- Shave away any chest hair where the pads will be placed.
- Dry the skin.

Procedure
- Apply the pads (there is a diagram on each pad indicating where it should be placed). One pad to the right of the sternum just below the clavicle, the other to the 5th/6th intercostal space in the left anterior axillary line (📖 see Fig. 20.9, p.593).
- Ensure all other monitoring is attached.
- Administer oxygen if not already commenced.
- Administer sedation.
- The energy to be delivered is selected—a low dose to begin with, usually 50–100 joules. This can be increased.
- ☻ In children an initial dose of 0.5–1J/kg is used followed by 2J/kg if a second shock is required.
- Activate the synchronized function on the defibrillator.
- All staff are instructed to 'stand clear'.
- The shock is delivered.

- The rhythm is reassessed. If the tachycardia has not been reverted a second highly synchronized shock can be delivered.
- If a second shock is administered **ensure** the synchronized function is activated.
- When the rhythm is stabilized, record the patient's vital signs.

Catheterization—female

Urethral catheterization is the introduction of a catheter into the bladder for the collection and/or measurement of urine. The catheter may remain in situ for a period of time or can be removed once the bladder is drained.

Indications

- To relieve obstruction to the outflow of urine.
- To accurately monitor urine output.
- To protect skin when its integrity is compromised through incontinence.

Equipment

- Two tier trolley—cleaned.
- Catheterization pack.
- Sterile gloves—2 pairs.
- Disposable apron.
- 0.9% sodium chloride for cleansing.
- ⊕ Female catheters: sizes 10 and 12 (shorter in length) with 10mL of water for injection (usually included in the pack). ⊕ 📖 See Table 20.3 for paediatric sizes.
- Drainable urine bag ± hourly measurement.
- Clinical waste bag.

Patient preparation

- Explain the procedure to the patient.
- Obtain informed consent.
- Undress if not already undressed.
- Ensure privacy by performing procedure in an area that will not have any interruptions.
- Position the patient supine with their hands by their side. Do not expose the perineum until necessary.

Procedure

- Place bed protection under the patient in case of any spillages.
- Ask the patient to bend their knees bringing both heels together. Ask the patient to let their knees flop apart exposing the perineum.
- Apply both pairs of sterile gloves.
- Place sterile towels on either side of the perineum. Using a saline-soaked swab, clean from the top of the labia down towards the patient's anus until clean.
- Remove outer pair of gloves.
- Bring the sterile kidney dish and catheter. Rest them on sterile towels.
- Dip the catheter tip into the sterile sodium chloride to provide lubrication.
- Open the labia and insert catheter into the urethra, urine should appear in the tube, Continue to insert the catheter approximately 10cm, keeping the open end in the kidney dish.
- Attach the drainage bag.
- Insert the water for injection into the additional port.
- Gently retract the catheter tube slightly until stopped by the inflated balloon.
- Dispose of waste and wash hands and trolley.

- Measure the amount of urine drained.
- Clamp after 12 drained release after 30 mins.
- Assist patient to dress and maintain their dignity.
- Document the catheter inserted, water used to inflate the balloon, and urine drained.

Table 20.3 Paediatric sizing for catheters (both male and female)

ⓘ Age of child	Catheter size (Fr)
Neonate	5*
0–2 years	6
2–5 years	6–8
5–10 years	8–10
10–16 years	10–12

* It is common practice to use 5 Fr feeding tubes in this age group.

Catheterization—male

Rationale
- To relieve obstruction to the outflow of urine.
- To accurately monitor urine output.
- To protect skin when its integrity is compromised through incontinence.

Equipment
- Two tier trolley—cleaned.
- Catheterization pack.
- Sterile gloves—2 pairs.
- Disposable apron.
- Sterile anaesthetic lubricating jelly.
- 0.9% sodium chloride for cleansing.
- Male catheters × 2 size 14 and 16 (longer than female) with 10mL sterile water for injection (included in pack). (See Table 20.3, p.597 for paediatric sizes.)
- Drainable urine bag ± hourly measurement.
- Clinical waste bag.

Patient preparation
- Explain the procedure to the patient.
- Obtain informed consent.
- Undress if not already undressed.
- Ensure privacy by performing procedure in an area that will not have any interruptions.
- Position the patient supine with their hands by their side. Do not expose the perineum until necessary.

Procedure
- Place bed protection under the patient in case of any spillages.
- Ask the patient to expose their genitals.
- Apply both pairs of sterile gloves.
- Place sterile towel over genital area with a tear in the middle to expose the penis.
- Place a sterile swab around penis retracting foreskin and clean the glans with a saline-soaked swab.
- Remove outer pair of gloves.
- Insert a small amount of lubricating gel to the opening of the urethra wait a few minutes.
- Bring the sterile kidney dish and catheter. Rest them on sterile towels.
- Hold the penis in a vertical position.
- Insert the tip of the anaesthetic gel tube into urethra and administer the rest of the gel. (Wait ~ 3–5min so that the gel is able to coat the urethra and anaesthetize it.)
- Continue to hold the penis vertically. Insert the catheter all the way into the urethra (if any obstruction is felt gently insert catheter while asking the patient to cough).
- Attach the drainage bag.
- Insert the water for injection into the additional port.

- Gently retract the catheter tube slightly until stopped by the inflated balloon.
- Ensure foreskin (if present) is pulled forward again over the glans.
- Dispose of waste and wash hands and trolley.
- Measure the amount of urine drained.
- Clamp after 12 drained release after 30 mins.
- Assist patient to dress and maintain their dignity.
- Document the catheter inserted, water used to inflate the balloon, and urine drained.

🔆 For paediatric catheter size see p. 597, Table 20.3

Central venous pressure (CVP) line insertion and monitoring

CVP lines are often inserted into critically ill or injured patients as they provide direct access to the central circulation. Central access enables drugs and/or fluids to be given rapidly and to act immediately, and also allows close monitoring of pressures within the central venous system. CVP lines can accurately monitor intravascular volume and assess hydration and levels of hypovolaemia. It is a common procedure prior to transfer to intensive care.

Indications for insertion and CVP monitoring
- Shock.
- Inotrope infusion.
- Fluid resuscitation.
- Cardiac arrest.
- Multiple trauma.

Equipment
- Central venous catheter pack with appropriate number of lumens.
- Sterile dressing field, gloves, and gown/apron.
- Pressure bag.
- 500mL bag of normal saline or heparinized saline.
- Transducer set (with blue stripe to indicate venous, if available).
- Suture pack.
- Appropriate sutures.
- 1% lidocaine.
- Variety of syringes.
- Heparinized flush.
- Skin cleansing equipment.
- Transparent dressing; CVP line label.

Patient preparation
- Explain procedure to the patient and/or family.
- Help position the patient, usually flat with 10° head down tilt.
- Support patient during procedure.

Procedure
- Place the saline/heparinized saline bag into the pressure bag.
- Run the saline/heparinized saline through the transducer set using the flush device to prime the line and ensure there are no bubbles.
- Inflate pressure bag to 300mmHg. This ensures that the infusion is under higher pressure than the patient's systolic BP and the fluid maintains the patency of the line.
- Prepare the equipment ensuring that there is a sterile field around the chosen insertion site.
- Following insertion of the catheter connect the set aseptically.
  ▶ **Ensure** that all cannula connections are securely fastened.
- Secure cannula with transparent dressing and label the line.
- Connect the transducer giving set to the distal port if more than a single lumen (this should be labelled clearly on the catheter).

- Connect the transducer cable to the transducer giving set and connect to the monitor. CVP transducers are usually connected to the P1 connection on the monitor.
- Tape the transducer device to the upper arm in line with the heart
- Ensure that a CXR has been ordered post-insertion.

Complications

- Haemothorax.
- Pneumothorax.
- Cardiac arrhythmias.
- Thoracic duct trauma.
- Brachial plexus injury.
- Air embolism.
- Haemorrhage.
- Misdirection or kinking.

Measurement of CVP using a transducer

In resuscitation rooms the CVP measurement is transduced to monitoring equipment to give a continuous reading. CVP measurements can be undertaken manually using a pressure manometer. This is usually done in non-critical care areas.

- Position the patient.
- Turn the 3-way tap off to the patient, open to the air, and remove the cap.
- 'Zero' the monitor and wait for calibration.
- When 'zeroed', replace the cap and turn the 3-way tap on to the patient.
- The CVP trace should produce a waveform on the monitor associated with right atrial contraction and a measurement displayed as a number on the monitor screen.
- Document the measurement.

Normal CVP ranges are 5–10mmHg or 4–8cmH$_2$O.

Nursing role

- Monitor the CVP readings and document the measurement.
- Report any changes.
- Ensure the site is observed for haemorrhage or loose connections.
- Monitor for complications.
- If a multi-lumen line is being used, ensure no drugs are given via the distal port where the CVP is being monitored. This lumen often gets flushed or primed and the patient may receive a sudden injection of a drug, which could have a dramatic effect.

Cervical collar application

Cervical collars are devices used to immobilize the necks of patients whose mechanism of injury may have caused a C-spine injury. Patients need to stay immobilized in a cervical collar until their C-spine has been 'cleared' of possible injury (📖 see p.606).

Indications (📖 see p.606.)

Equipment

- Selection of different sizes of hard collar.
- Measuring device (optional).
- 2 people to apply collar (person one to hold and stabilize the neck; person 2 to apply the collar).
- Head blocks and straps.

Application

- Explain the procedure to the patient and/or relatives.
- Check motor and sensory function of the hands and feet prior to collar application.
- Prior to collar application, the patient should be positioned with the spine in alignment. Using your hands to support the neck slowly move the head until the neck is straight and the head faces forwards.
- Person 1. Ideally approach the patient from behind placing both hands either side of the face and neck. Spread fingers out along the occipital ridge and hold firmly. Maintain this position until both the collar and head blocks are in place.
  - ▶ *Do not let go until procedure is completed*.
- Person 2. Measure the patient for the correct size of collar following the manufacturer's instructions.
  - ▶It is important that you are familiar with the types of collars available, how they are sized/measurement for the correct fit, and how they are put together
  - Ensure chin support is folded out on collar.
- Person 2. Slide the back of collar under the back of the neck taking care not to move the head or neck. Sweep the front of the collar under the chin so that the chin sits on the chin rest and fasten securely.
- Person 1. As the collar is applied carefully move hands out over the collar so that, when the collar is secured, your hands are not inside.
- If the patient has been sitting during collar application they can be sat on a trolley with the backrest upright. Gradually move the backrest to a flat position.
- At this stage the neck is stable in the collar but not fully immobilized until the head has been secured with some form of immobilization device, e.g. head blocks and tape, spinal board.
- In patients who are cooperative the care of the immobilized C-spine is usually uncomplicated. They should be managed in a well observed area with oxygen, suction, and a call bell to hand.

Considerations

- 🧒 ❶ In adults or children who are uncooperative/combative for whatever reason the continuous presence of a nurse is mandatory.

The airway is at risk from vomiting or secretions and the adult/child may try to remove immobilization devices.

- 🔆 ❶ The combative adult/child should be managed in whatever way is possible without using forcible restraint as this increases the risk of further injury to the C-spine. Children may be most settled on a parent's knee with a collar in situ.

Chest drains

A chest drain is used to drain or 'decompress' the contents of the pleural space. Most commonly air occupies the pleural space. Following trauma, blood is more likely. Occasionally, other fluids may be present such as chyle, pus, or gastric/oesophageal contents. As contents fill the pleural space the underlying lung expansion is restricted and the lung 'collapses'. Pneumothoraces are classified as:

- Spontaneous/simple pneumothorax is a non-expanding collection of air around the lungs/pleural space caused by an injury to the lung tissue or spontaneous rupture of a pleural bulla.
- Tension pneumothorax is an expanding collection of air in the pleural space, which can be life-threatening if left untreated.
- Open pneumothorax caused by penetrating trauma as air allowed into pleural space via a wound—classically an 'open sucking chest wound'.
- Haemothorax is a collection of blood in the pleural space usually caused by blunt or penetrating trauma or occasionally through the erosion of pulmonary vessels by tumour.

Indications Symptoms vary depending on amount of air/fluid in pleural space. A small pneumothorax may have relatively few symptoms. The larger the area of 'collapse', the more significant the respiratory distress and the need for intervention with chest drain ± needle thoracocentesis. Presenting symptoms may include:

- Respiratory distress: breathlessness; tachypnoea; confusion.
- Increased work of breathing, accessory muscle use.
- Pleuritic chest pain.
- Pallor, greyness progressing to cyanosis.
- Reduced air entry on the affected side.
- Unequal chest rise.
- Reduced SpO_2.
- Hyperresonance to percussion on the affected side in pneumothorax.
- Dullness to percussion on the affected side in haemothorax.
- Sucking chest wound in an open pneumothorax.
- Deviated trachea, distended neck veins, hypotension/shock in tension pneumothorax.

Equipment

- 2 tier trolley.
- Sterile dressing field, gloves, and gown/apron.
- Chest drain insertion pack: scalpel, instrument for blunt dissection.
- Handheld suture (e.g. 1.0 silk).
- 1% lidocaine.
- Syringes.
- Needles.
- Skin cleansing equipment.
- Transparent dressing.
- Chest drain. Size depends on whether air or fluid needs to be drained and on weight of patient. Wider bore tubes are needed to drain blood. To drain blood/fluid in an adult use a size 28cH tube or larger. It is increasingly common to use smaller bore Seldinger chest tubes

(usually size 12cH) to drain air. In children smallest possible tube should be used. ✚ Use Table 20.4 as guide for tube sizes in children.
- Bottle of sterile water.
- Chest drainage system with tubing.
- Dressing to secure the drain. A large dressing is not necessary.

✚ **Table 20.4** Paediatric chest drain sizes (for draining blood/fluid)

Weight of patient (kg)	Chest tube size (Fr)
< 3	8–10
3–5	10–12
6–10	12–16
11–15	17–22
16–20	22–26
21–30	26–32
> 30	32–40

Preparation
- Prepare the chest drain bottle. Connect to chest drain when inserted.
- Using sterile technique open the chest drainage system.
- Pour sterile water into drainage bottle until it reaches the prime level.
- Connect one end of the tubing to the drainage system.
- The other end of the tubing is inserted into the chest drain.

Patient preparation
- Explain the procedure to the patient and/or relatives.
- Assist with positioning the patient. This depends on site of chest drain.
- Ensure appropriate monitoring is attached.
- Ensure pain is scored and analgesia is given.
- Ensure oxygen therapy is administered as required.
- Ensure patient has patent IV access and IV fluids as required.

Care following insertion of the chest drain
- Continue monitoring cardiovascular/respiratory status. Record observations.
- Rescore pain and give further analgesia as indicated.
- Check chest drain bubbling (swinging) at regular intervals. (Air and water in chest drainage system move with each inspiration/expiration.)
- Bubbling chest tube only to be clamped under specialist supervision.
- Do not allow the chest drain or tubing to 'kink'.
- Ensure the chest drainage system is protected from accidentally being knocked over by securing on a stand to the ED trolley.
- Do not allow the chest drain to be lifted higher than the insertion site.
- Ensure a repeat CXR is ordered.
- Monitor and record any fluid drainage every 15min for the first hour, every half hour for the next 2h, and hourly thereafter.

▶▶ Alert clinician for patient if > 500mL of blood drained. May need: urgent cross-match; rapid IV infusion of warmed fluids/blood; ABG.

C-spine assessment

The assessment, protection, and clearance of a potential C-spine injury is critical as poor management can lead to significant morbidity and mortality. Most patients who require C-spine protection and clinical assessment are already immobilized with appropriate devices in the pre-hospital setting. However, patients will often self-present with a significant injury that must be suspected in the first instance and then managed correctly.

▶ There are potential pitfalls, especially when the mechanism is unclear or the patient is vague about their symptoms.
• **Always** have a high index of suspicion and, if in doubt, immobilize
• Patients who do not have GCS 15 should be immobilized

Indications for assessment and possible imaging of the C-spine

Step 1
• Clinical suspicion of a neck injury and GCS 15.
• Is there any paraethesia in the extremities?
• Are they ≥ 65 years?
• Is there a potentially dangerous mechanism?
  • Fall from ≥ 1m or 5 stairs.
  • Axial load to the head.
  • High speed motor vehicle collision (> 60mph).
  • Roll over or ejection from vehicle.
  • Bicycle collision or motorized recreational vechicle.
• Are there any prior neck problems (making the neck more vulnerable)
  • Ankylosing spondylitis.
  • Rheumatoid arthritis.
  • Spinal stenosis.
  • Previous cervical surgery.

If the answer is yes to any of the queries in Step 1, apply a hard collar and use an immobilization device. A C-spine X-ray will be required as a minimum.

Equipment
• Appropriately sized collar.
• Immobilization device.

Patient preparation Explain the procedure to the patient, ensuring they understand the need to remain still whilst the assessment takes place.

Collar application 📖 see p.602.

No If the answer is no to all of the queries in Step 1, the assessment continues to Step 2, to identify if there are any 'safe assessment features'.

Step 2 Are there any safe assessment features?
• Simple rear end collision.
• Comfortable in a sitting position.
• Ambulatory since the time of injury and no mid-line C-spine tenderness.
• Delayed onset of neck pain.

No safe assessment features ⚠ Apply a hard collar and use an immobilization device. A C-spine X-ray will be required as a minimum.

One or more safe assessment features The presence of one 'safe assessment feature' indicates that it is safe to assess the range of movement of the neck as in step 3.

Step 3 Range of movement assessment
Has the patient got 45° left and right lateral rotation?
- If the answer is **yes** patient does not require C-spine immobilization.
- ⚠ If the range of movement is limited or painful, apply a hard collar and use an immobilization device. A C-spine X-ray will be required as a minimum.

▶▶ If in doubt immobilize the neck and do not delay in providing protection!

Further information

See www.nice.org.uk

Defibrillation

Indications

Defibrillation is used in the treatment of ventricular fibrillation (VF) and pulseless ventricular tachycardia (VT). Prompt defibrillation offers the greatest chance of survival in cardiac arrest.

Equipment

- Defibrillator.
- Appropriate adhesive defibrillation pads.
- Towel to dry the chest.
- Razor for any chest hair.

Safety

⚠ Safety during defibrillation is of paramount importance. The clinician who delivers the shock has ultimate responsibility for the safety of the patient and the team.

Procedure

- Call for help.
- Ascertain that it is safe to approach.
- Confirm cardiac arrest: the loss of consciousness with the absence of carotid or femoral pulse.
- Switch on the defibrillator and select the appropriate energy level (this will be dependent on the monitor).
  - In adults the biphasic energy is 150J.
  - ❸ In children the biphasic energy is 4J/kg.
- Prepare the chest. Ensure that it is dry, that any chest hair that may prevent the adhesive pads from having good contact is removed, and that any jewellery or metal-based patches are removed.
- Ensure the monitor is reading the rhythm through 'pads'. Apply the pads (there is a diagram on each pad indicating where it should be placed). One pad to the right of the sternum just below the clavicle, the other to the 5th/6th intercostal space in the left anterior axillary line.
  - ▶ Pads must be placed at least 12.5cm away from a pacemaker (📖 see Fig. 20.9, p.593).
- Once the pads are in place, check the monitor and confirm the cardiac arrest rhythm. If the rhythm is pulseless VT or VF prepare to shock the patient.
- In a loud clear voice inform all other clinicians to 'stand clear' and that you are 'charging the defibrillator'.
- Simultaneousl,y perform a visual check of the immediate area and all the staff ensuring that no one is in direct or indirect contact with the patient.
- Instruct the person managing the patient's airway to 'take the oxygen away' if it is not a sealed unit. Ensure that this is done.
- As you are about to deliver the shock, shout 'stand clear'.
- Perform a further visual sweep of the patient and bed area to confirm that there is no direct or indirect contact with the patient.
- Finally, confirm that the patient remains in a shockable rhythm and deliver the shock.
- Immediately after the shock is delivered start/resume basic life support.

Diagnostic peritoneal lavage (DPL)

DPL is the introduction of a catheter into the peritoneum so that fluid can be instilled into the peritoneal cavity and drained out. DPL is infrequently performed in resuscitation rooms with the advent of bedside USS and the increased availability of CT scans. However, there may be occasions when USS and CT care not available and an injured patient requires an urgent diagnosis of any intra-abdominal pathology. Alternatively, peritoneal lavage with warmed fluids is indicated in the rewarming of hypothermic patients (📖 see p.502.)

Indications
- Re-warming in hypothermia.
- Blunt abdominal trauma. DPL is 98% sensitive but with a low specificity.

Equipment
- Peritoneal catheter.
- Scalpel.
- Local anaesthetic.
- Skin cleansing solution.
- Gloves, mask, gown, apron.
- Sterile drapes.
- 1L bag of warmed saline + giving set.
- Catheter drainage bag.

Patient preparation
- Explain the procedure to the patient.
- Ensure the patient has adequate IV access.
- Assist the patient into a comfortable lying position and expose the abdomen when the procedure is about to start.
- Obtain consent.
- NG tube: it is important to decompress the stomach.
- Urinary catheter: it is essential that the bladder is empty.

Procedure
DPL is usually performed by a surgeon.
- The skin is cleaned, local anaesthetic is used to infiltrate the area, and a scalpel is used to make a small incision below the umbilicus.
- The surgeon identifies the peritoneum and makes a small incision into it to introduce the peritoneal catheter. At this stage blood may ooze from the incision site, giving a positive result.
- If no obvious blood is seen, a giving set primed with warmed fluid is attached and 1L of saline is infused via the catheter into the peritoneum.
- The empty fluid bag can then be placed lower than the patient's abdomen and the fluid drains back into the bag.
- The fluid that has drained from the peritoneum is then observed for blood, bile, or faeces.
- If the DPL is negative, the incision will be closed in layers and a dressing applied.

- If the DPL is positive the patient is likely to go to theatre for a laparotomy.

Special considerations

- DPL will not diagnose a ruptured diaphragm or a retroperitoneal haemorrhage.
- In the obese it is technically difficult to perform.
- During the procedure air can be introduced to the peritoneal cavity. X-rays of the chest or abdomen may have air visible on them.

DPL for active rewarming in hypothermia

- The peritoneal catheter is inserted.
- 500–1000mL of warmed fluid is infused into the peritoneal cavity and left *in situ* for 10–20min.
- The fluid is then drained out and replaced with more warmed fluid.

Donway splint

The Donway splint is a pneumatic traction splint for use in patients with a fractured shaft of femur. It is washable, re-usable, and X-rays can be taken to demonstrate the position of the fracture after the splint is applied.

Indications Early splinting of a femur fracture has several benefits: pain relief; stabilization of the fracture site (which can help prevent the development of a fat embolism); prevention of further damage to muscle, vessels, and soft tissue from the fractured bone ends; and a reduction in blood loss.

Equipment
- An appropriately sized splint comprising:
  - 1 extended U-shaped ring;
  - 1 ischial ring (black padded semicircle with strap and buckle);
  - 2 leg supports (broad black perforated plastic straps);
  - 1 knee strap;
  - 1 foot plate;
  - 1 heel stand;
  - 1 ankle strap;
  - 1 pneumatic pump;
  - 1 pressure gauge.

Application of the splint
- Explain the procedure to the patient and/or relatives.
- Check the pedal pulse is present and distal sensation is intact.
- Ensure the patient has received adequate analgesia including a femoral nerve block. Entonox® may be required when the splint is fitted.
- Lie the patient on trolley exposing the injured leg.
- Place the ischial ring around the uppermost part of the injured leg and secure using belt.
- Place the affected limb in the U-shaped frame resting the limb on the leg supports.
- Ensure the patient's foot rests on the foot plate and secure the ankle tightly using the straps. Finish strapping the ankle with a figure of 8 over the back of the foot plate. It is important to spend time applying the ankle strap correctly and tightly or the splint will be ineffectual.
- Secure the ischial ring into the side arms of the U-shaped frame and ensure the screw-lock caps are released.
- Gently extend the splint by pumping air in using the pump to a pressure of 10–14 pounds/square inch (green area of pressure gauge). Once the splint has been extended, the patient's pain should diminish.
- Once the required traction has been achieved, lock the screw caps and release the pressure by pressing the air release valve (orange valve beside pressure gauge). The heel stand can be used but may cause the splint to topple over.
- Recheck the pedal pulse and distal sensation.
- Document splint application and neurovascular status of the limb.

ECG recording

Equipment needed
- ECG machine with 10 leads and clips for the adhesive tabs.
- Adhesive tabs.
- Clippers.
- Towel.

Preparation
- Check the ECG machine is set to the standard mode of recording, 25mm/sec, and the standard calibration of 10mm/mV.
- Explain the procedure to the patient and/or relatives.
- Inform patient that the best recording will be obtained when relaxed and still.
- Ensure the patient's privacy and dignity are maintained as the chest needs to be exposed.
- Position the patient reclined, either on a trolley or bed.
- There needs to be access to the skin of the chest, arms, and lower legs to allow correct placement of adhesive tabs. To maintain dignity the patient's chest can be covered once the leads are attached correctly.
- Remove any excess chest hair with clippers.
- Dry any damp skin with a towel. This gentle exfoliating motion also improves the contact of the adhesive tabs.

Placement of adhesive tabs and 10 leads

Limb leads (📖 see Fig. 8.2, p.209)
- Place the tabs on the four limbs e.g. shins or ankles, shoulders or inner wrists.
- Attach the limb leads which are either labelled or colour-coded:
  - red lead—right arm (RA);
  - yellow lead—left arm (LA);
  - green lead—left leg (LL);
  - black lead—right leg (RL).

Precordial or chest leads (📖 see Fig 8.1, p.209)
- The correct position for the placement of the chest leads is as follows.
- V1: 4th intercostal space (ICS) right sternal border.
- V2: 4th ICS left sternal border.
- V3: Midway between V2 and V4.
- V4: 5th ICS left mid-clavicular line.
- V5: Left anterior-axillary line at the same horizontal* level as V4.
- V6: Left mid-axillary line at the same horizontal* level as V4 and V5.
*at right angles to the mid-clavicular line.

Attach the chest leads, labelled V1–V6. When recording an ECG on a female patient it is conventional to place electrodes V4–V6 under the left breast. Although it is acknowledged that attenuation of the signal does not change when electrodes are placed over the breast there is insufficient published evidence to support this.

Right-sided leads are mirror image of normal left-sided leads and may be requested when ST segment elevation in V1 and V2 is noted on standard ECG. Right-sided leads can more accurately determine an RV infarction.

- The limb leads are placed in the standard position.
- V1r: 4th intercostal space (ICS) left sternal border.
- V2r: 4th ICS right sternal border.
- V3r: Midway between V2r and V4r.
- V4r: 5th ICS right mid-clavicular line.
- V5r: Right anterior axillary line at the same horizontal* level as V4.
- V6r: Right mid-axillary line at the same horizontal* level as V4 and V5.
*at right angles to the mid-clavicular line.

⚠ The ECG machine does not usually recognize that leads are not in standard position. Therefore the labelling needs to be clearly changed on all chest leads. The right-sided leads are usually labelled with an **'r'.**

Posterior leads indicated when there is a tall 'R' wave in V1, ST segment depression in V1 and V2, and tall upright T waves are noted on standard ECG. Posterior leads more accurately determine posterior infarct.
- The limb leads are placed in the standard position.
- All the chest leads are removed.
- Ask the patient to lean forwards as 3 tabs have to be placed on the posterior chest.
- Place the first tab at the same horizintal* level as V6 in the posterior axillary line: this is V7.
- Place the next tab between V7 and V9: this is V8.
- Place the final tab at the same horizontal* level as V6 next to the vertabral column: this is V9.
*at right angles to the mid-clavicular line.

⚠ The ECG machine does not usually recognize that the leads are not in the standard position. Therefore the labelling needs to be clearly changed. There will only be three chest leads on this ECG and they should be relabelled V7, V8, and V9.

❶ **Paediatric considerations** Use paediatric tabs. Pad position same as in adult.

Recording the ECG
- Enter patient's details, name, and other identifiers into ECG machine.
- Ensure patient is relaxed and still.
- Press the 'record" button.
- Avoid using any filter buttons unless interference from muscle movement makes it difficult to interpret the ECG.
- Ensure ECG is a good trace, disconnect the leads, maintain patient dignity.
- If any cardiac signs or symptoms, document them on the ECG.
- The ECG should be shown to a clinician able to interpret it to ensure any urgent medical treatment can begin.
- Ensure equipment is cleaned and tidied away ready for next use.
- Inform patient of the results.

Troubleshooting
- AC interference/artefact. Remove any electrical equipment if possible, ensure leads are untangled, check adhesive tab contact, and ensure patient is not touching metal.
- Wandering baseline. Check adhesive tab contact; check the patient is not moving, or that there is not 'pull' on the leads.
- Tremor. Usually due to patient movement. Ensure patient not cold and as relaxed as possible.

Eye irrigation

Eye irrigation is an urgent procedure and is indicated when there is any chemical splash in the eye/s. Patients with any chemical in their eye/s will be allocated a high triage priority for immediate irrigation. The most common irrigating fluid is normal saline (0.9%) but sterile water is also appropriate. When neither of these fluids is immediately available, tap water is an adequate substitute and is often used in the pre-hospital setting.

Equipment
- pH paper.
- Irrigation fluid, usually normal saline 0.9%.
- Wide bore giving set.
- Gloves.
- Receiver.
- Towels prescribed.
- Anaesthetic drops (reduce pain and enable to patient to cooperate).

Procedure
- Protect the patient's clothing with a towel. It may be easier for the patient to remove their top clothes and wear a gown.
- If immediately available, use pH paper to ascertain pH of the chemical.
- Remove contact lens.
- Instil local anaesthetic eye drops and repeat as necessary during the irrigation.
- Position the patient with the head inclined to the affected side.
- Ask the patient to hold the receiver close to their check to collect the irrigation fluid.
- Alternatively, if appropriate and a sink is available, patient can lean over sink.
- Hold patient's eye apart using your first and second finger against orbital ridge.
- Direct fluid from nasal corner outwards and ask patient to move their eye in all gaze directions.
- Evert the lid to ensure that any particles have been removed.
- Once thoroughly cleansed, a minimum of 1L of fluid should be used.
- Dry the eye/s and face.
- Recheck the pH.
- Dispose of equipment.
- Check the patient's visual acuity.
- Document the procedure and pH measurements in the patient's notes.

🛈 All but the most trivial of injuries should be referred to an opthalmologist.

⛨ Eye irrigation can be impossible in young children. Tap water is a reasonable substitute.

Eyelid eversion

Upper eyelid eversion is a routine procedure when examining a patient with an eye injury. It should also be done during eye irrigation, especially if there is particulate matter in the eye as some may remain under the lid despite copious irrigation. Lid eversion is a simple procedure once mastered and can be practised on willing colleagues or relatives. If the upper lid is very swollen lid eversion is much more difficult—document any failed attempts clearly in the notes.

Equipment
- Cotton bud.
- Local anaesthetic eye drops if needed.
- Good lighting.

Patient preparation Some patients become very anxious if you describe the procedure in detail and in those cases it may be wiser just to inform them you are checking under their upper eye lid.

Procedure (Fig. 20.10)
- Wear gloves. However, if the patient has very short eyelashes, it can be difficult to feel them with gloves on.
- Instil local anaesthetic eye drops if the eye is painful.
- Instruct the patient to 'look down' with their eyes as if trying to see their shoes. Keep the head in a neutral position.
- Dry the eye/eyelashes with a swab if they are wet.
- Grasp the eyelashes in the middle of the upper eyelid and pull outwards stretching the lid away from the globe.
- With the tip or side of the cotton bud, gently press down on the middle of the upper lid and 'flip' the tarsal plate over the bud.
- Inspect under the lid.
- Remove any FB with the cotton bud.
- Release the lashes and return the lid to the normal position.

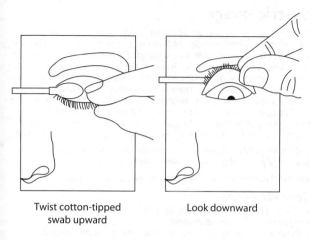

Twist cotton-tipped   Look downward
swab upward

Fig. 20.10 Eyelid eversion.

Gastric lavage

Gastric lavage is the passage of a tube via the orogastric route into the stomach so that small amounts of fluid can be administered and siphoned out with the intention of removing the gastric contents. Once a routine procedure in EDs, gastric lavage is now rarely performed. Following toxicology research the indications for gastric lavage in accidental and non-accidental ingestion are few. There is no certain evidence that it improves clinical outcome and it is associated with significant complications. The local poisons service should be contacted if there is doubt over whether to perform gastric lavage. If lavage is indicated, 50g of activated charcoal may be indicated. This is poured down the tube just before its is removal.

Indication Only indication is the ingestion of a potentially life-threatening amount of poison that presents within 60min of ingestion.

The instillation of warmed fluid in hypothermia (📖 see p.502).

Contraindications
- Loss of protective airway reflexes unless intubated and ventilated.
- Ingestion of a corrosive material.
- Patients with oesophageal varices or other pre-existing medical or gastrointestinal problem that may be adversely affected by lavage.

Complications
- Laryngospasm.
- Aspiration.
- Oesophageal perforation.
- Hypoxia.
- Hypercarbia.
- Trauma to the throat and larynx.
- Bradycardias.

❶ Combative patients are more at risk of complications.

❶ Because of the possible serious complications 2 members of staff with airway management skills and experience of performing lavage *must* carry out the procedure.

Equipment
- Gastric lavage tube with funnel-type attachment and mouth piece airway.
- 2 large buckets: one empty- the other with lukewarm water.
- pH paper.
- Jug.
- Oxygen.
- Suction.
- Lubricating jelly.
- Continuous monitoring. Ideally the procedure should be performed in a resuscitation room.
- Gloves, aprons, floor protection (sheets, towels). and shoe covers
- 50g of activated charcoal if prescribed.
- Towels to protect the patient, patient gown.

Patient preparation

Procedure must be explained to the patients and verbal consent gained. If consent is refused the procedure must not be performed; uncooperative patients are at significant risk and performing a procedure without consent is assault. Explain to the patient that a plastic tube will be passed into their stomach through their mouth so that the 'tablets' can be washed out with warm water. The procedure is not painful but is uncomfortable. patients often feel that they cannot breathe. Reassure them that the tube will be immediately removed if any problems are encountered.

The patient should be undressed and put in a gown as their clothing is likely to become wet. Transfer the patient to an appropriate area with oxygen, suction, and monitoring. Position them in the left lateral position with a 20° head down tilt; their left arm should be behind their back.

⚠ If the patient has an altered level of consciousness or loss of protective airway reflexes they **must** be intubated prior to the procedure.

Procedure

- One member of staff performs the procedure, the other has responsibility for holding patient's head/neck, managing the airway, and observing the vital signs. The patient is likely to vomit during the procedure as he/she 'gags' on the orogastric tube—airway management is vital.
- Protect floor with towels/sheet so that staff do not slip if spillages.
- Protect patient's bed sheet. Place plastic-backed pad under head/neck.
- Hold tube to the patient's nose and measure approximate length to epigastrium. This is approximate length of tube that should be inserted.
- Ensure the bed is at a reasonable height so that gravity assists in the drainage of the gastric contents
- Insert the mouth piece. This prevents the patient from biting down on the orogastric tube and occluding it.
- Lubricate the end of the tube with jelly.
- Insert the tube through the mouth piece and into patient's mouth. Tell them to swallow the tube when they feel it at the back of their throat.
- Push tube into the mouth/throat. Once patient swallows, continue to push tube into the stomach until you reach the measured length.
  - ⚠ Force must **not** be used.
- Once tube in place, hold 'funnel' end into empty bucket and wait until gastric secretions drain out. Drop pH paper into bucket; ensure it changes colour and confirms a pH < 4 to indicate gastric secretions. Alternatively, air can be instilled, whilst listening over the stomach with a stethoscope. 'Gurgling' over stomach confirms correct placement.
- Once correct placement of the tube confirmed, the lavage can begin. Slowly instill 200–300mL of warm water down the tube, tip funnel end into the bucket, and allow the water to siphon out. Repeat until the lavage fluid runs clear. This may take 5–10 instillations of water.
- Instil charcoal if prescribed.
- Remove lavage tube.
- Help patient into a comfortable position and assist with hygiene needs.

⚠ If patient shows any sign of airway compromise or respiratory difficulty tube should be immediately removed.

Inhaler technique

When adults and young people are discharged home after receiving emergency asthma treatment their inhaler technique should be checked. Poor technique and lack of knowledge about the importance of regular inhaled therapies can contribute to a worsening of symptoms and the need to seek emergency care.

There are many inhalers available and as many spacer devices. However, a metered dose inhaler (MDI) is the device most commonly used and stocked in emergency care areas to be given out at discharge.

Step-by-step use of an MDI

- Remove cap and shake inhaler.
- Breathe out gently.
- Place mouth piece in the mouth and, as you begin to breathe in, press canister down and continue to inhale steadily and deeply.
- Hold your breath for 10sec (or as long as comfortable).
- Wait for 30sec before taking any additional doses and follow the above steps again.
- ▶ Only use the inhaler for the number of doses stated on the label; then start a new inhaler.

 If a patient has difficulty using an MDI, a spacer can be used. This is routine in younger children.

Further information

 www.asthma.org.uk

❻ Intraosseous (IO) insertion

An IO needle is an alternative to IV access and is most frequently used in cardiac arrest and critical illness in children. In cardiac arrest (unless an IV is already established) the IO should be used. In other situations when a child is critically ill or injured, do not waste time trying to establish an IV line; IO should be used. IO needle insertion is not a skill limited to medical staff. ED nurses can learn and use it in an emergency (Fig. 20.11).

Equipment
- IO needle.
- Skin cleansing solution.
- 3 way tap with short 10cm extension.
- Fluid giving set.
- 20mL/50mL syringes.
- 500mL normal saline.
- Saline flush.
- First-line resuscitation drugs, fluid bolus.
- Splint for the limb if required.
- Tape.

Site selection
- The most common site is the proximal tibia 2.5cm below the knee (or 1 finger-breadth) on the flat anteromedial surface.
- Other sites include the calcaneum, distal tibia, distal femur, iliac crest, sternum and the clavicle.
- Limbs where there is a fracture above the chosen site must not be used.

Patient preparation
- Expose the site for insertion.
- Local anaesthetic can be used if the child is not unconscious.
- Clean the skin.
- Explain the need for the procedure to parents/carers.

Complications
- Infection.
- Fracture.
- Extravasation.

Procedure
- Flush a 3-way tap and 10cm extension with saline. Have 5mL syringe available and first-line resuscitation drugs.
- Support the limb but do not hold it underneath the site for insertion.
- Hold the IO needle firmly with the butt of needle in the palm of your hand and with 'gloved' fingers close to the tip of the needle. Holding the needle too near to the butt reduces the tactile control.
- Place needle on to the bone aiming at 90° or at an angle away from the knee if flat anteromedial surface of the tibia is your chosen site. Insert with a twisting action (or a rotating action if IO needle is based on a screw design). The twisting action resembles the 'bevelling' of a hole.

Continuous pressure is required until there is a loss of resistance as the IO needle enters the cortex.

- Remove stylet. Attach 5mL syringe and aspirate 'bone marrow' sample. Often this proves impossible. If sample obtained, send for U & E, FBC, or cross-match.
- Flush needle with 10mL of saline (use previously prepared 3-way tap with extension). Observe for leaking around the insertion site and/or swelling of local tissues.
- Attach the fluid giving set to the 3-way tap. Fluid boluses can be administered from the IV fluid via the tap.
- The IO needle is typically 'stable' within the cortex of bone. The use of a 3-way tap with a 10cm extension reduces the risk of accidental removal of the IO needle by reducing local movement as syringes are attached or removed. Application of tape and a splint can improve stability.
- All drugs can be administered via an IO needle.
- Insertion of IO needle with a power drill (e.g. EZ-IO) is similar to that described above but is generally easier and faster to achieve.

Nursing care of the IO needle

- Examining site and local tissues to identify leaking reduces adverse risk.
- Remove needle once IV access is reliable. This is best risk reduction strategy.

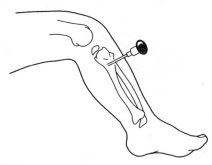

Fig. 20.11 Tibial intraosseous access (Reproduced with permission from Wyatt, J., et al. (2005). *Oxford Handbook of Accident and Emergency Medicine*, 2nd edn, p. 613. Oxford University Press, Oxford.)

Minor injury treatments

There are numerous 'minor' treatments that are completed each day in emergency care. The treatment of 'minor' injuries may seem very simple and sometimes even mundane. However, the injury may have a significant impact on the patient's daily life. The time taken to give a clear explanation of the injury, the expected recovery, and the important features of self-care are essential in shortening the recovery phase and preventing unplanned follow-up. Ideally all verbal advice should be given in written form so that it can be referred to at a later date. ⬤ The following minor treatments apply equally to adults and children.

Neighbour/buddy strapping

Indications

For fractures, or sprains of fingers and lesser toes. NB. The Gt toe should not be strapped to the second toe. Injuries to the great toe can be treated with a toe spica.

Equipment

- Gauze
- Adhesive tape (non-elasticated)
- Scissors

Patient preparation

- Explain the procedure to the patient
- Strapping toes can be painful

Procedure

- Expose injured fingers or toes.
- Fold one piece of gauze and cut to the length and width of fingers/toes.
- Cut two lengths of tape, use one piece of tape to strap the proximal phalanx together, the other to strap the middle phalanx.
- Ensure strapping is comfortable and not too tight, check capillary refill.

Discharge advice

- Advise the patient to keep the fingers/toes strapped for as long as the injury requires, most strains/sprain need early mobilisation
- If the digit is swollen advise about the importance of elevation
- Advise about pain relief
- Advise about work/school, contact sport and other activities that the patient may regularly undertake
- Advise about follow-up and how and when to seek further help if problems persist.

Slings

Broad arm sling

Indications To support an injured shoulder or arm or to elevate a swollen upper limb.

Equipment
- Triangular sling.
- Tape or nappy pin.

Patient preparation
- Explain the procedure to the patient.
- Place the arm in the correct position, usually with the shoulder and elbow at 90°.

Procedure
- Locate the 90° angle on the sling. Holding this with one hand, slide the sling under the injured arm so that 90°angle is at the patient's elbow.
- Put the uppermost corner of the sling over the opposite shoulder.
- Bring lower corner of the sling over the injured arm and tie the two ends behind the neck.
- Secure the elbow in the sling with tape or a safety pin.

Discharge advice
- Advise the patient about whether to wear the sling under or over their clothes (this will depend upon the injury).
- Patient do not usually have to sleep in a sling.
- Advise about the importance of elevation, especially if the limb was swollen.
- Advise about pain relief.
- Advise about work/school, contact sport, and other activities that the patient may regularly undertake.
- Advise about follow-up and how and when to seek further help if problems persist.

High arm sling

Indications To reduce swelling of hand, wrist, forearm, or fingers or to help control haemorrhage.

Equipment
- Triangular sling.
- Tape or nappy pin.

Patient preparation
- Explain the procedure to the patient.
- Place the arm in position with the shoulder and elbow at 90°.

Procedure
- Locate the 90° angle on the sling. Holding this with one hand, slide the sling under the injured arm so that 90°angle is at the patient's elbow.
- Put the uppermost corner of the sling over the opposite shoulder.
- Bring lower corner of the sling over the injured arm and tie the two ends behind the neck.

- Secure the elbow in the sling with tape or a safety pin.
- Place the hand of the injured arm on the opposite shoulder.
- Fold the now loose sling up and over the arm and secure with a nappy pin.

Discharge advice
- Advise about the importance of elevation.
- Advise about pain relief.
- Advise about work/school, contact sport, and other activities that the patient may regularly undertake.
- Advise about follow-up and how and when to seek further help if problems persist.

Collar and cuff

Indications
- Fracture of the humerus.
- Elbow injury/fracture.
- Post reduction of a dislocated shoulder.

Equipment
- Collar and cuff.
- Tie fastener.
- Elastic adhesive tape.
- Scissors.

Patient preparation
- Explain the procedure to the patient.
- Place the arm in position with the shoulder and elbow at 90°.

Procedure
- Cut the required length of collar and cuff foam by measuring against the patient.
- Encircle in a figure of eight around the neck and wrist of injured arm.
- Secure with a tie fastener; cut the unused end off.
- Cover tie fastener with elastic adhesive tape, so no sharp edges are exposed.
- Check for circulation by checking the radial pulse and observing the colour and sensation of the hand.
- Ensure patient can slip the collar over the head and hand.

Discharge advice
- Advise the patient about whether to wear collar and cuff under or over their clothes (this will depend upon the injury).
- Patients may have to sleep in the collar and cuff. Wearing a snug fitting T shirt over the collar and cuff will help keep the arm secure by the patient's side.
- Advise about pain relief.
- Advise about work/school, contact sport, and other activities that the patient may regularly undertake.
- Advise about follow-up and how and when to seek further help if problems persist.

Splints and thumb spica

Wrist splint

Indications
- Soft tissue injuries.
- Tenosynovitis.

Equipment Correct size splint (small, medium, large, or extra large and in right or left).

Patient preparation
- Explain the procedure to the patient.
- Expose the patient's forearm and wrist.

Procedure
- Position wrist brace with metal bar running along palmar aspect of wrist.
- Place velcro straps across the dorsum of the wrist and between thumb and index finger.
- Ensure wrist brace fits snugly around wrist allowing full movement of fingers and thumb. The patient may be able to adjust fit more easily.

Discharge advice
- Advise the patient about when to wear the splint and how long for (this will depend upon the injury)
- Advise about pain relief and NSAIDs if appropriate
- Advise about work/school, contact sport, and other activities that the patient may regularly undertake. If the patient has been prescribed the wrist brace for tenosynovisits they may have to wear it for prolonged periods.
- Advise about follow-up and how and when to seek further help if problems persist.

Thumb spica

Indications
- Fractures of the thumb.
- Soft tissue injuries of the thumb.

Equipment
- 5cm crepe bandage.
- Adhesive tape.
- Beware of possible allergy.

Elastoplast® tape can be used for a thumb spica but there is no evidence to support the use of crepe over Elastoplast®. Elastoplast® is more difficult to apply and painful to remove. Therefore, crepe should be used when there is no clear rationale for Elastoplasts®.

Patient preparation
- Explain the procedure to the patient.
- Expose the patient's wrist, hand, and thumb.
- Ask the patient to hold their wrist in a neutral position and extend their thumb.

Procedure
- Anchor the bandage around the wrist several times.
- Place the bandage, from the wrist to around the tip of the thumb in a figure of eight.
- Continue the figure of eight bandaging down the thumb until all the thumb and thenar eminence is supported.

Discharge advice
- Advise the patient about wearing the spica and how long for (this will depend upon the injury).
- Advise about pain relief and NSAIDs if appropriate.
- Advise about work/school, contact sport, and other activities that the patient may regularly undertake. Advise about follow-up and how and when to seek further help if problems persist.

Mallet splint

Indications Mallet deformity ± a fracture.

Equipment
- Gauze.
- Non-elastic tape.
- Mallet splints of various sizes.

Patient preparation Explain the procedure and the role of the mallet splint to the patient.

Procedure
- Wrap a thin layer of gauze around the finger. This provides padding and absorbs perspiration.
- Fit the appropriate sized splint. The splint should force the DIPJ into 10–15° extension and not be too tight. If there is swelling at the DIPJ the rest of the splint may appear loose. Several size splints may need to be fitted until the 'best fit' is found.
- Tape in place around the base of the splint over the middle phalanx.

Discharge advice
- Advise the patient about continually wearing the splint.
- Arrange follow-up and refer for splint care. Advise how to remove splint and keep the DIPJ in extension to wash finger and then reapply splint.
- Advise about work/school, contact sport, and other activities that the patient may regularly undertake.

Trephining

Indications Recent subungual haematoma causing pain and discomfort. Old haemotomas that have clotted under the nail will not drain.

Equipment
- Gauze.
- Trephining tool. Most tools generate intense heat to burn through the nail.
- Dressing.
- Eye protection is essential.

Patient preparation Explain the procedure to the patient reinforcing that it is not painful and will immediately relieve symptoms.

Procedure
- Lay the patient down.
- Place the hand/foot on a flat hard surface.
- Gently apply the trephining tool until a give is felt and blood escapes.
- Apply gentle pressure to the pulp of the digit until all the blood has been released.
- Apply a dressing.

Discharge advice
- Advise the patient about pain relief.
- Advise the patient about elevation of the limb if appropriate.
- Advise about work/school, contact sport, and other activities that the patient may regularly undertake.

Mobility assessment

Many patients who have accessed emergency care will require an assessment of their mobility prior to discharge. A comprehensive mobility assessment is usually done by a physiotherapist or occupational therapist. However, there are many instances when a brief assessment of mobility is made by the emergency care clinician.

Indications

- Prior to discharge in any patient who is known to have a mobility problem.
- Prior to discharge in any patient with an injury that has the potential to affect their mobility.

To assess

- Is the patient safe to mobilize independently (with or without the use of walking aids)?
- Is the patient safe to transfer from sitting/lying to standing position independently (with or without the use of mobility aids)?
- Is the patient able to stabilize themselves and walk around cubicle/bed area with no assistance needed (with or without walking aids)?

If there is doubt about the need for a comprehensive mobility assessment request physiotherapy/occupational therapy input.

Tips for observation

- Observe the patient transfer from bed/trolley to standing position.
- Observe the patient sitting down and standing up from an appropriately sized chair.
- Observe the patient mobilize around bed area for a distance of at least 2 metres.

▶ Two health care professionals should perform a mobility assessment. Both assessors should stand close to the patient to allow for support and stabilization if needed.

Key questions

- Will the patient be safe at home alone or with family members?
- Will the patient need a new walking aid? If so the patient must be trained on the appropriate use of such an aid.

Nasal packing

Indications

Nasal packing is frequently performed in emergency settings when simple first aid measures and/or cautery fail to stop an epistaxis. Both nostrils **must** always be packed so that pressure is applied the septum from both sides. It is rare to have to perform this procedure on children.

Equipment

- 2-tier, silver trolley.
- 2 × expanding foam tampons.
- Apron and sterile gloves.
- Sufficient light.
- Local anaesthetic spray: xylocaine.
- Dressing pack or sterile field and gauze.
- Receiver.
- 2 × syringes with 10mL of sterile water.
- Naseptin® or other antibiotic nasal cream.
- Tape.

Patient preparation

This is an unpleasant procedure for the patient. Whilst not usually painful, it can be distressing and some patients are not able to tolerate it. It's crucial that what needs to be done, why, and what it will be like is clearly explained so the patient knows what to expect. Reassure them that it will be over quickly and in almost all cases is successful in stopping the bleeding

Depending upon how much the patient is able to cooperate with the procedure, a second person may be required, i.e. to hold the receiver.

Procedure

- Position the patient sitting upright, either in a chair or on a trolley.
- Have a light positioned so that patient's face is well lit.
- Prepare the trolley, dressing pack, gauze.
- Prepare each tampon, coating each side liberally with antibiotic cream. This eases insertion and prevents infection.
- Ask the patient to blow their nose. This will remove any clots and allow the tampons to be more easily inserted.
- Ask the patient/second person to hold the receiver at the patient's mouth so that blood and/or clots can be spat out.
- Spray each nostril with LA spray.
- Insert the first tampon into the nostril that is bleeding. Push (the end without the cotton) horizontally along the floor of the nostril. This has to be done firmly and may cause the patient some distress. Push until it will not go any further; the end with the cotton should be just visible. (How much of the tampon is inserted will depend to some extent on the size of the patient's nose.)

- Put the tip of the a water-filled syringe directly on the exposed tampon and soak the tampon. The tampon will swell and fill the nostril.
- Insert a second tampon into the other nostril as above.
- Tape the cotton to each side of the face.
- Help the patient wash and clean their face.
- Prepare the patient for admission.

Nasogastric (NG) tube insertion

Indications

NG tube insertion is usually indicated in the following emergency situations: perforated peptic ulcer; bowel obstruction; multiple trauma; pancreatitis; and in some cases of persistent vomiting. Ventilated adults and children also need an NG tube to decompress the stomach, which can improve ventilation. 🕭 Some adults and children are managed at home with an NG tube for feeding and may attend ED if the tube 'falls out'.

Equipment

- Apron and sterile gloves.
- NG tube (select an appropriate size).
- Sterile 20mL syringe with connection.
- Drainage bag and spigot.
- Lubricant.
- pH indicator strips.
- Cup of water.
- Tape.

Cooling the NG tube in a fridge for 20min can sometimes ease its passage as it stiffens the tube.

Patient preparation

This is an unpleasant procedure. It makes the patient retch and feel as if they can't breathe. Many patients can't tolerate the procedure and may stop you proceeding. Explain the procedure to the patient and the reasons why an NG tube is required. Assist the patient into a comfortable position, ideally sitting upright on a trolley. Explain to the patient their role in the procedure, which is:

- to signal by raising their hand if they want the procedure to stop;
- to drink water and swallow when they are instructed to; this will be when they feel the tube at the back of their throat.

Procedure

- Measure the approximate length of the NG tube. Take the tip of the tubing and place at the epigastrium, place the tubing up the patient's chest, over the ear and to the bridge of the nose. At this point mark the tubing at the level of the nose with a marker pen. This is the length of tube that should be passed.
- Ensure the patient is ready to proceed and understands the procedure.
- Lubricate the tip of the NG tube.
- Insert the tip of the tube into the nostril. Pass the tubing along the floor of the nostril ensuring there is no resistance. If resistance occurs withdraw tubing slightly and advance again carefully at a slightly different angle.
- As the tubing advances and the patient feels it at the back of their throat (which is when you may feel some slight resistance) offer them water to drink. This should enable them to swallow the NG tube and ease its passage into the stomach.

- The patient may cough and retch. This is normal and you should continue to try to pass the tube. However, if the patient is distressed, raises their hand, or appears to have difficulty breathing, remove the tube immediately.
- Continue to pass the tube until the marker you have made is at the nostril.
- Secure the tube with tape to the nostril and side of the face.
- Check for correct insertion into the stomach by aspirating the NG tube and measuring the pH of the aspirate to make sure it is < 5.5.
- Ensure that a CXR is ordered to check the exact site of the tube.
- Spigot the tube or apply a drainage bag.

Complications

- Inadvertent passage down the trachea and into the pulmonary tree.
- Failure to pass into the stomach (sometimes the tube can coil up at the back of the throat).
- Epistaxis.

Needle thoracocentesis

Needle thoracocentesis is the initial procedure used to correct a tension pneumothorax. A tension pneumothroax is a potentially life-threatening condition and needs to be dealt with rapidly by this method. A needle thoracentesis is a temporizing measure and must be followed up by an immediate chest drain (📖 see p.604).

Signs and symptoms of a tension pneumothorax
- Respiratory distress: breathlessness; tachypnoea; confusion.
- Increased work of breathing, accessory muscle use.
- Pallor, greyness progressing to cyanosis.
- Little or no air entry on the affected side.
- Little or no chest rise on the affected side
- Reduced SpO_2.
- Hyperresonance to percussion on the affected side.
- Deviated trachea.
- Distended neck veins.
- Hypotension/shock

Patient preparation
This is an immediately life-threatening situation and the procedure has to be performed rapidly. The patient is critically hypoxic and in many cases comatose. A quick and brief description of the procedure should be given when and if appropriate.

Equipment
- Skin cleaning product as per local protocol.
- A 14 gauge cannula.
- Chest drain equipment.

The clinician will clean the skin and insert the cannula into the 2nd intercostal space, midclavicular line on the affected side. As the cannula needle is removed air will be released and a 'hiss' should be heard. A chest drain then needs to be inserted.

Nursing role
- To continuously monitor ABC.
- To monitor vital signs, especially oxygen saturations and respiratory rate, and inform the treating clinician of improvement or deterioration.
- Apply high flow oxygen.
- Ensure adequate analgesia has been provided.
- Prepare for a chest drain.

Neurological assessment: the Glasgow Coma Score

The Glasgow Coma Score (GCS) is a key component of a neurological assessment and, together with an assessment of pupils, limbs, and vital signs, can provide a bedside assessment of cerebral function. GCS assesses and monitors conscious level in patients who have an actual or potential neurological problem. It assesses the integrity of normal brain functioning and, when repeated at regular intervals, can identify if the patient's neurological function is improving or deteriorating. The GCS was developed for assessing the conscious level of adults. A modification has been developed for use in children the 'Children's Glasgow Coma Score' (CGCS).

The GCS assesses and scores 3 parameters:
- eye opening;
- verbal response;
- motor response.

How to record GCS

Eye response
- Score 4. Eyes open spontaneously. The patient is seen to be awake with eyes open. The patient should be aware of your presence.
- Score 3. Eyes open to verbal command. Don't touch the patient. Speak to the patient in a normal voice first. Then, if necessary, gradually raise the volume of your voice.
- Score 2. Eyes open to painful stimuli. Initially, to avoid distress, touch or shake the patient's shoulders. If there is no response to this inflict a painful stimulus (🕮 see Box 20.2).
- Score 1. No eye opening. There is no response to painful stimuli. Only score when satisfied that sufficient stimulus was applied.

Box 20.2 Painful stimuli

- Supraorbital pressure. Just below the inner aspect of the eyebrow is a small notch through which a branch of the facial nerve runs. The nurse should use their thumb to press this area for a maximum of 30sec.
- Trapezium squeeze. Hold the trapezium muscle between thumb and forefinger and apply gradually increasing pressure for a maximum of 30sec.
- Sternal rub. The sternum is rubbed firmly with a closed fist.

Verbal response
- Score 5. Orientated. The patient is orientated to time, place, and person.
- Score 4. Confused. The patient is unable to say who they are, where they are, and why, and the current year and month.
- Score 3. Inappropriate words. Words that are not understandable or things said in an incorrect context.
- Score 2. Incomprehensible sounds. More often making sounds in response to painful stimulus, rather than conversation. Moaning, groaning, or crying sounds instead of formed words.

- Score 1. No verbal response. Unable to produce any speech sounds in response to verbal or painful stimulus.

Motor response
- Score 6. Obeys commands. The patient accurately responds to instructions, e.g. stick your tongue out.
- Score 5. Localizes to pain The patient will move their hand to the point of stimulus, in an obvious coordinated attempt to remove the cause of the pain.
- Score 4. Withdrawal from pain. The patient will move in a purposeful way away from the stimulus but the response is not specific to the site of stimulus.
- Score 3. Flexion (decorticate posturing). The patient flexes their elbows and rotates their wrists inwards.
- Score 2. Extension (decerebrate posturing). The patient straightens their arms at the elbow and internally rotates their shoulders. Often the legs are also in extension with the toes pointing down.
- Score 1. No motor response. No movement at all.

▶ Important considerations
- Sometimes it is difficult to accurately assess GCS, e.g. in patients with learning disabilities. If you are unsure of the assessment, double check the GCS score with a colleague.
- Sleeping patients should always be woken, e.g. it should never be presumed that a child with a head injury is 'just sleeping'.
- Ideally, the same person should perform the GCS assessment; this ensures consistency in assessment.
- The painful stimuli used should be documented and consistently used in each assessment.
- When the patient is handed over to another nurse or transferred out of the emergency care area, there should be formal handover of the GCS and agreement between the 2 clinicians as to what the GCS is at that time.
- Establishing and documenting a normal baseline in patients who already have some degree of neurological abnormality is vital. Assessing GCS in patients with dementia and cerebral palsy, for example, can be difficult. Relatives and carers can give vital information about what is 'normal' for the patient and if they perceive any change in behaviour or functioning.

Neurological assessment: other tests

Assessing pupil reaction

Pupil size and reactivity are a measure for the function of cranial nerve (CN) III, the oculomotor nerve. Any raise in ICP will eventually put pressure on this nerve causing its function to be impaired and pupil reactions altered.

- Use a bright light. Covering one eye and shining the light in the other assess pupil response. Repeat for the other eye.
- The light should be brought in from the side of the patient's face twice.

In intubated and sedated patients this is one of the only ways of monitoring neurological status and any increases in ICP.

A sluggish pupillary response can indicate some CN III compression. A fixed and dilated pupil indicates CN compression on the affected side. When both pupils are fixed and dilated this indicates significantly raised ICP and brainstem herniation.

⚠ Be aware of effects of drugs on pupil response.

Limb response

Assessment of limb movement identifies if there is any upper or lower, unilateral or bilateral limb weakness. Each limb should be assessed separately.

- Arms. Tell patient to hold arms out in front. Look for signs of weakness or drift.
- Legs. Ask the patient to push and pull feet towards assessor or ask the patient to raise their legs off bed and hold them there for a short amount of time.
- If a limb doesn't move then a painful stimulus needs to be applied to that limb to assess if this elicits any response.

Vital signs

Hypertension, bradycardia, and respiratory irregularity are the cardinal signs of significantly raised ICP. Patients with a GCS < 15 should have their observations recorded half hourly for 2h, then one hourly for 4h, and then two hourly after that, if no significant changes occur.

☉ Neurological assessment in children

A neurological assessment including GCS has to be performed in children in emergency care areas frequently, most commonly in head injury. For children ~ 5 years and over the standard adult GCS assessment can be performed. However in preverbal/preschool age children the verbal and motor assessment elements have to be modified.

Children's GCS < 5 years

Eye response

- Score 4. Eyes open spontaneously. The child is seen to be awake with eyes open. The child should be aware of your presence.
- Score 3. Eyes open to verbal command. Don't touch the child. Speak to the child (or ask a parent/carer to do so) in a normal voice first; then if necessary gradually raise the volume of your voice.
- Score 2. Eyes open to painful stimuli. Initially to avoid distress, touch or gently shake the child's arm or shoulders. If there is no response to this inflict a painful stimulus (☐ see Box 20.2, p.642).
- Score 1 – No eye opening. No response to painful stimuli. Only score when satisfied that sufficient stimulus was applied.

Verbal response

- Score 5. Smiles. An alert infant, contented with their parent.
- Score 4. Cries. A child who will not settle with a parent.
- Score 3. Inappropriate cries. At times cries out; not related to being disturbed.
- Score 2. Occasional whimper. Less frequent cries; may be associated with occasional whimper.
- Score 1. No verbal response. Unable to produce any sounds in response to verbal or painful stimulus.

Motor response

- Score 6. Obeys commands; spontaneous movement. Spontaneous, normal movements for the child.
- Score 5. Localizes to pain. Withdraws to touch.
- Score 4. Normal flexion. Withdraws from pain.
- Score 3. Abnormal flexion (decorticate posturing). The child flexes their elbows and rotates their wrists inwards.
- Score 2. Extension (decerebrate posturing). The child straightens their arms at the elbow and internally rotates their shoulders. Often the legs are also in extension with the toes pointing down.
- Score 1. No motor response. No movement at all.

Oxygen delivery

Oxygen delivery is integral to many aspects of emergency care treatment in adults and children. Selecting the correct device to deliver supplemental oxygen ensures that the patient's oxygen needs are met.

❶ Head box oxygen Used for supplemental oxygen in neonates and infants. Supplemental oxygen fills a Perspex box placed over the baby's head. A gauge measures the concentration of oxygen in the box, which can be titrated against oxygen saturations.

Nasal cannulae can deliver 24–40% oxygen at flow rates of 1–5L/min. They are often used for patients who have oxygen at home. Nasal cannulae can also be useful for patients who only require low concentrations of oxygen and cannot tolerate a face mask. Flow rates > 4L/min are very drying to the nasal passages and can be uncomfortable.

Oxygen (Venturi) mask A Venturi mask mixes room air with oxygen through a flow valve and can deliver settings of 24%, 28%, 35%, 40%, and 60% depending on which valve is attached. Venturi masks are particularly useful when there is concern about CO_2 retention.

Simple face mask A simple face mask (often used in pre-hospital settings) delivers 40–60% oxygen at flow rates of 5–10L/min.

Non-rebreathing face mask with reservoir If patients require > 40% oxygen the use of a non-rebreathing mask should be considered. With a tight fitting mask and the reservoir bag inflated, 85–90% oxygen concentrations can be delivered with a flow rate of 10–15L/min.

Bag value mask (BVM) ventilation For patients who require more active respiratory support a BVM, with reservoir, good face mask seal, and flow rates of 10–15L/min, delivers ~ 90% oxygen.

Paediatric considerations

❸ Forcing oxygen therapy on a child should be avoided as this increases their work of breathing and oxygen demand. Various techniques using play and turning the therapy into a game can be used to gain a child's trust and cooperation. Parents are often key in enabling oxygen to be administered. Holding free flowing oxygen in the general direction of the child's face may be the only compromise possible in a distressed child.

▶ Oxygen should be prescribed.

Pain assessment and management

Pain assessment and its subsequent management are an integral part of every clinical assessment in emergency care and should be regularly reassessed. There are few emergency care presentations that do not have a painful element. Failure to adequately manage pain can have serious consequences: increased anxiety; violence; aggression; distress for patient or relatives; dissatisfaction with care; physiological deterioration.

There are many challenges to be faced when managing pain, the first being appropriate assessment, which is not an easy task. Pain assessment must take the following variables into consideration: age; culture; previous pain experiences; level of anxiety; ability to use pain assessment tools; and activity disruption.

The 4 'As' of effective pain management in emergency care are:
- assess: pain score;
- administer: give pain interventions promptly;
- appropriate: ensure the interventions are appropriate;
- assess again: reassess after a period of time.

Pain assessment

The effectiveness of pain management cannot be assessed without a baseline measurement, which is most commonly represented as a score out of 10. 0/10 = no pain and 10/10 = the worst possible pain. A pain assessment tool that combines a behavioural tool, verbal descriptor tool, and visual analogue scale can be used for adults and children in emergency care settings (Fig. 20.12(a)). 🔆 Face scales are also valuable for assessing pain younger children (Fig. 20.12(b)). 🔆 Assessing pain in children and those with cognitive problems is particularly challenging. Parents and carers are especially valuable in assisting with pain assessment in these situations.

Pain intervention

The 3 'Ps' for pain intervention are:
- practical: splinting; elevation; slings; pillows; wound dressings; relocation of dislocation; treatment of the cause, e.g. acute retention;
- psychological: distraction; explanation; reassurance; play;
- pharmacological: simple analgesia; compound analgesia; NSAIDs; opiate analgesia; local/regional anaesthetic; Entonox® nerve blocks.

Severity of pain Pain can be classified as either mild (a low score/10), moderate (a middle score/10), or severe (a high score/10). Linking pain scoring to triage priorities ensures that moderate/severe pain is dealt with swiftly.

All severities of pain will require practical and psychological interventions. For pharmacological intervention 📖 see Table 20.5.

Pain reassessment is the final element of pain management. It must never be assumed that pain interventions have been successful. The clinician must reassess the patient's pain after an appropriate time interval and provide further intervention if and when necessary.

Table 20.5 Pharmacological interventions in pain management

Severity of pain	Analgesia
Mild	Simple
Moderate	Simple/compound ± NSAID
Severe	Opiate

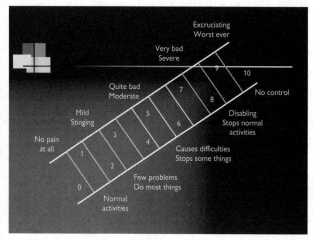

(a)

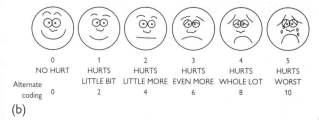

(b)

Fig. 20.12 (a) ♦ Manchester pain ladder. (Adapted with permission from Manchester Triage Group (2005). *Emergency triage*, 2nd edn. Wiley–Blackwell Publishing, Oxford.) (b) ♦ Face scale. (Reproduced with permission from Hockenberry, M.J., Wilson, D., and Winkelstein, M.L. (2005). *Wong's essentials of pediatric nursing*, 7th edn, p. 1259. Mosby, St. Louis.)

Peak flow measurement

Peak flow is an objective measure of lung function and is predominantly used for assessing patients with new onset of asthma or to monitor patients with known asthma. Patients with established asthma should regularly record their peak flow as a reduction can indicate early deterioration in lung function. Often patients do not know their baseline peak flow when well, or the 'best' peak flow they have every performed.

Measuring peak flow is a crucial assessment parameter in diagnosing the severity of an asthma attack and then monitoring the response to inhaled or IV therapies. The peak flow *must* be recorded, on arrival, in all patients attending with asthma. If patient know their 'best' peak flow, the % against their best can be calculated. If their usual peak flow is not known an estimate can be made using the chart in Fig. 20.13a.

Calculating the reduction in peak flow compared to the patient's 'best' or predicted 'best' is a key element in the diagnosis of asthma severity and guides subsequent treatment.

🕭 A peak flow can be performed, depending on individual ability, usually from age 6 upwards (🕮 see Fig. 20.13b), though some patients may need more practice than others. Good technique is essential in performing the peak flow for accurate recording and a demonstration may help achieve this.

Technique
- Put the pointer to zero.
- Ask the patient to stand upright if possible.
- Hold the peak flow horizontally to the mouth.
- Take a deep breath in and close lips tightly around the peak flow mouth piece making a good seal.
- Blow into the peak flow hard and fast. It should be like blowing out a candle rather than blowing up a balloon.
- 3 attempts should be made, with a check on technique each time. The best (highest) reading should recorded.

Poor technique is common. Often patients either fail to make a tight seal around the mouth piece with their lips or do not 'blow' quickly enough or hard enough.

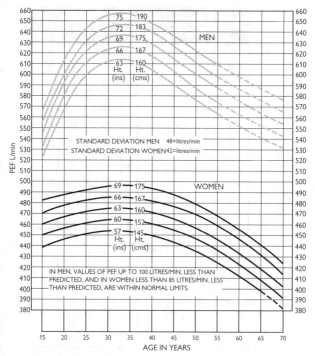

Fig. 20.13a Adult peak expiratory flow chart. (Reproduced with permission from Nunn AJ, Gregg I (1989). New regression equations for predicting peak expiratory flow in adults. *BMJ* **298**, 1068–70.

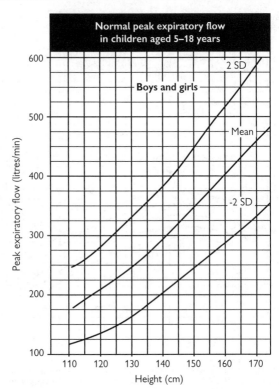

🔁 **Fig. 20.13b** Paediatric peak expiratory flow chart. (Adapted from Godfrey, S., Kamburoff, P.L., and Nairn, J.R. (1970). Spirometry, lung volumes and airway resistance in normal children aged 5 to 18 years. *British Journal of Diseases of the Chest* **64** (1), 15–24. ©1970, with permission from Elsevier.)

Pelvic fixation

Major pelvic fractures are a true orthopaedic emergency. They are often associated with massive blood loss, which can be life-threatening if the fracture is unstable. External fixation can control any further haemorrhage by preventing the movement of the pelvis. If an unstable fracture is suspected an orthopaedic surgeon must be involved early in the patient's care.

Indications
- Uncontrolled hypovolaemic shock from a pelvic fracture.
- Unstable pelvic ring fracture.

Equipment
- External pelvic fixator set.
- Scalpel.
- Local anaesthetic.
- Skin cleansing solution.
- Mask, gloves, gown/apron.
- Sterile drapes.
- Skilled operator, usually a orthopaedic surgeon.
- An image intensifier if available.

Patient preparation
- Explain the procedure to the patient and/or relatives.
- Obtain consent.
- Expose the pelvis.
- Continuous vital sign monitoring.
- Ensure adequate fluid resuscitation.
- Ensure adequate pain relief.
- Assess and document femoral and popliteal pulse.

Procedure
- The skin is cleansed and local anaesthetic infiltrated into the proposed sites for insertion.
- Small incisions are made into the skin at the insertion sites.
- The metal frame is inserted into the sites on the pelvis, under image intensifier if possible.
- The frame is then coupled together and the various pieces tightened together until the frame is complete and secure.

Considerations
If the patient does not require external fixation or a device is not readily available a sheet can be used. Place a sheet under the patient's pelvis and tie the ends together. There are various manufactured 'pelvic belts' available that can also be used.

Pericardiocentesis

Pericardiocentesis (also called pericardial tap or percutaneous pericardiocentesis) is used to remove excess fluid from the pericardial sac. When a pericardial effusion has developed over some time the procedure can be performed electively. In emergency situations the haemopericardium has to be drained immediately. The pericardial sac has filled rapidly with blood and cardiac filling and emptying are grossly impaired.

Increased amounts of pericardial fluid may result from:

- trauma (penetrating and non-penetrating): can result in life-threatening amounts of blood in the pericardial sac (cardiac tamponade);
- myocardial infarction, congestive heart failure;
- pericarditis caused by chest trauma, MI, infection, inflammation;
- surgery or other invasive procedures performed on the heart;
- cancer producing malignant effusions;
- renal failure.

In emergency care, the procedure is most commonly performed to remove blood from the pericardial sac and relieve the cardiac tamponade.

Signs and symptoms of acute pericardial effusion

- Beck's triad. Distant heart sounds, neck vein distension (due to compression on right atrium/ventricle), and hypotension.
- Tachycardia usually occurs due to ↑ venous pressure and ↓ BP, which indicates haemodynamically significant pericardial effusion.
- Tachypnoea will develop in acute situations.
- Narrow pulse pressure can occur in patients with significant pericardial effusion.
- Cardiac arrhythmias and PEA can occur if large effusions.
- Elevated CVP occurs from ↑ pressure in the pericardial space and the ventricles. This condition is usually associated with hypotension.

▶ In the busy resuscitation room clinical signs can be hard to isolate. An echocardiogram is an invaluable diagnostic tool.

Indications

- Cardiac tamponade.
- Haemodynamic compromise due to large/rapidly developing pericardial effusion.
- Management of large pericardial effusion (> 20mm separation of pericardial membranes on echocardiography).
- In cardiac arrest as a possible reversible cause of PEA.

Contraindications

- Small effusions do not require emergency needle pericardiocentesis.
- Haemodynamically stable patients can be managed conservatively.
- Aortic dissection as a cause for the pericardial effusion.
- Uncorrected bleeding disorder.
- Posteriorly located pericardial effusion.

Equipment

- 2 tier procedure trolley.
- An 18- to 20-gauge cardiac/spinal needle.

- A 3-way stopcock.
- Syringes (10mL, 20mL, and 60mL).
- Antiseptic skin cleansing solution.
- ECG monitor and defibrillator.
- Specimen collection tubes for fluid analysis and cultures.
- Small-gauge needle for LA and lidocaine.
- Sterile gloves, mask, gown, dressing materials, and gauze
- Resuscitation drugs.
- Sedating medications if required.

Patient preparation

- This emergency procedure has to be performed rapidly. Patients are critically ill with profound haemodynamic compromise. Explain the procedure clearly to gain consent if the patient is conscious.
- Sedation may be administered if the patient is restless or anxious.
- Position the patient upright at ~ 45° angle.
- Tell patient to remain still and support throughout if conscious.
- Cardiac monitoring and vital signs are recorded throughout procedure.

Nursing role

- Support the patient during the procedure. The patient may experience a sensation of pressure as the needle enters the membrane.
- Monitor vital signs and cardiac rhythm during pericardiocentesis. If the myocardium is stimulated by the needle, ST segment elevation will be noted on the ECG and the needle will need to be withdrawn slightly.
- When the needle is in the correct position, the clinician will withdraw blood from the pericardial sac with a syringe.
- A pericardial catheter may be attached to the needle to allow for continuous drainage of blood.
- After the cardiac needle is removed, pressure is applied to the puncture site for approximately 5min, and the site is then dressed.
- Continuous vital signs and cardiac monitoring.

▶ It is often reported that the blood aspirated from a haemopericardium does not clot in the syringe as the fibrin has been inactivated by the movement of the heart.

Patients often make a dramatic recovery immediately after pericardiocentesis; their conscious level, BP, and cardiovascular status improve.

Complications

- Laceration of coronary artery/vein.
- Acute left ventricular failure with pulmonary oedema.
- Puncture or laceration of any cardiac chamber.
- Bleeding.
- Ventricular/atrial ectopic beats.
- Arrhythmias.
- Hypotension.
- Pneumothorax.
- Pulmonary oedema.

Plastering skills

Applying a plaster of Paris (POP) or fibreglass cast is commonly done to immobilize a limb following a fracture or other significant injury. Plastering is one of the most common skills used in emergency care and a large range of casts may need to be applied. You may find that there are several ways of applying the same plaster and each clinician may have a slightly different approach. This section describes the general principles for applying common casts in adults and children.

Patient preparation

- Check you have the right patient and identify the correct limb.
- Check the patient notes and X-rays and ensure the plaster prescribed is appropriate for the injury.
- Inform the patient of procedure and rationale for applying the plaster.
- Obtain the patient's consent.
- Identify any allergies or sensitive skin conditions.
- Ensure adequate pain relief. This is crucial to enable the limb to be positioned correctly.
- Assist the patient into the most comfortable, appropriate position.
- Remove clothing as appropriate from the affected limb.
- Make sure you are at a comfortable height and have assistance to hold the limb if necessary.
- Remove rings, watches, and bracelets from the limb to be plastered.
- Check the skin is intact. If there are any wounds ensure they are cleaned, +/– closed and dressed as appropriate.
- Protect the patient's clothing from the wet plaster.
- Assess and document the neurovascular status of the limb (colour, sensation, capillary refill).

Plaster application—general principles

- Collect the correct-sized stockinette, padding, plaster, and bandages if a backslab is being applied.
- Apply adequate padding smoothly and evenly.
- Each plaster bandage should be soaked individually.
- Water should be lukewarm and the patient informed that when the plaster is applied it will feel warm and that this is normal (due to the thermogenic reaction of the setting plaster).
- Roll on the plaster bandage starting from one end of the limb. Cover 50% of the previous turn keeping the bandage smooth and without applying tension.
- When required number of bandages have been applied, smoothe with water so that each layer bonds together.
- Clean the patient's skin where any plaster has come into contact.

Discharge assessment and information

- Assess ability to perform ADLs, social circumstances, and available support. Refer to social services/intermediate care if necessary.
- Patients should be advised of the importance of elevation in reducing swelling, pain, discomfort, and complication.
- Give written and verbal 'plaster care instructions' (see Box 20.3).

- Ensure adequate discharge analgesia.
- Arrange follow-up.
- Supply necessary walking aids.

Box 20.3 Plaster care instructions

- Do not get the plaster wet
- Keep the limb elevated
- Do not walk on a lower limb plaster unless instructed to do so
- Keep the fingers/toes moving
- Return if your fingers/toes become painful, blue, numb, difficult to move or you experience pins and needles—the plaster may be too tight
- Return if the plaster becomes loose, cracked, or damaged in any way

---

Fibreglass casts

These are often used after initial swelling has settled or if a below-knee walking cast is required. The principles for application are similar to those for POP with several important caveats.

- Gloves must always be worn as the adhesive resin within the fibreglass does not wash off skin.
- Clothing must be protected as the resin will not wash off clothing.
- Great care should be taken around the edges of the cast and extra padding applied. As there is no 'give' in a fibreglass cast the edges remain hard and can be rough causing skin irritation, blistering, and even cuts.
- The importance of elevation should be emphasized as the fibreglass is a rigid structure and can quickly become too tight.

▶ Back slab casts are most commonly applied in the ED as the first cast because of the risk of swelling. Full casts are often applied a few days later.

Upper limb casts

Below elbow back slab

This plaster provides support yet allows for any swelling in the initial period post injury.

Equipment:
- Stockinette.
- Wool padding.
- Plaster of Paris (cut to reach from 1cm proximal to the MCPJ and 2cm from the elbow; folded to give 6–8 layers).
- Bandage.
- Scissors.
- Warm water (25–35°C).
- Gloves.
- Apron.
- Sling.

Application
- Apply stockinette to the limb cutting a hole for the thumb.
- Apply padding from knuckles to the elbow crease overlapping each previous layer by 50%.
- Trim plaster slab to round corners and cut out a triangle at one end to allow movement of thumb.
- Ensure the patient's elbow is resting on a firm surface, the wrist is in a neutral position, and the fingers and thumb outstretched.
- Wet plaster slab and apply to forearm; wrist should be in a neutral position.
- Smoothe to contours of the arm and fold over stockinette to a neat edge.
- Secure with pre-soaked bandage including securing through 1st web space.
- Finish with a small extra strip of plaster slab to secure final layer of bandage on top of the slab.
- Apply broad arm sling and advise patient on elevation.

Below elbow full cast

This cast is used to immobilize upper limbs, usually for fractures in the distal 1/3 of the forearm bones. This cast should extend from just above the knuckles at the back of the hand to allow full flexion/extension of the MCPJs to just below the elbow allowing full movement at the elbow joint. The thumb should be completely free.

Equipment
- Stockinette.
- Wool padding.
- Plaster of Paris bandage.
- Warm water.
- Gloves.
- Apron.
- Sling.

Application

- Apply stockinette to the limb cutting a hole for the thumb.
- Apply padding from knuckles to the elbow crease overlapping each previous layer by 50%.
- Position limb in required position for the type of fracture.
- Begin bandaging with the wetted plaster bandages at the elbow and down the arm towards the hand.
- Bring the bandage up through the 1st web space, fold down the stockinette, and catch with the 2nd layer of bandage.
- Mould the cast into the palm to allow the layers to bond.
- Ensure there is adequate room for the thumb to move without rubbing on the plaster.
- Apply broad arm sling and advise patient on elevation.

Scaphoid cast

This is a full below elbow cast but includes the thumb to the level of the IPJ but allowing movement of this joint.

Equipment

- Stockinette in two sizes.
- Wool padding.
- Plaster of Paris bandage.
- Warm water.
- Gloves.
- Apron.
- Sling.

Application

- Apply stockinette to the limb cutting a hole for the thumb. Cover the thumb with a slimmer length of stockinette.
- Apply padding from knuckles and around the thumb to below the elbow crease overlapping each previous layer by 50%.
- Position limb in required position for the patient (ask them to maintain a circle with the tips of the thumb and forefinger). The wrist should be in a neutral position.
- Begin bandaging with the wetted plaster bandages at the elbow and down the arm towards the hand.
- Bring the bandage up through the 1st web space, and go around the thumb.
- Fold down the stockinette on the hand and thumb and at elbow and catch with next layer of plaster. The tip of the thumb from the level of the IPJ should be exposed and the patient should be able to flex and extend the IPJ.
- Mould well into palm and around the thumb.
- Apply broad arm sling and advise patient on elevation.

Lower limb casts

Below knee back slab

This cast provides support and immobilization whilst allowing for any initial swelling post-injury.

Equipment

- Stockinette.
- Wool padding.
- Plaster of Paris bandage.
- Bandage.
- Warm water.
- Gloves.
- Apron.

Application

- Apply stockinette to the limb so that it extends beyond the toes and above the knee.
- Apply padding from below knee joint to base of toes overlapping each previous layer by 50%.
- Cut a plaster slab of 8 layers that extends from the back of the knee to the base of the toes.
- If applying the plaster without any assistance it will be easier to position the patient prone with their ankle bent over the edge of the trolley so it is at a 90° angle.
- Wet plaster slab and apply to lower limb. It should go posteriorly just below the knee, over the ankle, and to the base of the toes. The ankle should be at 90°.
- Smoothe to contours of the leg and fold over stockinette to create a neat edge.
- Secure with pre-soaked bandages.
- A long U-shaped slab called a stirrup may need to be added if the cast is immobilizing an unstable ankle fracture. The stirrup is applied down one side of the leg above the ankle, under the heel, and up the other side of the leg to the ankle. This is held in place with a pre-soaked stretch bandage.
- Finish with a small strip of plaster slab to secure final layer of bandage over the slab.

Below knee cast

This cast immobilizes the leg for lower limb injuries.

Equipment

- Stockinette.
- Wool padding.
- Plaster of Paris bandage.
- Bandage.
- Warm water.
- Gloves.
- Apron.

Application

- Apply stockinette to the limb so that it extends beyond the toes and above the knee.
- Apply padding from below knee joint to base of toes overlapping each previous layer by 50%.
- Soak plaster bandage and apply to lower limb starting just below the knee and extending to the base of the toes. The ankle should be held at 90°.
- Smoothe to contours of the leg and fold over stockinette to create a neat edge.
- Catch edges in with second layer of plaster bandage.
- Smoothe to allow layers to bond together.
- Advise patient on elevation.

Cylinder cast

This type of cast is used for leg injuries where the ankle does not need to be immobilized. It is usually used for injuries to the knee.

Equipment

- Stockinette.
- Wool padding.
- Felt padding.
- Plaster of Paris bandage.
- Stretch bandage.
- Warm water.
- Gloves.
- Apron.

Application

- Apply a 2 inch wide strip of orthopaedic felt around the ankle just above the malleoli.
- Apply stockinette to the limb so that it extends from the level of the ankle to the groin.
- Apply padding from the top of thigh to the ankle, overlapping each previous layer by 50%.
- The leg should be supported and the knee flexed at 10°.
- Soak plaster bandage and apply to limb. It should start distally just above the bottom edge of the felt padding.
- Smoothe to contours of the leg and fold over stockinette to create a neat edge.
- Catch edges in with second layer of plaster bandage.
- Smooth to allow layers to bond together especially around medial and lateral sides of the thigh.
- Advise patient on elevation.

Pulse oximetry

Pulse oximetry is a routine monitoring tool used in most if not all emergency care areas. It measures the amount of oxygen-saturated haemoglobin in the blood giving a bedside picture of oxygen requirements.
- 🔂 Probes are available for all ages and weights of children and neonates and can be attached to fingers, hands, toes, feet or earlobes depending on their design.
- ▶ For an accurate reading it is vital that the correct probe is used and it is attached to the right site.
- In health, oxygen saturations should be > 95%. 93–95% is often recorded in patients who smoke.

Equipment needed
- Pulse oximeter.
- Appropriately sized and type of probe.
- Oxygen and delivery devices if required.

Procedure
- Explain the need for the pulse oximetry to patient and/or parent.
- Remove any nail varnish as this may interfere with the reading.
- Ensure the probe is clean, attach to the patient's finger, ear, or toe depending on the probe design
- Observe the trace on the monitor. A poor trace may give a falsely low reading.
- When the trace and signal are of good quality record the oxygen saturation level.

▶ Reminders
Pulse oximetry is a quick, non-invasive method of measuring oxygen saturation. However it has many limitations.
- It is unable to differentiate between haemoglobin that is saturated with oxygen and haemoglobin that is saturated with carbon monoxide. In carbon monoxide poisoning pulse oximetry is of little value in establishing oxygen requirements.
- As the oxygen saturation falls there is a disproportionate fall in PaO_2. When saturations fall below 90% there is a dramatic fall in PaO_2.
- If the patient is cold, hypovolaemic, or peripherally vasoconstricted there may be an artificially low reading.
- In severe anaemia, saturations may be 100%. This is because all the available haemoglobin is saturated with oxygen. The probe does not identify when haemoglobin levels are low.
- The pulse oximeter does not detect the retention of carbon dioxide; this is measured by ABG sampling.

Rapid infuser

The rapid infuser enables the rapid infusion of warmed IV fluids and requires *one* dedicated member of staff to operate it. This is a commonplace piece of equipment in resuscitation rooms and other critical care areas.

Indication for use To provide rapid flow of warmed fluid, such as crystalloid or blood product, including red blood cells, as volume replacement for patients suffering from blood loss due to trauma or surgery.

Operation Please refer to operator's manual for in-depth instruction and alarms.

Equipment
- Disposable rapid infusor set.
- IV fluid.
- Fluid balance recording chart.

Set up
- Power off.
- Install disposable set.
- Prime disposable set.
- Power on.
- Fluid begins to warm.
- Activate pressure chambers.

Use of fluid warmer
- Ensure set up has been completed.
- Load the pressure chambers. Ensure solution bag is hanging on appropriate hook inside door.
- Pressurize the pressure chambers.
- Connect to the patient and begin infusion.
- Change fluid bag.
  - Release the pressure in the chamber.
  - Close clamp under empty bag.
  - Open door and remove used fluid bag.
  - Spike new bag.
  - Hang new bag and close and latch door.
  - Pressurize chamber.
  - Open clamp.
- Record times, types, and volumes of fluid delivered accurately.

After use
- Discontinue infusion.
- Turn fluid warmer off.
- Release chamber pressure.
- Remove disposable set.
- Discard set in biohazard container/sharps bin.
- Visually check condition of device, and report any problems.
- Clean with warm soapy water.

Sengstaken tube insertion

Sengstaken–Blakemore tubes are used as a salvage procedure. The tube acts as a temporary tamponade for any severe or life-threatening oesophageal bleeding. The tube has 3 lumens: one to inflate a gastric balloon; one to inflate an oesophageal balloon; and the third to aspirate the stomach.

Indication Severe/life-threatening haemorrhage from oesophageal bleeding when urgent endoscopy is not available.

Equipment
- Sengstaken–Blakemore tube (from the fridge).
- Lubricant.
- Manual sphygmomanometer.
- 50mL syringes.
- 1000mL normal saline.
- Local anaesthetic throat spray.

Patient preparation
- Explain the procedure to the patient. It can be unpleasant but is vital in the attempt to control the bleeding.
- Assist patient into left lateral position (unless intubated).

Procedure
- Check all the balloons inflate and do not leak.
- Hold the tube to the patient's nose and measure the approximate length to the epigastrium. This is the length of tube that should be inserted; note the marker on the side of the tube.
- Spray throat with local anaesthetic.
- The tube is inserted through the mouth. The patient is encouraged to swallow the tube.
- Insert approximately 10cm past the marker noted on the side of the tube when it was measured.
- Inflate the gastric balloon to the prescribed pressure (this is usually written on the packet). Withdraw the tube until resistance is felt. The tube should be sat below the oesophageal sphincter.
- The oesophageal balloon is not normally inflated.
- The stomach can be aspirated to remove any residual blood.
- The tube can be attached to a weight (1000mL saline). This helps to ensure the tube remains in situ.
- Monitor these pressures with the sphygmomanometer to ensure they stay inflated.
- Support the patient during the procedure as it can be very distressing.
- Monitor vital signs continuously.
- Give mouth care.

Complications
- Oesophageal rupture.
- Gastric rupture.

Skin traction: application

Skin traction is always applied prior to the use of a Thomas splint (📖 see p.670) or prior to Gallows traction in children < 2 years ●.

Rationale for use of skin traction

- To immobilize and maintain bone alignment by pulling the limb into a straight position.
- To reduce a fracture.
- To relieve muscle spasms.
- To relieve pain.
- To take pressure off the fractured bone ends by relaxing the muscle.
- To prevent further vessel or soft tissue injury.

Equipment

- Correct skin traction pack (adult or child).
- Razor.
- Scissors.
- Bandages.
- Tape.

How to apply leg skin traction

- Both sides of the limb should be shaved so that the fabric tape can adhere firmly to clean dry skin.
- Follow steps in Figs 20.14–20.18.
- Once the bandage is secured traction can be applied using standard 5–7lb weights. The pull of the cord must be level with the fabric tape; see picture 20.20.
- Assess the distal colour, sensation, and movement of the limb once the traction has been applied.

Precautions for use

- Avoid creases and wrinkles of the fabric tape as these could lead to pressure problems and cause ulcers.
- Patients with allergies to tape or elastoplast may have a reaction and their skin should be observed regularly.
- Avoid traction weight > than that which can be applied through the skin, i.e. not exceeding 7lb.

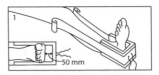

Fig. 20.14 With foot in dorsiflexion (toes pointing towards ceiling) place spreader plate with foam padding inwards towards sole of foot. It should be placed at distance of ~ 50mm from sole of foot. This allows free movement of ankle joint and protects ankle and side of foot from pressure.

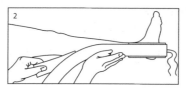

Fig. 20.15 Remove the backing material and unroll the full skin traction kit up either side of the patient's leg keeping the spreader plate 5cm from the foot. Smooth the adhesive surfaces of the fabric tape firmly up the leg.

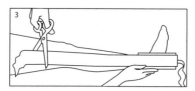

Fig. 20.16 The correct length of the adhesive tape can be determined and cut as desired depending on fracture site. Repeat procedure for opposite side of limb.

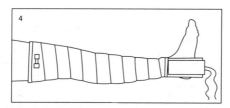

Fig. 20.17 Maximum adhesion can be obtained by application of the retention bandage. Commence bandaging at the ankle with one or two turns initially to secure the fabric tape. Use a firm but even tension along length of limb.

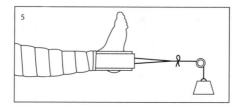

Fig. 20.18 Ensure patient is on a hospital bed prior to applying the weights as ED trolleys do not have the correct attachment to attach the weights.

Spinal boards

Spinal boards were originally designed as a pre-hospital extrication device used to transport patients with possible spinal injuries. They are not designed for the long-term management of patients with spinal injuries and patients should be taken off a spinal board as quickly as possible.

Uses

- The spinal board is a valuable tool for transfer and allows patients to be moved from one place to another without movement of their spine.
- Patients arrive at ED already on a spinal board. It is rare that patients are put on to a board in ED.

Equipment

- Hard collar.
- Spinal board and head blocks.
- 3 body straps.
- Suction.
- 5 persons.

Care of patient who arrives on a spinal board

- Explain to patient the need to stay on the spinal board until an examination of the neck and back has taken place.
- Instruct patient not to move.
- Ensure the collar is the correct size and fitted appropriately.
- Ensure the head blocks, straps, and body straps are secure.
- Ensure oxygen and suction are readily available.
- Assess and document limb movement and sensation. Ask the patient to gently wiggle their fingers and toes; check sensation in the upper and lower limbs.
- Ensure adequate pain relief.
- If the patient is nauseous arrange for an anti-emetic to be given.
- Give the patient and/or relative a call bell so they can immediately summon help.
- Any patient with GCS < 15, anxious, agitated, intoxicated, or with a potential airway problem should not be left unsupervised.

Cautions

- Pressure areas are at immediate risk once a patient is placed on a spinal board. Therefore, they should be taken off it as soon as possible.
- Any clothing under the patient can be uncomfortable and may contribute to pressure if it is wrinkled. Remove clothing to smooth out where possible.
- The airway is potentially at risk on any patient immobilized and strapped to a spinal board. A careful assessment must be made of the risk to their airway and it must be managed appropriately.

Log rolling on a spinal board

This is undertaken to examine the patient's neck and back.

- Assemble a team: one person to examine the patient, one team leader to take control of the head and neck, and 3 other people to perform the log roll.

- Ensure there is enough space to perform the log roll and that the trolley is at a comfortable height for the procedure.
- The team leader is responsible for coordinating the whole procedure and their commands **must** be followed at all times.
- Explain the procedure to the patient and reassure them that they will not fall.
- Any clothing that needs to be removed should be cut at this stage to enable easy removal when the patient is rolled.
- The team leader takes manual control of the head and neck after the straps and blocks have been removed. At no time is the head/neck left unrestrained. Depending on the patient's injuries and complaints of pain the collar may also be removed to allow examination.
- The 'log roll' team of three stand along one side of the patient. The patient should be rolled on to the side of least injury.
- The clinician examining the patient's neck and back stands on the opposite side from the team.
- The body straps are removed.
- The 'log roll' team position themselves. Person one stands at the level of the patient's shoulder with one hand over the far shoulder and the other over the far hip. The second person places one hand over the far hip next to person one's hand and their second hand under the far knee. The third person places both hands under the far leg.
- On the team leader's instruction (the team all have to be clear what the instruction is) the patient is rolled on to their side towards the team.
- The examining clinician removes clothing and examines the back and/or neck
- Once the examination is complete the spinal board and any clothing is usually removed
- The team leader give the command to roll the patient back on to their back
- Collar, head blocks, and straps may be reapplied.
- Depending upon the examination findings the patient may have to stay flat on the ED trolley with their neck immobilized until further investigations have been done.
- Movement and sensation of the limbs should be checked at the end of the procedure.

Thomas splint application

Indications

A Thomas splint is a traction splint, most commonly used to manage fractured shaft of femurs in adults and children > 2 years ❸. A Thomas splint provides:

- immobilization and stabilization;
- reduction of pain from muscle spasm;

Equipment

- Thomas splint (correct size and one size above and below).
- Tape measure.
- Calico slings.
- Safety pins (large).
- Skin traction kit.
- Crepe bandages.
- Padding (cotton wool rolls).
- Strong stretch tape (elastoplast).
- Two tongue depressors.
- Pillows.

Patient preparation

- Explain the procedure to the patient.
- Gain consent.
- Ensure adequate pain relief, ideally with a femoral nerve block. Use Entonox® as required.

Procedure

▶This procedure requires at least three people to ensure the comfort and safety of the patient.

- Identify that you have the correct patient.
- Assemble equipment needed for procedure.
- Identify the affected limb by confirming with the notes/X-rays and the patient.
- Measure the affected limb to determine the correct size of splint. Measure obliquely around the thigh at its highest point allowing an extra 1cm. Then measure from perineum to heel for the length of the splint allowing an extra 15–20cm for plantar flexion.
- Choose appropriate sized splint and one size above and below.
- Prepare the splint by attaching the calico slings with the safety pins ensuring that the pins are fastened at the back on the lateral aspect to avoid their contact with the patient.
- Check the status of the limb—pulse, colour, temperature, sensation, and movement—and document your findings.

An appropriately qualified person should apply gentle traction to the affected limb for the remainder of the procedure.

- Apply the skin traction kit (📖 see p.666).
- Gently place the leg through the Thomas splint, ensuring that the Achilles tendon is not lying on the calico slings. If the splint is the wrong size remove whilst still maintaining traction and reapply correct size. Ensure the splint is not rubbing against the genitalia or surrounding area,
- Place padding under the leg over the calico slings with extra padding under the back of the knee and, if required, under the site of the fracture.
- Attach the cords to the splint whilst the gentle traction is maintained.
  - Pass the tapes over the left and right bars one over and one under.
  - Whilst maintaining the gentle traction on the leg pull traction cords around the splint end over and under, then under and over.
  - Knot securely.
- Secure the leg to the splint with the crepe bandages and secure the bandages with elastic tape.
- Insert 2 taped together tongue depressors between the cords and gently twist to create traction.
- Elevate the leg on pillows.
- Check circulation and neurological function regularly.
- Re-X-ray the leg to determine the level of traction applied.
- Document application.
- Dispose of equipment.

Risks

- Increased pain to the patient.
- Pressure area formation if padding not applied appropriately.
- Damage to Achilles tendon if it lies over the calico slings.
- Damage to peroneal nerve if the knee not appropriately padded.
- Potential foot drop if not enough room to plantar flex foot.

Transporting the critically ill

Transporting patients to wards, X-ray, theatre, intensive care, and tertiary centres occurs regularly in emergency care. Transferring the critically ill/injured can be fraught with clinical risk if the transfer is poorly coordinated or lacks the right equipment or staff with the requisite training. Transfer-related mortality and morbidity is frequently reported with patients suffering from a wide range of problems, e.g. hypoventilation, hypotension, hypertension, ABG alteration, heart rate changes, changes in ICP, airway obstruction, disconnected IV lines, and abrupt stopping of medications.

Departmental policies and procedures should be followed to ensure that risk in minimized. Increasingly 'retrieval teams' from tertiary centres are used to retrieve patients, ensure they are stable, and transport them to their destination.

▶ Regardless of whether a patient is being transferred within the same hospital or across the country the same levels of preparation, supervision, and care must be ensured.

Preparation for transfer

Careful planning is required prior to transportation taking into consideration the following:
- pre-transport co-ordination and communication;
- mode of transport;
- personnel;
- patient stability;
- information for relatives;
- equipment for transport;
- drugs for transport;
- monitoring during transport.

Pre-transport communication

- The clinician responsible for the care for the patient should communicate directly with the receiving area and ensure that all the advice and instructions have been carried out.
- All notes, investigation results, and patient information should be copied for the transfer.
- The receiving area should be informed of the expected time of arrival of the patient.

Mode of transport

Out of hospital transfer could be undertaken by ground or air. Consider the following:
- patient problem/s;
- urgency;
- availability of various modes;
- geography;
- weather conditions;
- traffic;
- cost.

Personnel Clinical staff with appropriate training who are able to manage any eventuality on route should accompany the patient.

Patient stability

Patients must be fully resuscitated and stable prior to transfer in order to minimize any untoward occurrences. The main exception occurs when patients are being transferred to a tertiary centre for emergency surgery, e.g. vascular or neurological.

- Airway secured and maintained.
- Breathing adequately supported; intubation and ventilation may be required prior to transfer.
- Circulation stable, supported, and adequately monitored, e.g. arterial line, several secure venous lines, blood for transport if required, control of external bleeding, urinary catheter to monitor haemodynamic status.
- Neurological status. Maintain normal ICP; control seizure activity; preserve integrity of spinal cord.
- Musculoskeletal system. Prevent further blood loss; fracture immobilization; wound care; analgesia.
- All lines and tubes, e.g. ETT, chest drain, should be secure and protected from accidental dislodging.
- Care of the patient's clothing and valuables.

Relatives

- Informed of the need to transfer and approximate time span.
- Ensure that they see their relative prior to transfer.
- Give information about how to reach the destination and advise not to try to follow an ambulance.

Equipment

- Suitable trolley for transfer.
- Ability to keep the patient warm.
- Equipment that is reliable during transfer with fully charged batteries and an adequate supplemental oxygen supply.
- Additional equipment in full working order should accompany the patient; this is usually in some form of 'transfer bag'.

Drugs Appropriate drugs to treat any eventuality must be available.

Monitoring during transfer

- Secure monitors; easily visible.
- ECG, non-invasive or invasive BP, SpO_2, $EtCO_2$, temperature.
- Unhindered access to the patient during transfer.

Venepuncture

Venepuncture enables the collection of venous blood without the need to insert an indwelling device, e.g. cannula. The most widely used technique is with a closed 'Vacutainer®' system as this reduces needle stick injuries and the possible contamination of blood samples.

Equipment

- Needle or butterfly needle (often used in children) for use with Vacutainer® connection.
- Vacutainer® barrel.
- Appropriate blood collection bottles.
- Tourniquet.
- Non-sterile gloves and apron.
- Sharps bin.
- Alcohol-based cleansing swab.
- Gauze.
- Elastoplasts® (check patient allergies).

Patient preparation Explain procedure to patient, obtaining consent.

Vein selection

- Patients are often able to aid in the selection of a vein as they know which sites have previously been successful. Follow their advice.
- Usually the best site for venepuncture (unless the patient tells you otherwise) is in the antecubital fossa (ACF). Veins in the ACF have a large lumen, lie close to the surface of the skin, and there is minimal superficial nerve supply.
- Apply the tourniquet to the middle of the upper arm, 7–10cm above puncture site.
- With the arm in a downward position palpate the ACF to locate a vein.
- Identify the course and depth of the vein to distinguish nearby structures such as tendons and arteries. The vein should be bouncy, prominent, and refill easily when depressed.
- Release the tourniquet and observe the vein decompressing. A thrombosed vein will remain raised and should not be used.

Blood collection

- Wear gloves and an apron.
- Reapply the tourniquet.
- Clean the area over the selected vein with an alcohol swab and allow to dry.
- Connect the Vacutainer® to the needle.
- Without touching the chosen area of skin, apply manual traction with the thumb of the free hand 2–3cm below the chosen site to anchor the vein in position.
- Holding the needle at a 15°–30° angle to the vein with the bevel pointing upwards, advance into the skin. A sensation of resistance may be felt followed by the needle entering the vein.
- To stabilize the needle within the vein advance a further 1–2mm.
- Secure the needle by holding the Vacutainer® firmly in place.

- Using the other hand, advance the blood collection bottles into the Vacutainer® and over the rubber-sheathed needle one after the other.
- Blood will flow until the vacuum within the bottle is exhausted, ensuring an adequate sample size.
- Remove the final bottle and release the tourniquet.
- Cover the needle puncture site with the gauze and swiftly remove the needle from the skin at the same angle of insertion.
- Apply gentle digital pressure over the puncture site.
- Dispose of the needle within the sharps collection bin.
- The patient/relative can then apply digital pressure until bleeding stops (~2min).
- Check the puncture site and apply the plaster.
- Ensure that patient is comfortable.
- Check the patient's details, name, date of birth against the notes and label the blood samples.
- Transport samples to the laboratory.

Ventilation: mechanical

All patients on a mechanical ventilator need close monitoring, ideally one nurse to one patient. The nurse must have training in use of ventilators or immediate access to staff with adequate training.

Equipment
- Mechanical ventilator.
- Monitoring equipment, including capnograph.
- Oxygen supply.
- Suction.
- Bag/mask/valve (in case of ventilator failure).
- Stethoscope.

Procedure
- Secure endotracheal tube to patient.
- Ensure ET tube has been sited correctly with X-ray.
- Attach capnograph to appropriate monitoring equipment.
- Regular auscultation of chest to ensure air entry to both lungs.
- Suction if secretions are impeding gas exchange.
- Ensure patient maintains satisfactory body temperature.
- Tape patient's eyes closed.

Risks
- Hypothermia.
- Foreign body in patient's eye.
- Low pressure.
- Inadequate ventilation.
- Build up of secretions.
- Ventilator failure.

Actions
- Ensure patient is adequately warmed.
- Tape patient's eyes closed.
- Check all connections are closed and appropriate ports are closed.
- Discuss with the doctor whether ventilation pressures are appropriate.
- Suction patient as appropriate.
- Manually ventilate patient until ventilator is replaced.
- Ensure a comprehensive handover is given to receiving area staff.

Dräger Oxylog 2000/3000 transportable ventilator
The Oxylog ventilator provides advanced ventilation for both breathing and apnoeic patients by delivering consistent ventilation by control or synchronization.

Equipment
- One large full O_2 cylinder with a Schrader valve.
- One Oxylog 2000/3000.
- One breathing circuit.
- One bacterial filter.
- Full patient monitoring.
- One charging lead.

Ventilator safety checks

- Turn ventilator on to ensure that the charging light is illuminated, connect breathing circuit to ventilator, and connect to oxygen source.
- Set the ventilator to IPPV mode, P_{max} 40mmg, I: E ratio 1:2, freq. breaths 14, Vt 0.6L.
- Connect the test lung to the breathing circuit after 15 seconds ensure that the LCD is reading mV of 8.4
- Compress the test lung and hold this should activate the Pmax alarm.
- Remove the test lung after 5 second this should activate the apnoea alarm.
- Checks are now complete.

Ventilating the patient

- There must be an anaesthetist/experienced ED clinician present who will prescribe the ventilator settings.
- Ensure full monitoring.
- Plug the ventilator into a piped oxygen source and mains electricity.
- Connect the breathing circuit with bacterial filter to the ventilator.
- Set the prescribed ventilator settings before attaching to patient.
- Set mode of ventilation, e.g. IPPV.
- Set air or non-air mix (60% oxygen and 40% air in mix setting)
- Set prescribed frequency of breaths (dependent on patient condition/age)
- Set maximum pressure (Pmax), which depends on patient's condition/ age.
- Set PEEP (dependent on patient condition)..
- Set I:E ratio (dependent on patient condition)
- Set tidal volume (Vt) based on 7mL/kg.
- Connect to the patient.
- Ensure patient has 15-30min observations including recording minute volumes (mV). Minute volumes should be Vt × frequency of breaths.
- Take an ABG every hour.
- Only disconnect the ventilator from piped oxygen and mains electricity immediately prior to transfer. On arrival at the destination reconnect to piped and mains supplies.

Glossary of terms

- IPPV, intermittent positive pressure ventilation.
- CMV, controlled mandatory ventilation.
- SIPPV, synchronized intermittent positive pressure ventilation.
- CPAP, continuous positive airway pressure.
- SIMV, synchronized intermittent mandatory ventilation.
- PEEP, peak end expiratory pressure.
- I:E, ratio of inspiration time to expiration time.
- Pmax, maximum pressure exerted.
- Vt, tidal volumes.
- mV, minute volumes.

Ventilation: non-invasive (NIV)

NIV is the delivery of ventilatory support without the need for an invasive artificial airway, i.e. ETT. NIV plays a significant role in the management of acute and chronic respiratory failure in adults and children. NIV often eliminates the need for intubation or tracheostomy and preserves normal swallowing, speech, and cough mechanisms. The use of non-invasive positive-pressure ventilation (NIPPV) in hospital settings and at home has been steadily increasing. The two most common types of NIV are continuous positive pressure ventilation (CPAP) and bi-level positive airway pressure (BiPAP).

CPAP maintains the alveoli in an 'open' state by applying pressure at the end of expiration. CPAP reduces alveolar collapse with a resulting improvement in lung volumes and gaseous exchange. CPAP is effective in type I respiratory failure associated with conditions such as pulmonary oedema or pneumonia and is generally associated with the provision of high oxygen concentrations.

BiPAP modes IPAP (intermittent positive airway pressure) and EPAP (end positive airway pressure) provide positive pressure when the patient starts to breath in until they start to exhale. BIPAP is synchronized with the patient's respiratory cycle (i.e. the machine complies with the patient). IPAP is applied as the patient breathes in and functions by reducing the patient's work of breathing and increasing the tidal volume allowing greater CO_2 removal (normally set at 12–18). EPAP is the background or CPAP pressure that is on constantly, improving alveoli recruitment.

BiPAP is generally administered with controlled oxygen therapy. It is used in patients with type II respiratory failure associated most commonly with COPD/pneumonia/pulmonary oedema.

Absolute contraindications

- Coma
- Agitation
- Inability to protect airway

Relative contraindications

- Severe acidosis (pH < 7.1).
- Excessive bronchial secretions.
- Haemodynamic instability.
- Pulmonary TB.
- Recent upper GI surgery.
- Orofacial abnormalities.

▶ If a pneumothorax is present a chest drain must be in situ or there is a high risk of a tension pneumothorax developing.

Setting up

Assemble the machine/circuit away from the patient and ensure it is working properly. The initial settings are usually an IPAP of 12 and an EPAP of 4. If higher settings are likely to be required starting the patient on the lower setting indicated above can help with compliance.

- BiPAP machine.
- BiPAP circuit.

- NIV facemask. Must be measured to fit patient using guide provided.
- Filter.
- Attach circuit to machine and mask (usually only 1 way to do this).
- Attach oxygen tubing to port on mask and set at prescribed flow rate.
- If transfer (internal or external) on the machine is a possibility, ensure the transfer battery is on charge.

Patient preparation

The patient's first experience of BiPAP can be distressing but its effective use may be life-saving and greatly alter patient outcome.

- Explain clearly to the patient and/or relatives what the machine does and how it will help them.
- Let patient feel air pressures with their hands before applying to face.
- When applying mask to the face hold it gently in place, allowing the patient to become accustomed to the feel of it.
- Gradually apply more pressure to obtain the snug fit required.
- When the patient is ready apply the straps.
- Avoid strapping too tightly or unequally but try to minimize leakage (a small amount of leakage may be unavoidable).
- Try to avoid leaks into the eyes as this may precipitate drying.
- Dressing such as granuflex may need to be applied to the bridge of the nose and other pressure points if the patient has friable skin.
- Alterations to settings should be prescribed by clinician responsible and in response to patient's tolerance and ABG concentration.
- Provide continued support and encouragement reminding patient that the machine works with their breathing to make it easier.
- If necessary make an agreed time for short breaks if it aids compliance and will not be detrimental to overall respiratory function.
- Ensure suction, BVM, and resuscitation equipment are immediately available.
- Ensure chest X-ray has been undertaken to exclude pneumothorax or other pathology.

Continued care

- Full continuous monitoring should be maintained and documented every 15min at the beginning of treatment. The commencement of treatment as positive airway pressure may alter thoracic pressures and venous return to the heart and cause hypotension.
- Observe for any signs of increased respiratory effort, cyanosis, distress, anxiety, or reduced consciousness.
- Drying of the mouth and nasal passages may be reduced with petroleum jelly and regular mouth care.
- Nutrition and hydration should be managed by planned breaks and IV fluids where indicated.
- An NG tube and anti-emetics may be required if there is nausea and vomiting. If the patient's airway is at risk, e.g. vomiting, or the patient becomes acutely distressed use the quick release section to the front of the mask.

Visual acuity (VA)

Visual acuity is an objective assessment of visual function and **must** be recorded in all patients attending with an eye problem. Normal vision is 6/6: the eye can see at 6 metres what a *normal* eye can see at that distance.

Procedure

- Test the affected/injured eye first.
- Occlude the other eye using an occluder or the patient's hand.
- Distance glasses should be worn as the test is of the *best corrected* visual acuity.
- The test should begin at the top of the Snellen chart, the patient reading down and making an attempt to read all letters.
- The VA should be recorded as [distance at which eye is being tested (usually 6 metres)]/[number on last line read by the patient].
  - The number for the last line read by the patient is indicated on the Snellen chart, just above, or just below the letters.
  - If only part of a line is read this can be recorded as the line above plus the extra letters, or the line below minus the missed letters. For example, if the patient reads the '18' line except for 1 letter, at 6 metres, it should be recorded as 6/(18 − 1).

Considerations

- If the patient's vision is less than 6/9, VA should be assessed with a pinhole (a small hole in a card or a commercial pinhole) held in front of the eye. This corrects for reduced VA caused by refractive error.
- If the patient is unable to read the top letter of the Snellen chart, the distance should be reduced until the patient can see the top letter on the chart, i.e. 5/60, 4/60, etc. to 1/60.
- If top letter cannot be seen at 1 metre, the next possible level of vision is to count fingers (CF), see hand movements (HM), or perception of light (PL) at one metre.
- Lack of light perception is recorded as NPL.
- It is important to ascertain if the level of subnormal vision is **normal for the patient**.
- Strategies to overcome language difficulties may include: using a recognition chart so that the patient may match letters or shapes; obtaining the services of an interpreter or family member to translate for the patient.
- Children are often cooperative if picture tests (such as the Kay picture test) are used and the procedure is made into a game.

❸ Vital signs in children

Assessing vital signs in children can be challenging for the clinician without specific paediatric training or experience. Normal parameters are vastly different than in adults and alter with increasing age (Table 20.6).

▶ The accurate interpretation of vital signs in children relies on the clinician knowing what is normal for the age of the child, having the right equipment, and, of equal importance, knowing how to undertake an accurate assessment.

Child's behaviour Parents usually bring their child to an emergency care facility because of a change in behaviour. It is crucial to listen to the parent and document their concerns. An objective assessment should be made of the child's behaviour and if it is normal for them.

Weight A child's weight should be considered a vital sign. It enables assessment of growth, development, and hydration status. All medications are given according to weight so an accurate weight in kilograms should be taken at the earliest opportunity. If a child is critically ill and cannot be weighed, weight for children aged 1–10 years can be estimated as 2 × (age + 4) kg.

Temperature Parents know when their child has a temperature without the need for a thermometer. An objective assessment of temperature needs to be made and a device and route appropriate for the age of the child should be used, e.g. axilla, oral, or tympanic. Manufacturer's instructions should be checked to ensure the device is appropriate for the age of the child.

Respiratory rate Children rely primarily on their diaphragm for breathing as their intercostal muscles are immature. It is not easy to see a child's chest rise and fall as the diameter of their thorax does not alter greatly with respiration. What does alter is the degree to which their diaphragm contracts and flattens when their work of breathing is increased. It is for this reason that a child's chest and abdomen should be exposed when assessing the respiratory rate. The movement of the abdomen as it is pushed down by the diaphragm indicates the respiratory rate. Alternatively, the child's chest can be auscultated and their respiratory rate counted. The child's neck, clavicular area, chest, and abdomen should also be assessed for signs of recession. Recession indicates work of breathing and is significant.

Oxygen saturations The right sized probe attached correctly to the right site will ensure accurate assessment.

Heart rate A term baby's heart rate is approximately 160bpm which would be considered a tachycardia in an adult. A child's heart rate can be assessed by listening at the apex. Alternatively, the brachial pulse can be easily palpated in children < 1 year and in children > 1 year the carotid or radial are ideal sites to use.

Blood pressure Assessing a child's BP can be a falsely reassuring sign if the clinician is merely assessing it against normal the parameters for the age of the child. Children have an amazing ability to maintain a normal BP despite profound volume losses of up to 45%. A normal BP in the absence of other assessments such as capillary refill and conscious level can lead to cardiovascular abnormalities going undetected. Trends in BP measurements can be much more meaningful. The right sized BP cuff is essential for the accuracy of any assessment.

Capillary refill (CRF)

In early cardiovascular compromise a CRF time can be increased beyond 2sec. A CRF time together with the presence of other signs of cardiovascular compromise e.g. tachycardia, pale, cool mottled peripheries and altered conscious level requires prompt intervention.

- Use a thumb/finger and depress the skin of the sternum for 5sec, let go, and count how many seconds it takes the blanched skin to return to a normal colour.

Table 20.6 Normal values of respiratory rate (RR) and pulse in children at different ages

Age (years)	RR (breaths/min)	Pulse (beats/min)	Systolic BP (mmHg)
Infant <1 year	30–40	110–160	70–90
Toddler 1–2 years	25–35	100–150	80–95
Preschool 3–4 years	25–30	95–140	80–100
School 5–11 years	20–25	80–120	90–110
Adolescent 12–16 years	15–20	60–100	100–120

Further information

RCN standards for assessing, measuring and monitoring vital signs in infants, children and young people. ᐟ www.rcn.uk_data/assets/pdf_file/0004/114484/003196.pdf

Wounds: stages of healing

A huge variety of acute and chronic wounds present to emergency care areas each day. There is no single treatment or wound care product that meets all the criteria for the 'ideal dressing' for each different wound type, during each phase of healing. This section of the skills chapter provides evidenced-based information on the principles of traumatic wound management, which will support the clinician in making clinically and cost-effective dressing choices.

▶ When faced with a wound it is important to assess its stage of healing (Box 20.4). There are several points to be considered when approaching wound management at each stage.

> **Box 20.4 Wounds: stages of healing**
>
> *Vascular stage* The most common stage of healing seen in emergency care. A dressing needs to be able to absorb bleeding and help control it. Some wounds bleed profusely (that's why the patient has attended), e.g. skin loss to a finger tip. An alginate dressing is homeostatic and can help promote clotting. Bleeding should be checked to ensure it is not arterial in origin and can usually be controlled simply with a dressing, pressure, and elevation. If wounds are bleeding a simple dressing is all that is needed with redressing planned for 2–3 days later
>
> *Destructive migratory stage* Wounds at this stage may have a lot of exudate, e.g. burns, and will require a dressing that can absorb the wound 'ooze'. Dead/devitalized tissue needs to be removed. A product to remove slough/eschar may be required, e.g. hydrogel
>
> *Proliferative stage* A very fragile stage of healing as new tissue is being formed. Cooling a wound by exposing it for long periods or cleansing with cool solutions will slow or even stop epithelialization for several hours. Wound care products must not adhere to the wound surface at this stage as removing an adhered dressing is not very painful but will tear away new skin cells and blood vessels from the wound bed—the wound could even be returned to the vascular phase and healing significantly delayed
>
> *Maturation stage* Advice about scar care and keeping healed burns from the sun is relevant at this final stage of healing

Wound care

Healing by 'intention'

Wounds heal by either primary or secondary intention. Wounds that heal by primary intention, where the skin edges are brought together by suture, glue, or Steri-Strips™ will heal relatively quickly (5–14 days). Wounds that heal by secondary intention are wounds that extend into the dermis with skin loss. They heal as new cells are formed and the defect is filled, e.g. burns. These wounds can take 10–21 days to heal.

Ideal dressing criteria

Dressing products in emergency care areas may be limited and access to specialist treatments difficult. If a more appropriate dressing is required, early wound review where the dressing is available is required. There is no one product that has all the qualities of the 'ideal dressing'; compromises always have to be made. Depending on the wound type, characteristics, and stage of healing some of the following criteria will be more important than others.

- Maintain high humidity at the wound/dressing interface (to keep the wound moist).
- Remove excess exudate and toxic components (to keep the wound moist but not saturated and remove contaminants).
- Allows gaseous exchange (lets the wound breathe).
- Provide thermal insulation (to keep the wound warm).
- Is impermeable to bacteria.
- Is free from particulate and toxic contaminant, i.e. does not introduce anything toxic or leave anything behind.
- Allows removal without causing additional trauma; easy to remove.
- Is non-allergenic so it does not cause allergic reaction
- Is comfortable, conformable, and protective, i.e. it is comfortable for the patient, protects vulnerable skin, and bends over joints.
- Is cost-effective and available in the right size. It comes in an appropriate size and does not require frequent changes if dressing is expensive.
- Is acceptable to the patient. Some dressings have an odour; explain to the patient.

Table 20.7 describes the different traumatic wounds encountered in emergency care and suggests what should be taken into consideration when selecting a dressing.

Table 20.7 Dressing considerations for different types of wounds

Wound	Mechanism/definition	Dressing considerations
Abrasion	Friction force	Varying depth; can be contaminated; painful
Bite wounds	Human; animal; insect	Infection possible; may swell
Burn	Scald; flame; chemical; electrical	May cover large area; may be difficult to dress; painful; heavy exudate during 1st 72h
Contaminated wound	Contamination with: soil; gravel; mud; clothing. Industrial; sport/ recreation	Clean to remove contamination prior to dressing or use product that removes contamination. May need X-ray to rule out radio-opaque FB
Crush wounds	Blunt force	May swell
Cut/incised wound	Sharp object: glass/knife	Oppose wound edges with sutures/glue or steristrips. Heal quickly
Degloving injuries	Tissue torn from underlying attachments	Usually needs Plastics referral
Flap wounds	Blunt or penetrating	May be contaminated under flap. If poor blood supply to flap may become necrotic. Undue tension will compromise flap blood supply further
Fingertip wounds	Crush	Painful. Nailbed may be lacerated & need repair
Lacerations	Blunt force causes skin to split	May swell. Possible contused/ devitalized tissue
Pre-tibial lacerations	Wound to pre-tibial area; usually in the elderly	If poor blood supply to flap, may become necrotic. Undue tension will compromise flap blood supply further. In elderly blood supply compromised further & healing delayed
Puncture wound	Penetrating injury	Can't adequately clean base of wound. May be contaminated or have FB
Skin loss/ avulsion	Skin lost due to crush injuries or incised wounds	May bleed profusely. Prolonged healing by 2° intention
Abscess	Pocket of infection: retained FB; infected sebaceous cyst	Painful. After incision keep open to heal by 2° intention

Other wound characteristics at different stages of healing will require a different approach (囗 see Table 20.8).

Further information

Detailed data card information on all dressings can be found at *www.dressing.org* or read the manufacturing information leaflet that accompanies the dressing.

Table 20.8 Other wound characteristics affecting dressing choice

Type	Characteristics	Considerations
Necrotic	Black, hard, dry	Remove necrosis or wound will not heal. Once removed assess true depth & extent of wound. Use product that rehydrates wound & removes necrotic tissue
Sloughy	Yellow, or green, or grey. Slough may be soft & easily removed	Wound won't heal as slough prolongs inflammatory phase. Use desloughing agent
Infected	Red, hot, swollen, pus, painful, delayed healing	May have excess exudate. Some products not licensed for use on infected wounds
Granulating	Red, shiny, 'bumpy' in appearance	Fragile; easily damaged by adherent dressing. Bleeds easily. Use a low-adherent dressing
Epithelializing	Pale red/pink areas of new epithelial cell growth	Fragile new epithelial cells easily damaged. Use low-adherent dressing

Wound cleansing

Wound cleansing is an integral part of wound management and is the mainstay of treatment. Emergency care staff often underestimate the importance of this simple skill and how vital it is in preventing infection and promoting healing. All traumatic wounds should be considered contaminated with debris. Some patients may require a general anaesthetic for the adequate cleaning of wounds.

▶ An inadequately cleansed wound will have delayed healing, possible wound infection and scarring, and, on occasion, permanent tattooing that may require surgery.

Indications All traumatic wounds.

Equipment
- Tap water.
- 20mL syringe.
- Warmed cleansing fluid.
- Gloves.
- Eye protection.
- Apron.
- Scrubbing brush/tooth brush.
- Local anaesthetic.

There are also various commercial devices available to irrigate wounds under pressure.

The following points are important to note.
- ▶ There is a strong body of evidence to suggest that when wounds are cleansed with tap water there is no higher incidence of wound infection.
- ▶ 'Scrubbing brushes' of various types may have to be used. The risk of causing further trauma to the tissues is outweighed by the benefits of removing debris and preventing permanent tattooing of the wound.

▶ Cotton wool or gauze should be avoided in the cleansing of wounds as fibres can be shed into the wound. This method does not remove debris—it just moves it around the wound.

Patient preparation
- Explain the procedure to the patient.
- Remove any clothing that may become wet.
- Assist the patient into a comfortable position.
- Ensure adequate pain relief. The wound may need infiltration with local anaesthetic or the application of a topical anaesthetic gel.

Procedure
- Using the 20mL syringe push fluid through the wound to dislodge any dirt or debris. Take care not to cause further damage to the tissue if the water is forced under high pressure.
- Copious amounts of warm tap water are ideal for cleaning dirty wounds. Run the water for ~ 15sec; then cleanse the wound.

- Use a scrubbing brush if there is engrained debris.
- Close and dress the wound as appropriate.

Discharge advice

▶ Prophylactic antibiotics are not used routinely. Patients should be advised to seek further treatment if the wound is:

- hot;
- red;
- swollen;
- painful;
- odorous;
- not healed in the expected time;
- discharging.

Wound closure: tissue adhesive

Tissue adhesive is a means of closing smaller wounds by the application of specially formulated glue used for medical purposes. It is particularly useful for the management of small wounds in children and wounds where hair is present (scalp and eyebrows). The technique for glue application is relatively easy, providing the right type of wound is selected. There are several products available and the manufacturer's instructions should always be consulted.

Indications

Wounds suitable for glue:
- clean;
- not over a joint surface or area prone to excessive movement;
- relatively small, 4–5cm;
- superficial;
- not bleeding;
- edges easily opposed.

Equipment

- Wound cleansing solution.
- Dressing pack; gauze, sterile gloves, gallipot.
- Glue.
- Sterile dressing.

Patient preparation Explain the procedure to the patient. There may be a slight sting when the glue is applied.

Procedure

- Hold away any hair that may interfere with the glue application (sometimes the droplet of adhesive can track down the hair shaft).
- Clean the wound, remove any haematoma, and dry it thoroughly.
- Oppose the skin edges.
- Dry the wound again.
- Apply according to manufacturer's instructions, which will depend on the type of glue applicator.
- Do not apply the glue into the wound.
- Hold the edges of the wound in apposition for 30sec to allow the adhesive to dry.
- Apply sterile dressing if appropriate.

Precautions

- Do not apply too much glue as excessive adhesive will reduce the tensile strength of the glue.
- ▶ If your glove becomes stuck to the wound **do not worry**. Trim the glove so that only the area that is adhered is left. Advise the patient/parent that the glove will fall off as the wound heals.

Discharge advice

- Keep clean and dry for 4–5 days for a scalp wound; 5–7 days elsewhere.
- A larger scab may form; this in normal.
- The scab/glue will fall off after the wound is healed.

Steri-Strips™

Steri-Strips™ or 'butterflies' are adhesive strips (usually manufactured in 2 different widths) that can be used to close superficial wounds of varying lengths.

Indications

Wounds suitable for closure with Steri-Strips™:

- superficial;
- not bleeding profusely;
- edges easily opposed;
- not under tension or excessive movement, i.e. not over a moving extensor surface;
- do not require layered closure (although internal sutures can applied and the skin closed with Steri-Strips™).

Equipment

- Wound cleansing solution.
- Dressing pack: gauze; sterile gloves; gallipot.
- Steri-Strips™ of appropriate width.
- Sterile dressing.
- Friar's balsam/tincture of benzene. When this is applied to the skin surrounding the wound with a cotton bud, the skin becomes tacky enabling greater adherence of the Steri-Strips™. (Do not put into the wound or on grazed skin as it will 'sting' until dry.)

Patient preparation Explain the procedure to the patient.

Procedure

- Clean the wound, remove any haematoma, and dry it thoroughly.
- Paint the skin around the wound with friar's balsam if appropriate.
- Oppose the skin edges.
- Dry the wound again.
- Apply the Steri-Strips™ anchoring corners of the wound first, where appropriate.
- Apply with even tension, leaving gaps between each strip to allow serous fluid to drain from the wound. Ensure that the wound edges are not under too much tension. Undue tension will compromise the blood supply to this part of the wound and may compromise healing.
- Dress with appropriate dressing. If the Steri-Strips™ have been applied about a joint, immobilize the joint to prevent tension on the wound.

Discharge advice

- Keep clean and dry.
- Leave Steri-Strips™ in situ for 5–10 days depending on the site and type of the wound.
- Peel or soak off when requisite time has elapsed.

Local anaesthetic infiltration of wounds

Local anaesthetic (LA) causes a reversible loss of nerve conduction. Lidocaine is available in 1% and 2% concentrations and is very safe providing a toxic dose is not given. Allergic reactions are rare.

- The safe maximum dose of lidocaine is 3mg/kg.
- Overdose can occur if > 3mg/kg is given, or if there is inadvertent direct intravascular injection. The weaker the solution the more lidocaine that can be given.
  - 1% lidocaine contains 1g of lidocaine in 100mL.
  - 2% lidocaine contains 2g of lidocaine in 100mL.
  - Therefore 1mL of 1% contains 10mg of lidocaine (0.1mL = 1mg); 1mL of 2% contains 20mg of lidocaine (0.1mL = 2mg).

There are two techniques for infiltration of the wound with LA infiltration through the wound edge (Fig. 20.19(a)) or a field block (Fig. 20.19(b)). Infiltration should be done under the wound edge as patients cannot usually feel a 25G needle. Pain is felt with tissue distension and therefore infiltration should be slow and deliberate.

Ensure you have adequate anaesthesia before continuing with the procedure. Onset of action is usually within seconds and lasts 20min.

Digital nerve blocks

It can be painful to inject finger wounds and local anaesthetic often distorts the wound margins. A digital nerve block is required. There are a number of techniques that are commonly practiced. One technique is described below.

Place the hand flat, palm down with fingers abducted. Insert 22 gauge needle at the level of the base of the web. Angle the tip of the needle towards the palmar side. You may feel the needle against the proximal phalanx. Aspirate to ensure that the needle is not in a vessel and inject 1 to 2mLs of lidocaine. Repeat the procedure on the other side of the finger. Wait 5 minutes for the anaesthesia to develop.

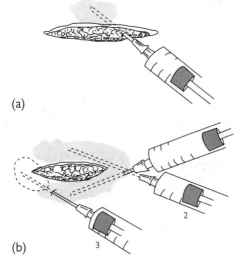

(a)

(b)

Fig. 20.19 (a) Infiltration through wound edge. (b) Field block.

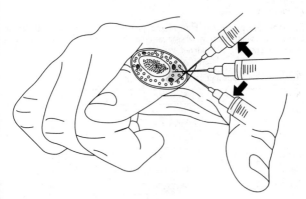

Fig. 20.20 Digital nerve block.

Suturing

Suturing with local anaesthetic is used to close a wide variety of wounds. Small simple wounds may require suturing for cosmetic reasons, e.g. small vermillion border lacerations. Large wounds, deep wounds, those that will be under some degree of tension, and wounds that can't be closed with glue or Steri-Strips™ will also require suturing.

There is a vast array of suture material available. The selection is based on the size of the suture material required to close the wound (📖 see Table 20.9). Absorbable materials are used for deep sutures or where there is no cosmetic concern over the scar, e.g. scalp. Rapidly dissolving sutures are also ideal for use in children as they avoid the need for potentially distressing suture removal.

Commonly used sutures
- Ethilon: non-absorbable
- Vircryl rapide: absorbable in 7–10 days.
- Monocryl: absorbable in 7–21 days.

Equipment
- Wound cleansing solution.
- Dressing pack: gauze; sterile gloves; gallipot.
- Suture set: needle holder; non-toothed forceps; scissors.
- Suture material.
- Sterile dressing.
- Needle.
- Syringe.
- Lidocaine.

Patient preparation Explain the procedure to the patient. Advise them that the infiltration with local anaesthetic can be painful but once complete suturing is pain free.

Table 20.9 Choosing correct size of suture

Site	Size	Removal in
Subcutaneous tissues	6.0	—
Scalp	3.0 or 4.0	Removal in 7 days
Face	6.0	≤ 5 days
Hands	4.0 or 5.0	7–10 days
Other area	Dependent on wound	7–10 days
Site over joints	Dependent on wound	10–14 days

Simple sutures

Simple sutures (Fig. 20.21) are the most commonly used sutures. The aim is to accurately oppose the skin edges and completely close the wound. Deeper wounds may require layered closure (📖 see p.702) to ensure that there is no 'dead space' where a haematoma can develop and act as a focus for infection. Take care not to insert the needle deeper than the visible base of the wound, in case the suture accidentally catches a deep structure, e.g. a tendon or nerve.

Tying knots

This skill is best demonstrated slowly by a competent practitioner.

- Pull the suture through the wound (as shown in Fig. 20.22) and wrap the long end of the suture (the end with the needle attached) around the tip of the needle holder 2 or 3 times.
- Grab the other end of the suture with the needle holder and pull this end through, pulling the knot tight
- Repeat 2 or 3 more times wrapping the suture in the opposite direction 2–4 times.

Discharge advice

- Advise about wound care: signs of wound infection; care of the wound; keeping it clean and dry.
- Written and verbal advice about removal of sutures and any follow-up.
- Advise about pain relief and NSAIDs if appropriate.
- Advise about work/school, contact sport, and other activities that the patient may regularly undertake.
- Advise about how and when to seek further help if problems persist.

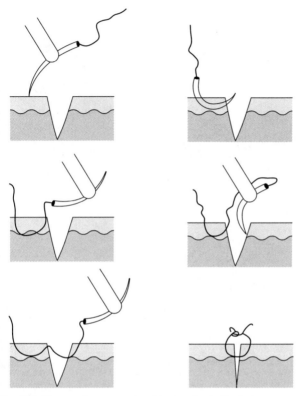

Fig. 20.21 Diagrammatic representation of the stages involved in a basic suture. (Reproduced with permission from Thomas, J. and Monaghan, T. (eds.) (2007). *Oxford handbook of clinical examination and skills*, p. 633. Oxford University Press, Oxford.)

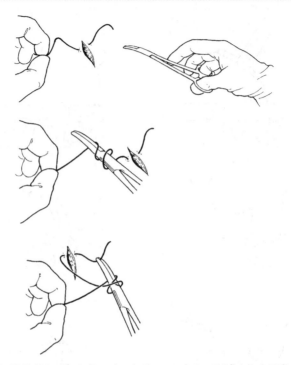

Fig. 20.22 Instrument tie (Reproduced with permission from Wyatt, J., et al. (2006). *Oxford Handbook of Emergency Medicine*, 3rd edn, pp. 406–7. Oxford University Press, Oxford.)

Deep sutures and mattress sutures

Layered closure for deep wounds

If the wound is deep it may require closure in layers to ensure there is no 'dead space' within the wound (Fig. 20.23). If all the layers of the wound are not closed an indentation beneath the scar may affect the final cosmetic outcome. Inserting an accurate layer of deep sutures may also enable the skin to be closed with Steri-Strips™, leading to an improved final result. Tie knots as in 'Simple sutures', 📖 see p.698.

Mattress sutures

Mattress sutures (Fig. 20.24) are very useful as they enable inverted skin edges to be more accurately opposed. They are contraindicated on facial wounds. If after inserting a simple suture the skin edges are inverted, this indicates that a mattress suture may be more appropriate.

Discharge advice

- Advise about wound care: signs of wound infection; care of the wound; keeping it clean and dry.
- Written and verbal advice about removal of sutures and any follow-up.
- Advise about pain relief and NSAIDs if appropriate.
- Advise about work/school, contact sport, and other activities that the patient may regularly undertake.
- Advise about how and when to seek further help if problems persist.

Coventry University Library

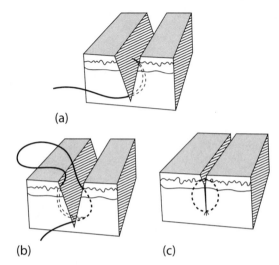

Fig. 20.23 Layered wound closure.

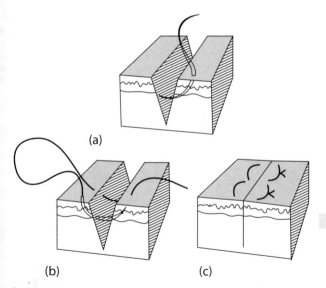

Fig. 20.24 Mattress suture.

Index